MEASUREMENT AND STATISTICS IN PHYSICAL EDUCATION

MEASUREMENT AND STATISTICS IN PHYSICAL EDUCATION

N. P. Neilson
University of Utah

Clayne R. Jensen
Brigham Young University

Wadsworth Publishing Company, Inc.
Belmont, California

ISBN–0–534–00054–1
L. C. Cat. Card No. 76–167906
Printed in the United States of America

1 2 3 4 5 6 7 8 9 10—76 75 74 73 72

Preface

Among the significant changes in physical education that have taken place in recent years are increased facilities, increased time, better preparation of teachers, improved teaching methods, and greater emphasis on sound testing procedures and useful statistical techniques. To be adequately prepared, today's physical education teachers must complete a basic course in physical education measurement. Such a course requires a preliminary understanding of elementary statistics. Because statistics and measurement are closely related and interdependent, they are often included in a single course in the physical education professional program. When this is done, it is logical to devote the first part of the course to selected statistical techniques and the second part to learning how to conduct a program of measurement and how to use the results.

An important advantage of giving a combined course in statistics and measurement is that the statistical techniques are immediately used in connection with the instruction in measurement, rather than forgotten by the time a later course on measurement is given. Also, students in physical education find it especially helpful to work problems in statistics using such scores as those for high jump, endurance, and strength rather than scores that do not relate to motor performance.

This book is designed for a combined course in statistics and measurement in physical education, taught at the upper-division college level. The book includes carefully selected statistical techniques which have frequent application in the educational setting. The techniques are presented in logical sequence for learning and explained in a simplified fashion. The numerous problem-solving situations included help students learn how to apply the techniques effectively. Also, the book includes valuable information about selecting, constructing, and administering tests and using test results. Many useful tests are described; scoring tables are included.

Measurement and Statistics in Physical Education should be interesting and meaningful to students majoring in physical education and related fields, to teachers, coaches, and school administrators.

The authors acknowledge the contributions of professors James Bosco, San Jose State College, and Peter Everett, Florida State University, who reviewed the manuscript and provided valuable suggestions, and professors Cyntha Hirst, Brigham Young University, and Barbara West, University of Utah, who offered suggestions relative to the book's content. The valuable assistance of Richard Greenberg, Wadsworth Publishing Company, is also acknowledged.

Contents

ONE
Introduction

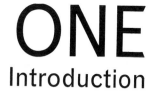

This section is designed to give the reader general insight into the field of measurement in physical education: the origin, development, and present status of this field as well as the classification, selection, and administration of various measurements.

1

The Need
for Measurement

Measurement is not new. From the beginning of recorded history man has devised and used tests of one sort or another to determine human ability in those factors considered important in the particular society. Crude measurements of strength, speed, and skill, for example, date back to antiquity.

Conversely, educational measurement, as we know it today, is relatively new. It has developed as a part of the elaborate and complex mass education system, and like other aspects of that system it is of recent origin. The qualities we measure today are numerous and precisely defined, and our techniques are more exact than ever before. Many of the measurement techniques and instruments used today have been developed during recent years. Likewise, the techniques we use to analyze measurement results are relatively new.

The measurement program in physical education is only a portion of the total measurement program within a school. In the modern educational system physical education measurement is concerned with such factors as knowledge, interests, attitudes and aptitudes, anthropometric traits, strength, endurance, power, agility, and specific skills.

Meanings

Test, measurement, and evaluation are commonly used terms with certain similarities and differences.

A *test* is an instrument requiring a performance by an individual being tested. The performer receives a score representing how well he has performed. The quality or quantity of an individual's strength, speed, jumping ability, knowledge, IQ, and so on are determined by the use of specifically designed tests.

The term *measurement* includes all tests but is not necessarily confined to the concept of testing. Some measurements do not require a performance by the person. For instance, such measurements as distance, weight, and time are not tests.

Evaluation is broader and more inclusive than either of the other terms. It is a process of determining the status of something and of relating that status to some standard in order to make a value judgment. For example, evaluations are made of teaching methods, program content, and teacher effectiveness. Evaluation is often based on information secured from observations, interviews, questionnaires, and measures.

Reasons for Measuring

Physical educators are vitally concerned with student development and adjustment resulting from participation in activity. They are specifically concerned with the development of knowledge, concepts, and judgments; interests, attitudes, and ideals; strength and skill; and the development of the organic systems.

To design a high quality instructional program and to teach effectively, the teacher must obtain considerable information about his students. The more information a teacher has about his students' performances, abilities, and needs, the better he can design and conduct an effective program. He must gather much of the needed information by the use of measurements. The need for precise measures calls for a well-designed program including carefully selected and well-constructed tests.

There seems to be rather general agreement on two major purposes for testing in physical education: to increase the knowledge of the teacher and students, and to improve instruction. Little is gained by increasing the knowledge of the teacher and students unless the increased knowledge is used to improve learning.

There are six important purposes of measurement:

1.   *Diagnostic.* Measurement is necessary to diagnose the differences in abilities, interests, and needs of students in order to plan and conduct adequate programs for them. Objective knowledge about specific student deficiencies is essential to provide remedial programs.

2.   *Classification.* Sometimes it is an advantage to classify students into homogeneous or heterogeneous groups, whichever is desired for a particular type of instruction or competition. Such classification is often based on the results of appropriate tests.

3.   *Measurement of Achievement.* It seems important to obtain objective measures and to keep accurate records of student achievement and progress, for these records form the basis for the selection of program content and the assignment of student grades.

4.   *Administrative.* Objective information obtained from testing can serve as a basis for determining the best methods of instruction and for guiding students. Accurate measurements help to determine the success of students and to learn whether students are ready to progress to the next higher level. In the absence of success, parents desire to know the reasons. Properly administered tests can help provide information needed and desired by students, teachers, parents, and school administrators.

5.   *Supervisory.* Objective test results are valuable in the evaluation of teachers and their teaching efficiency.

6.   *Research.* The field of physical education is rich with opportunities for valuable research. For example, additional research is necessary on the efficiency of various methods of instruction, on the rate of progress of students, on the physiological, psychological, and sociological values of the different activities, and on the evaluation of the entire school program in physical education. Certain kinds of research can be performed effectively only with the use of appropriate tests.

With the present emphasis on education there is a strong demand for teachers to measure student traits on a mass scale and with increased accuracy. In light of this need the selection and effective use of sound methods of measurement is an important problem for physical educators. Tests should be selected to meet the specific purposes of measurement.

2
Origin and
Development of Measurement

Familiarity with the historical development of a subject frequently results in a better appreciation of the subject and an understanding of its significance. In this light let us consider the major developments of measurement that have led to its present status in the field of physical education.

Physical education measurement is only one phase of educational measurement, since each subject in a field calls for evaluation techniques unique to that subject. Physical education tests frequently measure motor performances.

Measuring the structure and function of the human body is not new. Early civilized man used measures of strength, running speed, endurance, specific skills, and body size and proportions. At first the measures were crude, but gradually they became more refined and more numerous until today a large number of useful measures of structure and function are available.

The history of measurement in physical education has occurred with the development in five distinct areas: anthropometric, strength, cardiac function, athletic ability, and fitness.

Anthropometric Measurements

Measures dealing with structure and proportions of the body can be traced to ancient India where a treatise entitled "Silpi Sastri" describing the division of the body into 480 parts and explaining the structure and proportions of each part was written. In an attempt to find one body part which would serve as a standard for measurement of all other parts, the ancient Egyptians divided the body into 19 equal segments, each of which was the length of the High Priest's middle finger (Meyer and Blesh 1962).

Two ancient Greek sculptors, Phidias and Polyclitus, fashioned models in an attempt to demonstrate perfection in human proportions. Later, Roman sculptors developed human forms somewhat different from those created by the earlier Greeks. The Greek and Roman ideals of the perfect body form prevailed for centuries, during which time little was done in developing new ideas about human structure.

In 1770 Joshua Reynolds, an English painter, placed new emphasis on anthropometric measures. He called attention to the idea that body size and proportions are largely hereditary, that the individual has limited control over them, and that they change considerably from childhood to adulthood (Meyer and Blesh 1962).

7

In about 1850 anthropometric measures began to be important in organized physical education programs. In 1860 Cromwell, an Englishman, studied the growth patterns of Manchester school children from ages eight to eighteen. He found that from ages eleven to fourteen girls were taller and heavier than boys at the same age. In 1861 Edward Hitchcock, at Amherst College, took careful measurements to establish standards of age; height; weight; girths of the chest, arm, and forearm; and strength of the upper arm. Later, on the basis of his findings he developed more than 50 standard measures of body proportions.

Soon after Hitchcock's studies Dudley A. Sargent at Harvard University began a systematic anthropometric measurement program. The data he gathered, published in 1893, created a wider interest in growth and structure. As a result of his report several other universities initiated measurement programs.

At about the turn of the century Street developed the idea of a weight–height index. Later other researchers built on his idea and developed extensive weight–height indexes. These indexes became useful to educators and also to the public in general. They indicated how much a person ought to weigh in relation to his height and body type. In 1902 D. W. Hastings at Springfield College made a study of the rate of growth of the human body from the fifth to the twenty-first birthday.

Following the turn of the century the use of anthropometric measures lagged, but in the late 1920s a new interest developed. In 1928 Clifford Brownell of Columbia University presented a series of posture silhouettes with which to detect postural deviations in boys, soon after which Charlotte G. MacEwan and Eugene C. Howe provided a more extensive set of posture silhouettes. Two years later R. C. Quimby developed his weight analysis scale for man, and subsequently Helen B. Pryor of Stanford University constructed the Pryor Width–Weight Tables. Then, William H. Sheldon published his rather elaborate system of somatotyping of the human body.

In 1947 Thomas Cureton at the University of Illinois devised a simplified somatotyping system, and Howard V. Meredith published his height–weight charts. In 1948, Norman Wetzel published the widely used Wetzel Grid. Other significant events occurred along the way, but the aforementioned seem to be the milestones in the development of anthropometric measurements.

Interest in anthropometric measures has lessened during the last two decades. While the use of previously developed measures has declined, little productive work has been done toward improving existing anthropometric measures. However, some measures still serve worthwhile purposes, especially those used as screening devices to identify the more extreme structural types.

Strength Tests

The idea that strength is fundamental to vigorous athletic performances has long been recognized, and for this reason strength testing has interested physical education teachers, including athletic coaches. The actual origin of strength testing is not known.

The first wave of enthusiasm for strength development and testing in the United States reached its peak in the period from 1860 to 1875 during which time George Winship toured the eastern part of the country lecturing on exercise and giving exhibitions of weight lifting. In about 1880 Sargent began his strength studies of Harvard University students in an attempt to determine standards for American college men. The studies resulted in Sargent's Intercollegiate Strength Test, which received extensive use.

In 1890 Francis Galton devised a test to measure physical efficiency, especially for business and civil service use. Among other items Galton's test included strength measures. Late in the 1880s and early in the 1890s J. H. Kellogg did work emphasizing the importance of exercise as a therapeutic measure. His work led to the invention of the universal dynamometer in 1896. With this instrument he could test the strength of different muscle groups.

During the early part of the twentieth century a brief lapse occurred in strength testing. It was generally thought that strength tests did not lend enough emphasis to measures of endurance and especially to heart and lung development. Also the idea that muscle boundness hindered an athlete's performance led to the temporary abandonment of strength testing.

While studying the aftereffects of the Vermont Polio epidemic in 1915, E. G. Martin recognized the need for a strength test that could be used for comparing normal and affected muscle groups. He developed the Martin Resistance Test based on the principle of resistance to a pull in contrast to the idea of voluntary strength exertion. The original test measured 11 muscle groups, but a shorter test was devised involving four muscle groups.

In 1925 Frederick R. Rogers revived interest in strength testing by developing the Strength Index and the Fitness Index. Rogers' work brought forth new evidence that strength correlates significantly with athletic ability.

After Rogers' work several new tests appeared. J. H. McCurdy developed his so-called Physical Capacity Test in which strength was an important item. In 1931 Charles H. McCloy revised the Rogers' Strength Index by devising his own formula for estimating arm strength. Rump's studies on strength testing indicated that pull-up and dip strength were good indicators of total strength.

During the 1940s Thomas DeLorme did considerable strength testing and strength building among wounded war veterans under rehabilitation treatment. He is often referred to as the father of modern isotonic weight training, for largely under his leadership the value of strength in athletic performance was established. More recently H. Harrison Clarke developed tests to measure the strength of muscle groups responsible for 38 different joint movements. In the late 1940s Lenard A. Larson developed his Dynamic Strength Test, consisting of pull-ups, dips, and vertical jumps. The test was designed to measure ability to do work against the resistance of one's own body weight.

Currently strength is recognized as a major contributor to athletic performance, and some leaders claim it is the most important contributor to performance. The present popularity of strength testing stems from the extensive concentration on strength development in athletic conditioning. Most strength tests now used require a tensiometer and strap-and-cable arrangement to test strength of specific muscle groups. Also, tests that measure a combination of strength and endurance are often used. These tests consist of performances such as pull-ups, dips, and push-ups, in which the performer works against the resistance of his body weight.

Cardiac Function Tests

Angelo Mosso, the inventor of the ergograph, pointed out in 1884 that the ability of muscles to perform is related to the efficiency of the circulatory system. Thus attention turned toward more satisfactory methods of measuring cardiovascular condition. Subsequently significant strides were made in the development of procedures to measure blood pressure. In 1905 C. Ward Crampton used this knowledge to establish a rating scheme in order to obtain information about the general condition of a person by noting changes in cardiac rate and arterial pressure upon assuming the erect position.

In 1910 McCurdy devised a simple test of what he termed physical condition. He concluded that if the change in heart rate from the reclining to the erect position exceeded 15 to 18 beats per minute, the individual should be advised to consult a physician.

The next significant steps in cardiac function testing began in 1914 when G. L. Meylan, W. H. Foster, and J. H. Barach each reported a physical efficiency test. Meylan's test measured blood pressure, the reaction of the heart to exercise, the character of the pulse rate, and some other elements of general condition. Foster's test was similar to Meylan's test. Barach's test indicated the efficiency of the individual by means of the pulse rate and measures of diastolic and systolic blood pressure.

In 1916 T. B. Barringer attempted to show that physically deficient individuals displayed a delayed rise in blood pressure after completion of vigorous exercise. During and after World War I Campbell, an Englishman, developed a cardiovascular adjustment test involving breath holding and recovery of normal breathing rate after exercise. This test was later shortened to a pulse rate recovery test known as Campbell's Pulse Ratio Test.

In 1920 E. C. Schneider developed a test of physical efficiency to measure the effect of exercise on the cardiovascular system. The test was used extensively in aviation during World War II to determine the physical condition of flight personnel.

In 1931 W. W. Tuttle developed his Pulse Ratio Test. The pulse ratio was interpreted as the ratio between the pulse rate at rest and the pulse rate after a given amount of exercise, with a low ratio indicating efficiency of the circulatory system. Soon after the publication of Tuttle's test, McCloy presented his Test of Present Condition. In 1935 the McCurdy–Larson Test of Organic Efficiency became available. Attention increased toward almost all types of organic function tests with the advent of World War II.

In 1943 Lucien Brouha at Harvard University developed the Harvard Step Test designed to indicate the ability of the body to adapt to strenuous work and to recover quickly after work. In this test the efficiency of the circulatory system is indicated by the increase in heart rate during exercise and the speed with which the heart rate returns to normal after exercise. The test is based on the principle that the rate at which the heart slows down after it has been accelerated by a standard amount of exercise gives a correct measure of a person's condition. Brouha also worked with J. R. Gallagher on two other tests which measure essentially the same qualities as the Harvard Step Test. These tests are the Gallagher and Brouha Test for High School Boys and the Gallagher and Brouha Test for High School Girls.

During World War II the Pack Test was developed by Craig Taylor for testing large groups of men on their ability to sustain heavy work. This test, also similar to the Harvard Step Test, was used extensively during the war. In 1945 H. C. Carlson reported the Carlson Fatigue Curve Test, ten-second bouts of in-place running followed by pulse counts taken at specific times after the exercise. The underlying principle of this test is essentially the same as the Harvard Step Test.

Since the end of World War II little has been done to develop new cardiac function tests. Currently cardiac function tests receive limited use except in research projects.

Athletic Ability Tests

Strength tests were criticized as indicators of athletic ability because they measured strength primarily. Cardiac function tests were also considered inadequate as measures of athletic ability. Therefore, some physical educators felt the need for a different type of test, one which would measure several qualities important in athletic performance. General athletic (or motor) ability tests were designed to measure a combination of speed, power, agility, strength, endurance, and other important aspects of performance ability.

The beginning of athletic ability tests can be traced to the Normal School of Gymnastics at Milwaukee, where in 1894 the abilities of the students were measured in nine different test items and compared with their performances in athletic sports. In 1901 Sargent devised a test of six simple exercises which were continued for a period of 30 minutes. Those who completed the test were considered athletically fit. Three years later Meylan at Columbia University developed tests which incorporated items such as running, jumping, vaulting, and climbing. These tests were used widely in universities.

Use of athletic ability tests in the public school curriculum began in 1908 in the New York City and Cleveland schools. In 1910 the Cincinnati schools used the Button Test to measure all-round efficiency in athletic events. The Playground and Recreation Association of America (now the National Recreation and Park Association) published the Athletic Badge Test in 1913 to stimulate interest in achieving minimum athletic performance standards. These early tests aroused the interest of people in the public schools throughout the country.

The Decathlon Test, which originated with Hetherington and H. R. Stolz in

California, soon spread throughout the nation. This test for high school boys gave a choice of 20 activities including such events as the sit-up, push-up, rope climb, pull-up, high jump, broad jump, 100-yard dash, shot put, and throws for accuracy and distance. Tests were also available for high school girls and for elementary school children. In 1927 the Brace Test of Motor Ability was published and became widely used in the public schools. This test consisted of 20 stunts, which were easy to administer to groups of students.

Between 1900 and 1930 the development of athletic ability tests in college paralleled the development of those for public schools. Sigma Delta Psi, a national athletic fraternity, was established in 1912. To gain membership a candidate had to pass a general performance test. In 1915 the University of California Classification Test gained acceptance. It measured agility, defense ability, and swimming ability. In 1921 the University of Oregon began using athletic ability tests as a basis for prescribing the physical education courses for students. Other colleges used similar tests.

In 1924 McCurdy, chairman of a national committee on motor ability tests, pointed out the desirability of extending testing to the various games and sports, particularly to the so-called major sports. He developed general ability tests for football, soccer, field hockey, basketball, and tennis. These developments, along with others, led to the Cozens–Neilson books containing achievement scales for individual athletic events and to a study by Frederick W. Cozens which resulted in the Cozens Test of General Athletic Ability. Cozens' test, developed in 1929, consisted of a battery of seven tests especially selected to measure the seven components which he and other experts thought most important in athletic performance. The test has been used extensively and is still considered one of the better tests of its type.

The Humiston Motor Ability Test for college women, published in 1937, consisted of seven items which correlated highly with athletic performances. Larson's Motor Ability Test originated in 1941 and included five items in the indoor version and four items in the outdoor version. Lenard A. Larson's test has also been widely used.

In 1954 McCloy at the State University of Iowa used a rather complex approach in what is known as McCloy's General Motor Ability Test. This prescribed battery is different for various ages. It consists of a combination of strength tests and performances in track and field events. In 1957 Barrow developed a general motor ability test for college men which consists of an indoor version of three test items and an outdoor version of six items.

Several other general athletic ability tests have been developed and used in the schools. Some of these are Newton's Motor Ability Test, Scott's Motor Ability Test, Carpenter's Motor Ability Test, Olympic Motor Ability Test, Oberlin College Test, and the Emory University Test. Some other tests are closely related to general athletic ability but have been given other names. Among these are Johnson's Test of Motor Educability, Metheny's Revision of the Johnson Test, Carpenter's Test of Motor Educability, and McCloy's Test of General Motor Capacity. The validity of measuring educability and capacity has been seriously questioned.

Almost all general athletic ability tests are similar in nature. They consist of several short test items selected to measure specific qualities considered important in a variety of athletic performances.

Fitness Tests

The term *physical fitness* became popular during and following World War II and is used to refer to the individual's ability to perform multiple tasks requiring vigorous muscular activity. The emphasis is on the efficiency of the organic systems.

During World War II much emphasis was placed on the fitness of military men. This emphasis resulted in the development of fitness tests designed specifically for military personnel. Most prominent among these tests were the Army Physical Efficiency Test, the Navy Standard Physical Fitness Test, and the Army Air Force Physical Fitness Test. These tests were designed to measure strength, endurance, agility, speed and neuromuscular coordination. All three tests have been used extensively by the military and also in areas outside the military.

In 1943 Karl W. Bookwalter constructed the Indiana Physical Fitness Tests for high school boys and girls and for college men. These tests were designed to measure fitness with particular emphasis on administrative feasibility for large groups. They have been included in the Indiana Department of Public Instruction Bulletin on Physical Education and have also been used outside the state of Indiana. Two years later the Division of Girls' and Women's Sports of the American Association of Health, Physical Education and Recreation developed a test consisting of activities selected to measure power, agility, speed, strength, endurance, and coordination of high school girls. The test was used extensively until more recent tests became available. In 1947 Bernath E. Phillips reported the JCR (jump, chin, run) test which proved to be a popular test. In 1948, C. C. Franklin and N. G. Lehsten adapted the Indiana Physical Fitness Test for use in grades four through eight and developed norms for this age group.

In 1954 Hans Kraus and Ruth P. Hirschland used the Kraus–Weber Test of Minimum Strength to compare the fitness of American children with the fitness of children in other countries. The results indicated that the American children were relatively unfit. These findings caused a great upsurge in the development of fitness programs and in fitness testing in the United States.

Because of this emphasis on fitness, the American Association for Health, Physical Education and Recreation appointed a special committee in 1958 to develop a comprehensive fitness test. The test consists of six items especially selected to measure strength, endurance, agility, speed, power, and coordination. Two sets of norms, one based on the Neilson–Cozens Classification Index, were established. Probably this test has been more widely used in the schools than any other physical education test.

In 1961 the President's Council on Youth Fitness constructed the Youth Physical Fitness Test, consisting of pull-ups, sit-ups, and squat thrusts. This easy-to-administer test has been used in schools and in recreation and scouting programs.

In addition to the fitness tests already mentioned, other tests that have had less national appeal but have been used in certain localities include the Oregon Motor Fitness Test, University of Illinois Motor Fitness Test, Elder Motor Fitness Test, New York State Physical Fitness Test, California Physical Performance Test, and the AAU (Amateur Athletic Union) Junior Olympics. Currently, fitness testing is the most popular type of testing in physical education.

Selected References

Clark, H. Harrison, *Application of Measurement to Health and Physical Education*. Englewood Cliffs, N.J.: Prentice-Hall, 4th ed., 1967, pp. 3–8.

Meyer, Carlton R., and Blesh, T. Erwin, *Measurement in Physical Education*. New York: The Ronald Press, 1962, pp. 5–8.

Research Council, "Measurement and Evaluation Materials in Health, Physical Education and Recreation." Washington, D.C.: American Association for Health, Physical Education and Recreation, 1950.

3
Classification
of Measurements

When a field of study is in its first stages of formulation, confusion frequently results from a lack of clearly defined relationships among the areas of knowledge. Well-established sciences are bodies of analyzed, systematized, classified knowledge. In botany, for instance, plants are classified, and in zoology animals are classified. Physical education consists of a number of areas which are in various stages of classification, so one might contend that physical education is in the process of becoming a science. One of the first steps to avoid confusion in the study of physical education measurement is to view and study the various ways in which measurements may be classified.

Measurements are designed to examine, test, measure, and evaluate human traits. All human traits may be classified under two general categories: structural traits and functional traits. Structure and function are dynamic, that is, subject to change. They are closely related and affect each other to some degree throughout the whole period of a person's growth and development. Both structural and functional traits may be analyzed, synthesized, and hence classified from the general to the specific and from the specific to the general.

Differences in Traits

People exhibit differences in many structural and functional traits. In general these differences may be classified according to race, sex, age, and individual traits. When they fall outside the range called normality, these differences are classified as divergencies, or anomalies. Six fingers on one hand, one arm rather than two, a broken leg, mitral insufficiency, and typhoid fever are examples of divergencies in structure or function. Difficulties in testing may often be avoided by using tests constructed specifically for one sex, or for one age, when such groupings are important. Likewise, tests may be designed for children in elementary school, for boys or girls in junior or senior high school, for college men or women, or for the middle-aged or even older adults.

Method of Classifying Measurements

All measurements in physical education are of either structural or functional traits. Anthropometric measurements deal with structural traits. Tests of functional traits fall into four categories: interpretive traits (knowledge, concepts, beliefs, and so on), impulsive traits (feelings, interests, attitudes, and so forth), neuromuscular traits (nerve–muscle coordinations), and organic traits (functions of the organic systems).

Anthropometric Measurements

Anthropometric measurements are objective measurements of the structure of the body. Height, weight, hip width, chest depth, and girth of the upper arm are examples of anthropometric measurements. Long before the Christian era the people of India, China, and Greece measured the size, form, and symmetry of the body and related these traits to beauty and function. Sculptors in Greece searched for a unit of measurement that could be used to find the correct proportions of the perfect man and woman.

Measurement in objective units is possible with such tools as scales, tape measure, calipers, stadiometer, and silhouetteograph. Helen B. Pryor's Width–Weight Tables and the Wetzel Grid have proved to be useful standards for finding the lower and upper limits of normal weight in terms of growth rate. Sheldon classified physique, or body type, as endomorphic, mesomorphic, or ectomorphic. Body build assumes importance as a facet of measurement because of its effect on motor performance. Certain body builds are advantageous to certain activities; a heavy build may help a football tackle, but is a hindrance to a distance runner.

Tests of Interpretive Traits

Interpretive traits include perceptions, ideas, concepts, understandings, knowledge, and judgments. Information or knowledge tests about the history of physical education; about the rules, techniques, and strategies which govern performance; about the environment which influences performance; and about oneself as a performer may be classified as tests of interpretive traits. These tests may be given orally, or they may require writing an essay or answering true–false, matching, multiple-choice, or completion questions. Tests of interpretive traits have been and may be constructed in a great variety of physical education activities.

Tests of Impulsive Traits

Tests, or ratings, of the degree of interest in physical education activities, of attitudes toward activities, of maturity of emotions, and of the quality of ideals held may be classified as tests of impulsive traits. These kinds of measurements are usually in the form of rating scales or check lists. They become subjective estimates of the traits under consideration. The rating scales relating to interest may use such headings as *excellent, above average, average, below average,* and *poor.* Relating to attitudes the headings may be *always, usually, sometimes, rarely,* and *never*; or, *strongly agree, agree, undecided, disagree,* and *strongly disagree.* While little has been done to date, possibilities exist for the development of tests to measure the ideals and the emotional maturity as these factors relate to physical education.

Tests of Neuromuscular Traits

Neuromuscular tests include measurements of strength, specific skills, agility, power, reaction time, speed, balance, flexibility, and other qualities of performance which depend primarily upon the effective functioning of the nervous and muscular systems.

Individual strength tests have been devised for specific muscle groups, such as strength of arm and shoulder girdle, hand, back, abdomen, and legs. A general strength index may be determined with a battery of strength tests. Tests of other neuromuscular traits have also been developed, including tests of muscular (explosive) power, flexibility, speed, agility, reaction time, and balance.

Many tests of specific skills are available in the areas of individual events (100-yard run, long jump), elements in games (football kick for distance, softball throw for accuracy, base running against time, putting accuracy), individual sports (archery, bowling, golf, swimming), dual activities (badminton, handball, tennis), and team sports (baseball, basketball, field hockey, American football, rugby, softball, soccer, speedball, and volleyball).

Tests of Organic Traits

Organic traits include the physiological functions of internal organs and systems of organs (circulatory, respiratory, digestive, eliminative, and heat regulating mechanisms). Physical educators are primarily interested in the efficiency of the circulatory and respiratory processes of organic systems.

There are two kinds of tests of endurance: tests of muscular endurance (static and dynamic) and tests of circulatory–respiratory endurance. Some activities emphasize muscular endurance (the ability to repeat muscular contractions many times) while other activities emphasize circulatory–respiratory endurance.

Batteries of Tests

Two or more different tests administered to a person within a short time is called a *battery of tests.* The tests might measure several traits, and the intercorrelations of the traits may be relatively low. A battery of tests may be given in one activity, such as soccer, it may include two or more activities, or it may test a series of traits within one aspect of development. The results of batteries of tests may be interpreted in relation to achievement, ability, and progress. Skill tests in individual athletic events may be combined into a pentathlon (five events) or a decathlon (ten events).

Batteries of tests have been developed to measure such traits as general athletic ability, total body strength, and flexibility. In recent years several test batteries, labeled Tests of Physical Fitness, have been introduced.

Summary

Physical educators are concerned with the anatomical structure of the body and the function of the interpretive, impulsive, neuromuscular, and organic processes. Interpretive fitness means ability to comprehend and remember. Impulsive fitness refers to a variety of wholesome interests, desirable attitudes, emotional maturity, and beneficial ideals. Neuromuscular fitness is the ability to do coordinated movements—to perform skillfully. Organic fitness refers to the ability of the organic systems to function efficiently. Although they are related, structure and function are nevertheless distinct from each other. In addition functions of different systems, although interrelated, are somewhat separate. Therefore, tests should be specific to the particular aspect of structure or function which they are designed to measure, and the tests should be labeled accordingly. Much confusion exists at the present time because of the improper naming of tests.

Other Methods of Classification

Physical education measurements may also be classified according to kind of activity (such as basketball tests or swimming tests), type of test structure (such as true–false or essay), purpose of test (such as diagnosis or motivation), and traits to be measured (such as ability, achievement, or progress). A given test may fall under all four categories, for example, a *true–false* test of *ability* to remember certain rules of *basketball* given for *diagnostic* purposes to discover which rules need to be reviewed.

Kind of Activity

Tests named after specific physical education activities have been constructed and used in football, gymnastic activities, archery, badminton, baseball, basketball, bowling, dance, diving, fencing, golf, swimming, tennis, individual events in track and field, volleyball, wrestling, and a great variety of other activities appropriate for students in the elementary schools, secondary schools, and colleges.

Type of Test Structure

Written tests may consist of essay questions which are to be answered in paragraph form, statements which are to be answered true or false (true–false test), statements which are to be matched (matching test), several statements from which the most appropriate one is to be selected (multiple-choice test), and statements which are to be completed by inserting the missing words (completion test). A given test may be composed of one or more of these type questions.

Tests may be given for different reasons, that is, for diagnostic, classification, administrative, motivational, supervisory, or research purposes. Tests given by physical education instructors to determine the needs of students for specific kinds of development serve a diagnostic purpose, and the results may be used to guide individuals. Tests may also be used to classify students into homogeneous groups for purposes of instruction or competition. Tests have an administrative use when grading students and when evaluating methods of instruction. They have a supervisory use when evaluating the efficiency of teachers, and they may serve the purposes of research when the data obtained are needed for the solution of specific problems.

Tests may be designed to measure performance, progress, achievement, ability, and capacity. The basic tool in determining values in any aspect of function (behavior) is the performance record. Scores representing progress, achievement, ability, and capacity are only interpretations of performance records. A given performance record cannot be used as an achievement score, ability score, or capacity score without proper conversion.

Measurement of Performance.   A sample performance record of a student is not necessarily his present ability or his capacity to perform. Performance may depend upon a number of factors including motivation, emotional status, effort, organic condition, time of day, and even weather. Performance may also be influenced by sex, age, height, weight, body build, innate capacity, and degree of maturation. An individual's performance is what he does on a particular occasion, for example, five feet in the high jump.

Measurement of Progress.   Two or more measures, separated by a period of time, are necessary to measure progress. For example, performance tests may be given at the beginning and again at the end of a course for the purpose of measuring the amount of progress made during the intervening time. Measuring progress is important because the results indicate whether certain kinds of development have occurred and at what rate.

Measurement of Achievement.   When a student does a standing long jump of seven feet and then asks the instructor whether this performance is poor or good, the instructor may give a subjective evaluation (his judgment based on past experience) or an objective evaluation if he has an achievement scale at hand. Measures of achievement are simply evaluations of performance in terms of what other students in a classified group can do. Measuring achievement is of primary value in motivating students to perform better.

Achievement scales may be constructed in individual games or sports (archery), in individual events (high jump), and in elements of games or sports (volleyball serve for accuracy). The necessary requirement is that the individual perform alone; that is, his performance should not depend upon the performance of others.

Measurement of Ability.   In physical education the terms *ability* and *capacity* have sometimes been used interchangeably without regard to the differences in meaning. Capacity means potential, or the limits within which ability may be developed. Ability indicates the actual amount (expressed overtly in performance) to which capacity has been developed. Hence, an individual will probably always have a greater capacity to perform in a given activity than he has ability to perform. At any given time a person's ability is represented by his best performance record taken from numerous trials. Ability in activities may be modified considerably as a result of learning, practice, and conditioning.

Measurement of Capacity.   The capacity to perform an activity is limited in part by heredity and in part by the development that occurs during the period of maturation. To some extent capacity is dynamic, a result of a number of factors. To illustrate, one's capacity to high jump at age two years, 20 years, and 80 years is not the same. Capacity is different from ability in that capacity represents the limits within which ability may be developed. At present it is doubtful whether there are any valid tests of capacity to perform in motor activities. Perhaps the best approach to estimating capacity is to study learning and achievement curves represented by improved performances. It seems logical to assume that motor aptitude and motor educability are aspects of motor capacity.

4

Selection and
Administration of Tests

Measurements range from highly subjective to highly objective tests. Objective measures are based largely on fact, while subjective measures are primarily a result of personal judgment. Subjective measurement, such as a teacher's evaluation of a student's character, includes some degree of objectivity but also involves a large amount of judgment. Objective measurement is based on more precise information. A measure is objective to the extent that it will produce the same results when conducted by different people under similar conditions—in other words when the subjectivity of the test administrator is eliminated. No measure in physical education is completely objective, and no measure ought to be completely subjective. Teachers should strive for a high degree of objectivity in measurement but still realize that not all important traits can be measured objectively.

Selection of Tests

The physical education teacher is confronted with the problem of selecting good tools to be used in measurement. Successful selection of tools demands a knowledge of measurement in general and of the characteristics of good tests. Tests may be selected for classifying pupils, measuring achievement, diagnosing defects, grading, or motivating students.

In the selection of tests to be incorporated into the physical education program, validity, reliability, and objectivity of each test should be considered. Validity is the most important characteristic of any measure. It is the degree to which the test actually measures what it is supposed to measure. For instance, a test of strength is valid to the extent that it actually measures strength. Tests are usually validated for only one purpose, and a valid measure of one characteristic is not necessarily a valid measure for any other characteristic.

Not every quality can be measured with the same degree of accuracy. For example, ability to perform in the vertical jump can be measured accurately, while ability to perform in soccer is more difficult to measure. Although there is no general rule concerning the degree of validity necessary for a measure to be useful, the most valid measure available should be used, and high significance should not be attached to results from tests which are not highly valid.

Reliability is the extent to which a test consistently measures the same thing each time. A test can be reliable and still not be highly valid, but a test that is valid is also reliable. Lack of reliability may result from variations in the behavior of the examiner and to causes inherent in the test or external to the test.

Objectivity is the degree to which consistent results are obtained from the use of the same method of measurement by different persons. Essentially, objectivity is the precision of the instruments and techniques used. Since it contributes to consistency, objectivity can add or detract from the reliability of a measure.

Administrative economy, educational application, and existence of norms and standard instructions are also important factors in the selection of tests. Administrative economy is determined by the time and money needed to administer the test. A practical and useful test must be economical in terms of time and cost. It is difficult to say how much time and money should be devoted to the administration of any test, but in every case, before he decides to use a test, the instructor should weigh the value of the results in comparison with the expenditure of money, time, and effort.

Educational application is the degree to which the testing experience is educational in itself and the degree to which it motivates the students to learn. In the selection and construction of tests educational application should serve as an important guide. In other words, the experience of taking the test should be educational. The tests used should be harmonious with and supplement the course content.

Norms are standards against which raw scores may be compared. The availability of norms may lead to the selection of one test in preference to another. Standard instructions are important for the administration of standardized tests if the results are to be reliable. Hence, some good tests may be rejected because standardized instructions are not available. Test instructions should be as brief, complete, and clear as possible; they should also include an example or demonstration.

In general, authorities on testing agree that, except for research, only valid measures that can be administered to a group of students at one time and require little equipment are highly useful in physical education. Measurements are of value only if the results can be accurately interpreted and practically applied.

Administration of Tests

Careful attention should be given to the administration of tests. Poorly administered tests can produce results which are misleading and useless to both the teacher and the students. The following guides are helpful in administering tests.

1.   Select and administer a test for a specific purpose, and be certain that it is administered in such a way that it accomplishes that purpose.

2.   Become familiar with the test and the procedures involved before attempting to administer it.

3.   Make early arrangements for all necessary facilities and equipment, and be sure the equipment is in usable condition.

4.   Determine the layout of testing stations and have needed equipment in place at the required time. The layout for testing should permit the test items to be given in correct sequence and still result in easy flow of traffic.

5.   Be sure those being tested appear in appropriate clothing, especially in appropriate footwear.

6.   Make early arrangements for necessary assistant leaders to help administer the test. In some cases a short period of training the assistants may be desirable.

7.   Conduct the test exactly as explained in the instructions.

8.   Teach the students to perform the test item correctly.
      a.   State the purpose of the test item (what it measures).
      b.   Give a description of the test item and the way to perform it.
      c.   Demonstrate the item. (Either the teacher or a trained student may demonstrate.)
      d.   Answer any questions to clarify procedure.
      e.   Lead the students in the practice of items for which pretest practice is appropriate.
      f.   Describe briefly the method of scoring and the way results will be interpreted and scored.

9.   Have the necessary score sheets, pencils, and scoring scales available.

The test results should be interpreted and used to the advantage of the students and the program. Teachers should constantly be aware that the exactness and correctness with which they administer a test influences its reliability. Measures that might have been valuable become useless when they are improperly administered and incorrectly interpreted.

Selected References

Barrow, Harold M., and McMee, Rosemary, "Evaluation of Tests" and "Administration of Tests," *A Practical Approach to Measurement in Physical Education.* Philadelphia: Lea & Febiger, May 1966.

Clarke, H. Harrison, "Test Evaluation," *Application of Measurement to Health and Physical Education.* Englewood Cliffs, N.J.: Prentice-Hall, 1967.

Johnson, Barry L., and Nelson, Jack K., "Test Evaluation and Construction," *Practical Measurements for Evaluation in Physical Education*. Minneapolis: Burgess Publishing Company, 1969.

Mathews, Donald K., "Test Selection," *Measurement in Physical Education* (third ed.), Philadelphia: W. B. Saunders Company, 1968.

TWO
Basic Statistics
Applied to Physical Education

To select tests, construct tests, and use the results of tests effectively, it is necessary to understand certain statistical techniques. This section includes explanations of the techniques which are often useful to physical education teachers. The more advanced statistical techniques used primarily in research are not included.

Recording
and Presenting Data

This chapter deals with basic mathematical procedures, recording data (scores), organizing data, and presenting data in tables and graphs.

Mathematical Review

The following is a review of basic mathematical procedures. (Refer to a mathematics textbook for a more extensive review.)

Addition. For numbers of like signs, add the numbers and use the sign common to both of them: $(15) + (10) = 25$; $(-15) + (-10) = -25$. For numbers of different signs, find the difference between the numbers and apply the sign of the larger number: $(15) + (-10) = 5$; $(-15) + (10) = -5$.

Subtraction. Change the sign of the number to be subtracted and then add the numbers algebraically: $(15) - (10) = 5$; $(-15) - (10) = -25$; $(-15) - (-10) = -5$; $(15) - (-10) = 25$.

Multiplication. When numbers of like signs are multiplied, the answer is positive: $(15) \times (10) = 150$; $(-15) \times (-10) = 150$. When the two numbers are of different signs, the answer is negative: $(15) \times (-10) = -150$; $(-15) \times (10) = -150$.

Division. As in multiplication, when two numbers are of like signs, the answer is positive: $(15) \div (10) = 1.5$; $(-15) \div (-10) = 1.5$. When the two numbers are of different signs, the answer is negative: $(15) \div (-10) = -1.5$; $(-15) \div (10) = -1.5$.

Percentage: Divide the total into the portion, or divide the larger number into the smaller number: 15 is what percent of 30? ($15 \div 30 = .50 = 50$ percent); 29 is what percent of 80? ($29 \div 80 = .36 = 36$ percent); 687 is what percent of 1560? ($687 \div 1560 = .44 = 44$ percent).

Squares. To square a number, simply multiply it by itself: $25^2 = (25) \times (25) = 625$; $2.5^2 = (2.5) \times (2.5) = 6.25$. To check the answer, divide it by the original number: $625 \div 25 = 25$; $6.25 \div 2.5 = 2.5$.

Square Root. Square roots of many numbers are found in the Table of Square Roots in Appendix E. But the square roots of some numbers not in the table may be needed; therefore, it is important to recall the procedure for computing square roots. Following is a description of how to extract the square root of the number 4854.60:

$$
\begin{array}{r r r}
 & & 6\ 9.\ 6\ 7 \\
 & & \overline{4854.6000} \\
6 & & 36 \\
\hline
129 & & 1254 \\
 & & 1161 \\
\hline
1386 & & 9360 \\
 & & 8316 \\
\hline
13927 & & 104400 \\
 & & 97489 \\
\hline
 & & 6911 \\
\end{array}
$$

a.   Begin at the decimal point and mark off two places at a time to the left and to the right.

b.   Estimate the root of the first number, or pair of numbers (48), and place the root (6) as the divisor and also in the answer.

c.   Multiply the divisor (6) by the answer (6) and subtract the result ($48 - 36 = 12$).

d.   Bring down the next pair of figures (54).

e.   Multiply the present answer by 2 and add a zero to represent another digit ($2 \times 6 = 12$, add a zero $= 120$). This figure is the new divisor.

f.   Place the next root in the answer and replace the zero in the divisor by that same number (9). The divisor is now 129.

g.   Multiply 9×129 and subtract the result (1161) from 1254.

h.   Repeat the procedure until the answer appears in as many decimal places as desired.

Assignment 1

1.   Addition
   $(26) + (-92) =$
   $(-93) + (-13) =$
   $(56) + (112) =$
   $(-16) + (63) =$

2.   Subtraction
   $(-62) - (-26) =$
   $(-47) - (32) =$
   $(113) - (-47) =$
   $(23) - (17) =$

3. Multiplication
    $(-13) \times (43) =$
    $(-28) \times (-69) =$
    $(93) \times (-12) =$
    $(67) \times (10) =$

4. Division
    $(-73) \div (12) =$
    $(-69) \div (-30) =$
    $(24) \div (-6) =$
    $(36) \div (14) =$

5. The following chart contains the season won–lost records for four professional baseball teams. Express the season record for each team in a percentage:

Team	Won	Lost	Percentage
A	101	51	_____
B	70	90	_____
C	78	83	_____
D	109	53	_____

6. Express the batting percentage of the following players:

Player	At Bat	Hits	Percentage
A	491	149	_____
B	432	135	_____
C	544	170	_____
D	540	132	_____

7. Squares
    $16^2 =$
    $132^2 =$
    $44^2 =$
    $220^2 =$

8. Square Roots
    $\sqrt{1} =$
    $\sqrt{144} =$
    $\sqrt{10.46} =$
    $\sqrt{1224} =$

Recording Data

A number of important considerations should be understood in the recording of data.

1. The exact unit of measure to be used is determined to a large extent by whether the data are *continuous* or *discrete*. A series which is capable of any degree of subdivision is defined as continuous data. For example, height can be measured in yards, feet, inches, and so on. Conversely a series which cannot be subdivided without destroying the unit is called discrete data. The number of people in a class or the number of balls in a storeroom are examples of discrete data. Continuous data may be recorded in units as refined as one chooses; discrete data may only be as refined as its whole unit of measure.

2.   The unit of measure to be used and its refinement must be determined. For example, the weight of an object may be computed to the nearest pound, half pound, or ounce.

3.   Whether the recorded measures will represent the next unit, the nearest unit, or the last unit is decided. Age is customarily measured to the *last* (lowest) whole year. Height is usually measured to the *nearest* whole inch, and weight to the nearest pound. Centuries are recorded to the *next* unit; for example, we are now in the twentieth century.

4.   The real limits of a recorded score are the highest and lowest values which are represented by that score. Where age is recorded to the *last* whole year, a recorded age of 21 years actually represents any age between 21.000 years and 21.999 years. Where height is recorded to the *nearest* inch, a height of 5 feet 2 inches actually represents all heights between 5 feet 1.500 inches and 5 feet 2.499 inches.

Frequency Distributions

Anyone who has worked with test scores knows the difficulty of making meaningful interpretations from a group of unordered scores. Scores need to be presented and arranged in some meaningful fashion so that they are easy to work with and easy to interpret. One possibility is to place them in order from the highest to the lowest scores (rank order). If the number of scores is small such an arrangement is adequate, but with a large number of scores a rank order arrangement presents an awkward situation. Therefore, a better procedure is to construct a frequency distribution.

Frequency distributions may be either simple or grouped. In a *simple frequency distribution* data are organized with all possible score values listed in order of size; the number of frequencies of each score value is then indicated. A simple frequency distribution greatly facilitates interpretation; the more frequently occurring scores stand out clearly so that the high and low scores and the total number of scores become apparent. The simple frequency distribution gives a graphic impression of the distribution of scores. Table 5-1 is an example of a simple frequency distribution.

To establish a simple frequency distribution:

1.   Indicate the distribution as a table and assign it a number.

2.   Give it a title which identifies it as a simple frequency distribution and describes its contents.

Table 5-1
Simple Frequency Distribution of Scores Made by 50
High School Girls on the Sit-up Test (Data I)*

x (score)	t (tally)	f (frequency)
21	//	2
20	//	2
19	////	4
18	⊬⊬ /	6
17	⊬⊬ ⊬⊬ /	11
16	⊬⊬	5
15	////	4
14	////	4
13	////	4
12	/	1
11	///	3
10	/	1
9	//	2
8		0
7	/	1
		N = 50

* Data I appears in Appendix A.

3.   Establish three columns and label them score (x), tally (t), and frequency (f).

4.   In the x column record all possible score values from the highest to the lowest score.

5.   In the t column tally each score by recording a tally mark opposite that score value.

6.   Total the tally marks for each score value and record that total in the f column.

If the scores are numerous and cover a large range, the simple frequency distribution becomes bulky; therefore, a more compact arrangement is desirable. Such an arrangement can be accomplished by a *grouped frequency distribution*, an organization of scores with all possible score values included within equal intervals and with the score values within each interval indicated. The grouped frequency distribution may give a better concept of the shape of the distribution of scores than a simple frequency distribution, but in a grouped distribution the identity of the individual scores is lost. Table 5-2 is an example of a grouped frequency distribution.

Table 5-2
Grouped Frequency Distribution of Scores Made by 75
High School Boys on the Right Grip Test, Measured to the Nearest
Pound, and Recorded in Intervals of 5 Units (Data II)*

Intervals	t	f
135–139	//	2
130–134	/	1
125–129	ЖЖ	5
120–124	ЖЖ ////	4
115–119	///	3
110–114	ЖЖ ////	9
105–109	ЖЖ /	6
100–104	ЖЖ ЖЖ //	12
95–99	ЖЖ ЖЖ	10
90–94	ЖЖ //	7
85–89	ЖЖ	5
80–84	//	2
75–79	ЖЖ	5
70–74		0
65–69	/	1
60–64	///	3
		N = 75

* Data II appears in Appendix A.

To construct a grouped frequency distribution:

1.   Give the table a number and a descriptive title.

2.   Establish three columns and label them intervals (steps), t (tally), and f (frequency).

3.   Determine the range of the scores (highest score minus lowest).

4.   Determine the approximate number of intervals desired (usually not more than 25 intervals nor less than 12).

5.   Divide the range of scores by the desired number of intervals to determine the approximate size of the intervals.

6.   Make a final decision on the number and size of intervals on the basis of convenience and purpose.

7.   Record the interval limits, tally the scores, and record the frequencies.

Certain points concerning the construction and interpretation of a grouped frequency distribution are important.

1. Two, five, and multiples of five are preferred sizes of intervals because these numbers are easy to handle mathematically. Usually odd numbers, such as three, five, seven, are preferred over even numbers because odd numbers yield a whole number as the midpoint of each interval.

2. The upper limit of one interval is always separated from the lower limit of the next higher interval by one unit of measure. The unit of measure for the data in Table 5-2 is one pound. Therefore, the step intervals are separated by one pound (60–64, 65–69, 70–74, and so on). Had the data been recorded to the nearest half pound, the step intervals would have been separated by that unit of measure (60–64.5, 65–69.5, and so on).

3. When data are recorded to the nearest unit, the real limits of a step interval extend one half unit above and one half unit below the recorded limits of the interval. For example, in Table 5-2 the recorded limits of the second and third intervals are 65–69 and 70–74 respectively. The real limits of the two intervals are 64.5–69.499 and 69.5–74.499 respectively. (74.499 represents 74.5 reduced.)

Recorded Limits (separated by one unit of measure)	Real Limits (includes all values actually represented by the interval)
75–79	74.5–79.499
70–74	69.5–74.499
65–69	64.5–69.499
60–64	59.5–64.499

4. The scores within a given interval in a grouped frequency distribution are assumed to be spread evenly over the entire interval. The midpoint of the interval is the most logical choice to represent all scores within a given interval by a single value. To compute the midpoint of the interval 100–104 in Table 5-2, the following formula should be used:

$$\text{midpoint} = \text{lower real limit of interval} + \frac{\text{upper real limit} - \text{lower real limit}}{2}$$

Hence, $\text{midpoint} = 99.5 + \dfrac{104.5 - 99.5}{2} = 102$

Assignment 2

1. Using Data III from Appendix A, make a frequency distribution for each factor under the following conditions:

	Interval	Highest Interval
Height	1	70
Weight	5	155–159
Leg strength	20	760–779
High jump	2	58–59
100-yard run	.5	10.0–10.4*

* In races the lowest time is the best (highest) score.

2. State the range for each distribution prepared under number one above.

3. In leg strength what is the midpoint of the third step from the top?

4. In the 100-yard run what is the midpoint of the second step from the top?

5. N = the number of scores. What does N equal for weight? for high jump?

Graphical Methods

Graphs reveal the same information found in frequency distributions, but in graphs the information is conveyed pictorially. There are certain advantages of graphs over frequency distributions: (a) In some graphs the shape and characteristics of the distribution become more obvious, and (b) for people unfamiliar with the data the information in a graph is more easily understandable. Basic graphs are based on the coordinate system which involves two axes: Y, the vertical axis (ordinate); and X, the horizontal axis (abscissa).

Any point can be plotted on the coordinate system when its X and Y values are known. For example, locate point P when $X = +2$ and $Y = +2$.

The histogram, frequency polygon, and cumulative frequency curve are standard graphs. Variations of these standard forms are often used. These three graphs have the following points in common:

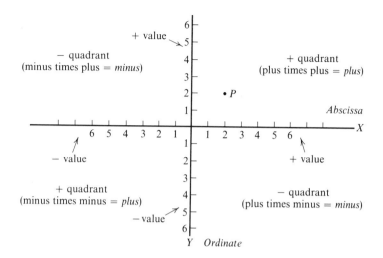

Figure 5-1. Coordinate System. Any point can be plotted on the coordinate system if its *X* and *Y* values are known. For example, point *P* is plotted when *X* = +2 and *Y* = +2.

1. In all cases the score values are recorded on the horizontal axis (abscissa), and the frequencies are represented on the vertical axis (ordinate).

2. The score values are recorded from low to high, moving from left to right.

3. When the data are grouped, the midpoint of each interval is used to represent all scores in the interval. Hence, all values on the horizontal scale are midpoints of intervals.

4. Each graph must carry a title and should be labeled "Figure" with a number (for example, Figure 5-1). The title is usually placed below the graph.

5. Both axes (ordinate and abscissa) are labeled.

Histogram

A histogram is a graph in which the score frequencies are represented by a series of adjacent columns. The base of each column corresponds to the size of the interval, and the height of each column is proportional to the frequencies in the interval. The middle of the column is at the midpoint of the interval, and the edges of the column represent the upper and lower real limits of the interval. Figure 5-2 is an example of a histogram.

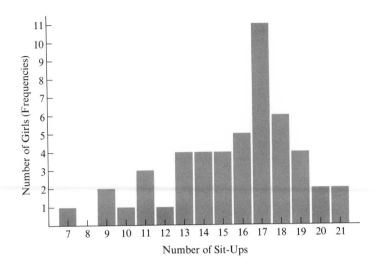

Figure 5-2.   Histogram of scores made by 50 high school girls on the sit-up test (see frequency distribution in Table 1).

To construct a histogram:

1.   Leave a space of one-half column between the ordinate and the first column and between the last column and the end of the abscissa.

2.   Be sure that all columns are exactly the same width because they represent intervals of equal size. (They need not be separate as in Figure 5-2).

3.   Decide on the size for the length and height of the graph. (The height is generally about two thirds of the length.)

4.   Label both the vertical and horizontal scales and assign a title describing the content of the graph.

5.   After establishing the vertical and horizontal scales, plot the upper and lower limits of each interval along the abscissa, plot the upper and lower limits of each interval at the height of the frequencies in that interval, and draw the necessary lines to complete the columns (see Figure 5-2).

Frequency Polygon

A polygon is a line graph in which the midpoints of the intervals are joined by straight lines at the height of the frequencies in the intervals (see Figure 5-3).

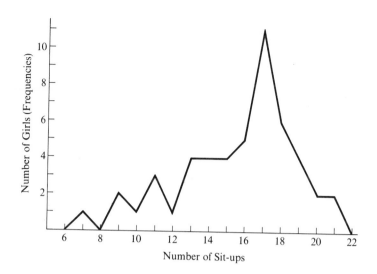

Figure 5-3. Frequency polygon of scores made by 50 high school girls on the sit-up test (see frequency distribution in Table 1).

To construct a frequency polygon:

1.   Place the first number along the horizontal scale at a distance of one interval from the ordinate.

2.   Plot a point directly above each interval midpoint which appears on the horizontal scale and directly opposite the appropriate point along the frequency (vertical) scale. After the points have been plotted in the correct positions draw connecting lines between the points.

3.   Close the graph line at both ends to a point one interval above the highest number and one interval below the lowest number on the horizontal scale.

Cumulative Frequency (Ogive) Curve

A cumulative frequency curve is made up of the total frequencies in the distribution which have been added cumulatively, beginning at the bottom of the column (see Table 5-3). Each cumulative frequency point is plotted at the upper limit of the step in which it falls. After being plotted, the points are connected with straight lines to form the curve. The slope of the curve indicates the concentration of scores; for example, the steeper the line the greater the concentration of scores.

Table 5-3
A Simple Frequency Distribution of Scores Made by 50
High School Girls on the Sit-up Test (cf column added)

x	f	cf (cumulative frequencies)
21	2	50
20	2	48
19	4	46
18	6	42
17	11	36
16	5	25
15	4	20
14	4	16
13	4	12
12	1	8
11	3	7
10	1	4
9	2	3
8	0	1
7	1	1
		$N = 50$

For a more meaningful curve a percentile scale may be added to the right-hand side of the graph. The scale is labeled and marked off in equal units covering a range of 0 to 100 percent. When the percentile scale is added, the curve is called an "ogive." (Percentiles are described in Chapter 6.)

To construct a cumulative frequency (ogive) curve:

1.   Add a cumulative frequency column to the frequency distribution (see Table 5-3).

2.   Devise the *left-hand scale* to cover the range of the total number of frequencies in the distribution. (This scale is equal to the cumulative frequency (*cf*) column in a frequency distribution.) Devise the *horizontal scale* to cover the total range of scores, and the *right-handed scale* to include the complete percentile range (0–100). (The right-hand scale should correspond to the cumulative frequency scale in height and proportion.)

3.   Plot a point above the upper limit of each score at the height of the cumulative frequencies of the score. Then draw lines connecting the points.

4.   Label each of the scales and assign a descriptive title to the graph.

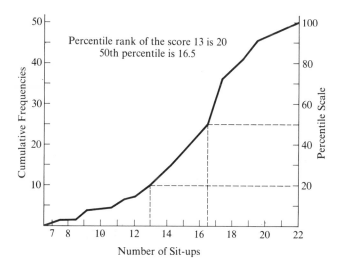

Figure 5-4. Combined cumulative frequency curve and percentile scale (ogive curve) of scores made by 50 high school girls on the sit-up test (see frequency distribution in Table 5-3).

Once the cumulative frequency curve and percentile scale have been constructed, the percentile rank of any score can be determined by drawing a line vertical to the curve line and then a line horizontal to the percentile scale. The opposite procedure may be followed to find the score equal to any given percentile (see Figure 5-4).

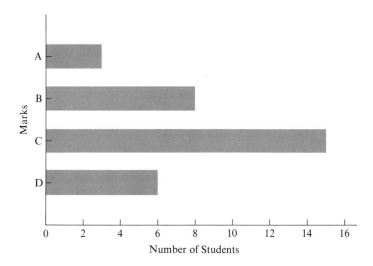

Figure 5-5. Horizontal bar graph of marks given to 32 students in a basketball class (A—3, B—8, C—15, D—6).

Horizontal Bar Graph

A horizontal bar graph (Figure 5-5) is a variation of a histogram. Sometimes the bars are made of figures representing the content of the graph. For instance, if the graph were about population trends, the bars might be made of figures of people.

Pie Graph

A pie graph is simply a complete circle divided into pie-shaped portions with each portion proportionate to the amount that it represents (see Figure 5-6). Each portion is usually labeled with the percentage of the whole that it represents. This type of graph is easy to read and is, therefore, often used to present information to laymen and to the masses.

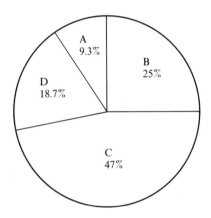

Figure 5-6.   Pie graph of marks given to 32 students in a basketball class.

Assignment 3

1.   Using the height scores in Data III from Appendix A, construct a histogram and give a verbal interpretation of what the graph tells you.

2.   Using Data II as it is organized in Table 5-2, construct a frequency polygon and give a verbal interpretation of what the graph tells you.

3.   Using Data II as it is organized in Table 5-2, construct an ogive curve and answer the following questions. (A *cf* column will need to be added to Table 5-2.)
(a)   Which score is at the 60th percentile? the 30th percentile?
(b)   What is the percentile rank of the score 75? of the score 115?

4. In connection with Data II from Appendix A the following ratings are given: excellent 125 and above, good 110–124, average 95–109, fair 80–94, poor 79 and below. Construct a pie graph showing the proportion of students who scored excellent, good, average, fair, and poor.

6
Basic
Statistical Methods

Central tendency measures, variability measures, percentiles, distribution curves, correlation, and reliability measures are statistical techniques useful to teachers.

Measures of Central Tendency

Measures of central tendency are points on a scale of scores which give a single measure that best represents the whole group. The three measures of central tendency used most frequently are the mean, the median, and the mode.

The mean is the arithmetic average. It is the sum of the scores divided by the number of scores.

The median is the middle measure in a series in which all scores have been arranged in order of their size. It is the point on the scale, above and below which 50 percent of the scores fall.

The mode is the most frequent score. When the scores are plotted on a curve, the mode is at the highest point of the curve.

Uses of Measures of Central Tendency

Generally measures of central tendency are used as convenient representative measures of a group; they can be used to make comparisons among groups. Each measure of central tendency has a specific use, but for the best interpretation of the distribution all three measures should be used.

Characteristics of Each Measure

The mean is the arithmetic average and is affected by the numerical value of each score. It is highly stable; that is, only when many scores are changed or when a few scores are changed a great amount does the mean vary appreciably. It is highly reliable, arithmetic, algebraically sound, and it is the only measure of central tendency derived from the actual score values. On the other hand it is the most difficult of the three measures to determine, and it is a poor representative measure of a skewed distribution because it is affected by extreme scores.

The median is a measure of position only. It is easy to calculate and the best

43

representative measure of a skewed distribution since extreme scores do not affect it. However, no further calculation may be made from it because it is a nonarithmetic measure. It is not highly stable since it can be changed with the alteration of only a few scores (depending on which scores are altered).

The mode is the most frequent score in a distribution and is easy to calculate. Yet it is extremely unstable, may be a poor representative measure of the group, and may not be used as a basis for further calculations.

Computing the Mean

The mean may be computed by any of the following formulas, each of which has certain advantages. In the formulas: M = mean; Σ = sum of; X = scores; N = number of scores (cases); f = frequency; GA = guessed average (arbitrary reference); d = deviation; SI = step interval; $\overline{M}$ = midpoint; and $\cdot$ = multiply.

Formula A $\quad M = \dfrac{\Sigma X}{N}$ (to be used when data are not ordered)

Formula B $\quad M = \dfrac{\Sigma(f \cdot X)}{N}$ (to be used when data are not grouped)

$\quad M = \dfrac{\Sigma(f \cdot \overline{M})}{N}$ (to be used when data are grouped. $\overline{M}$ is substituted for X in grouped data.)

Formula C $\quad M = GA + \left(\dfrac{\Sigma fd}{N} \cdot SI\right)$ (to be used with either simple or grouped data)

The following chart is an example of the application of formula A, using the unordered scores in Data I from Appendix A.

Scores

15	20	9	15	16
7	17	17	18	11
10	16	19	17	17
11	14	17	13	15
19	21	14	12	13
15	16	11	14	18
17	17	17	18	21
15	19	17	18	16
13	17	16	20	14
18	19	9	17	18

$\Sigma X = 781$
$N = 50$

$$M = \frac{\Sigma X}{N}$$

$$= \frac{781}{50}$$

$$M = 15.62$$

The following chart is an example of the application of formula B using a simple frequency distribution of Data I.

X	f	fX
21	2	42
20	2	40
19	4	76
18	6	108
17	11	187
16	5	80
15	4	60
14	4	56
13	4	52
12	1	12
11	3	33
10	1	10
9	2	18
8	0	0
7	1	7
	N = 50	fX = 781

$$M = \frac{(f \cdot X)}{N}$$

$$= \frac{781}{50}$$

$$M = 15.62$$

The following example shows the use of formula B with a grouped frequency distribution of Data II.

Interval	$\overline{M}$ (midpoint)	f	$f \cdot \overline{M}$
135–139	137	2	274
130–134	132	1	132
125–129	127	5	635
120–124	122	4	488
115–119	117	3	351
110–114	112	9	1008
105–109	107	6	642
100–104	102	12	1224
95–99	97	10	970
90–94	92	7	644
85–89	87	5	435
80–84	82	2	164
75–79	77	5	385
70–74	72	0	0
65–69	67	1	67
60–64	62	3	186
		$N = 75$	$\Sigma f\overline{M} = 7605$

$$M = \frac{\Sigma(f \cdot \overline{M})}{N}$$

$$= \frac{7605}{75}$$

$$M = 101.40$$

The following chart is an example of the use of formula C with a grouped frequency distribution of Data II.

Interval	f	d (deviation)	fd
135–139	2	7	14
130–134	1	6	6
125–129	5	5	25
120–124	4	4	16
115–119	3	3	9
110–114	9	2	18
105–109	6	1	6
GA 100–104	12	0	0
95–99	10	−1	−10
90–94	7	−2	−14
85–89	5	−3	−15
80–84	2	−4	−8
75–79	5	−5	−25
70–74	0	−6	0
65–69	1	−7	−7
60–64	3	−8	−24
	$N = 75$		$\Sigma fd = -9$

$$GA = 102 \text{ (midpoint of the interval)}$$

$$SI = 5$$

$$M = GA + \left(\frac{\Sigma fd}{N} \cdot SI\right)$$

$$= 102 + \left(\frac{-9}{75} \cdot 5\right)$$

$$= 102 + (-.60)$$

$$= 101.40$$

When the data are grouped and formula C is used:

1. Arrange the data into a frequency distribution.

2. Guess an average near the center of the distribution. (The GA is the midpoint of that interval.)

3. Record the deviation (d) of each interval in terms of step intervals from the GA.

4. Multiply the d of each interval by its corresponding f to get the fd.

5. Find the algebraic sum of the plus and minus fds and divide this sum by the number of cases (N).

6. Multiply $\dfrac{\Sigma fd}{N}$ by the size of the step interval.

7. Add the answer in Step 6 algebraically to the GA to get the mean.

Uses of Each Formula

Formula A is the basic formula for calculating the mean. It is used when there is a small number of scores and no need to construct a frequency distribution. This formula produces accurate results.

Formula B is the *long method* formula for calculating the mean from a simple or grouped frequency distribution. It produces accurate results from a simple frequency distribution, but because the midpoint of each interval is used to represent all the scores in that interval, slight error may occur with grouped data.

Formula C is the *short method* formula for calculating the mean from a simple or grouped frequency distribution. It produces accurate results from a simple frequency distribution but may produce slight inaccuracies when used with grouped data. The short method formula eliminates extensive addition, greatly simplifies multiplication, and, in cases for which further calculations are to be made from the frequency distribution, saves time because of the columns added to the distribution. When the mean is calculated from a sample frequency distribution, the *SI* (step interval) serves no purpose since it always equals one.

Basic Assumptions in Calculating the Mean

When data are grouped, the identity of individual scores is lost. Therefore, when the mean is calculated from a grouped frequency distribution, the assumption is made that within each interval the mean of those scores is equal to the midpoint of the interval. Errors, although usually negligible, may result if the assumption is not true. Yet with extensive data the convenience of the method outweighs the possibility of error, unless the data are to be used for exact research, in which case accuracy cannot be sacrificed for convenience.

Assignment 4

1.   Using Data III from Appendix A, and formula *A*, compute the mean for each of the six factors.

2.   Using Data III, formula *B*, and the groupings suggested under Assignment 2, compute the mean for height and the high jump.

3.   Using Data III, formula *C*, and the groupings suggested under Assignment 2, compute the mean for strength and the 100-yard run.

Computing the Median

The median is the middle measure on a scale in which all measures have been arranged in order of their size. The median of the following scores is nine.

4   5   6   7   8   9   10   11   12   13   14

↑

median

To compute the Median from a Simple Frequency Distribution:

1.   Arrange the data into a simple frequency distribution.

2.   Add a cumulative frequency (*cf*) column by successively adding the frequencies of each score beginning at the bottom.

3.   Divide *N* by 2 and locate the step in which that number occurs in the *cf* column. The score in that step is the median.

Note the following example using Data I.

X	f	cf
21	2	50
20	2	48
19	4	46
18	6	42
17	11	36
16	5	25
15	4	20
14	4	16
13	4	12
12	1	8
11	3	7
10	1	4
9	2	3
8	0	1
7	1	·1
	$N = 50$	

$$Mdn = \frac{N}{2} = \frac{50}{2} = 25\text{th score}$$

The median is the score in the step which includes the 25th score from the bottom in the cf column.

$$Mdn = 16$$

To compute the Median from a Grouped Frequency Distribution, use the any-percentile formula:

$$P = LL + \frac{np - n'}{f'} \times SI$$

where

$P =$ desired percentile (Mdn $=$ 50th percentile)
$LL =$ lower real limit of the interval in which P will lie
$n =$ number of cases
$p =$ percentage desired
$n' =$ number of cases included up to the lower limit of the interval in which P lies.
$f' =$ frequencies in the interval in which P lies
$SI =$ size of the step interval

Note the following example using the any-percentile formula and Data II.

X	f	cf
135–139	2	75
130–134	1	73
125–129	5	72
120–124	4	67
115–119	3	63
110–114	9	60
105–109	6	51
100–104	12	45
95–99	10	33
90–94	7	23
85–89	5	16
80–84	2	11
75–79	5	9
70–74	0	4
65–69	1	4
60–64	3	3
	$\overline{N = 75}$	

$$Mdn \text{ (50th percentile)} = LL + \frac{np - n'}{f'} \times SI$$

The interval in which P will lie is found by taking $n \times p$; that is, $75 \times .50 = 37.5$ (rounded to 38). The interval in which P will lie is the one corresponding to the 38th score in the cf column. The 38th score lies in the interval 100–104, of which the lower real limit is 99.5. Therefore,

$$Mdn = 99.5 + \frac{37.5 - 33}{12} \times 5$$

$$Mdn = 101.38$$

By use of the same formula the 10th, 20th, or any other percentile can be determined. Again, because with grouped data the identity of individual scores is lost, it must be assumed that the scores are evenly distributed within the interval in which the median is found. If the assumption is not met slight error may result.

Computing the Mode

The mode is the most frequent score in the distribution. If there are two most frequent scores, then there are two modes and the distribution is said to be bimodal. If there are three or more most frequent scores, the distribution is multimodal.

If the data are grouped, the mode is at the midpoint of the interval containing the highest number of frequencies. Because this midpoint may vary from the real mode, it is referred to as the crude mode.

Assignment 5

Problems

1. Using Data III from Appendix A, the any-percentile formula, and the groupings suggested under Assignment 2, compute the median for height and the high jump.

2. Using Data III and the groupings suggested under Assignment 2, determine the mode or modes for the 100-yard run, strength, and weight.

Practice Questions

1. A physical education teacher gave a performance test to determine the number of sit-ups each student could perform. After all students were measured, the mean score was found to be 20, but the median was only 15. The teacher reasoned that since the average student could do 20 sit-ups, 20 should be the standard number expected of all students after a short training period. He thought that 20 sit-ups would work a hardship on only a few students. What was wrong with his reasoning?

2. You gave a standardized strength test to your students and found that the median score was seriously below the national norm. The school principal asked you to do something about it. After a little thought you realized that you could raise the median considerably by concentrating on a few students. (a) Which students would you concentrate on? (b) Which measure of central tendency would not be raised appreciably by concentrating on a few?

3. A test is given to two groups of students, A and B. The following statistics are found:

	Mean	Median
Group A	20	25
Group B	25	20

If any score above 20 is considered as good, which group has more good students in terms of this test?

4.   Which is the least stable of the three measures of central tendency?

5.   Which measure should be used to avoid the influence of extremely high or extremely low scores?

Measures of Variability

Variability refers to the extent of differences. The term is commonly interchanged with the words *dispersion, spread, scatter,* and *deviation.* Measures of variability are distances along the scale of scores. Except for range and equidistant percentiles a measure of variability should be thought of as a unit of distance along the scale by which any measure in the distribution may be described with a measure of *central tendency* as the reference point. By knowing measures of central tendency, one is able to visualize the concentration of scores. By knowing measures of variability, one can visualize the amount that scores spread or deviate from the central tendency.

The different measures of variability are the range, equidistant percentiles, interquartile range, semi-interquartile range, average deviation, variance, and standard deviation.

Range (R) may be expressed as the distance from the highest score to the lowest score in the distribution, for example, from 100 to 50. It may also be stated as the difference between the extreme scores (100–50; range $=$ 50).

Equidistant percentiles are percentiles which occur on opposite sides of the median and are equal distances in terms of percentage of cases from the median. For example, the 10th and 90th percentiles are equidistant percentiles as are the 25th and 75th percentiles.

Interquartile range is the distance between Q_1 (25th percentile) and Q_3 (75th percentile).

Semi-interquartile range (Q) is half the distance between Q_1 and Q_3. It is the interquartile range divided by two.

Average (mean) deviation (AD) is the average amount by which all the scores deviate from the mean of the distribution. It is the arithmetic average of the absolute deviations.

Variance is the average of the squared deviations taken from the mean of the distribution.

Standard deviation (SD or σ) is the square root of the average of the squared deviations.

Equidistant percentiles, interquartile range, and Q are based on the percentile scale. They are nonarithmetic (not affected by score values); therefore, they relate to the median, which is a nonarithmetic measure of central tendency. The average deviation, variance, and standard deviation are arithmetic measures based on score values. They relate to the mean, which is the arithmetic average of the scores. The range, average deviation, and standard deviation are highly useful to a teacher, and only those measures of variability will be discussed further.

Range (R) is a nonarithmetic measure which indicates the difference between the highest and lowest scores. This measure gives the total spread of the scores and is easy to calculate. However, since it gives a limited amount of information (highest score, lowest score, and difference between the two), the range is a rough measure.

Average deviation (AD) is an arithmetic measure which is the average of the absolute deviations of the scores from the mean of the distribution. It can be used when extreme scores should be deemphasized. The average deviation is easy to calculate and understand, yet because it is not algebraically sound, this measure should not be used as a basis for further calculations.

Standard deviation (SD) is an arithmetic measure which is algebraically sound, highly reliable, and stable; therefore, it may be used for additional calculations although it is somewhat difficult to compute.

The AD is the average amount by which all the scores deviate from the mean. The basic formula is

$$AD = \frac{\Sigma d}{N},$$

where no account is taken of $+$ and $-$ signs in the summation of deviations. For example, suppose we have seven scores: 9, 10, 13, 16, 18, 19, and 20. The mean is 15. To find the deviation of each score, we subtract the mean from the score:

X	M	d

$$
\begin{aligned}
20 - 15 &= +5 \\
19 - 15 &= +4 \\
18 - 15 &= +3 \\
16 - 15 &= +1 \\
13 - 15 &= -2 \\
10 - 15 &= -5 \\
9 - 15 &= -6 \\
\hline
\Sigma d &= 26
\end{aligned}
$$

(when signs are ignored)

where

$$d = X - M$$

$$AD = \frac{\Sigma d}{N}$$

$$= \frac{26}{7}$$

$$AD = 3.71$$

To compute the AD from a simple frequency distribution, we use the formula

$$AD = \frac{\Sigma fd}{N} \text{ or } AD = \Sigma \frac{(f \cdot d)}{N}$$

The following is an example of computing AD from a simple frequency distribution, using Data I from Appendix A.

X	f	d	fd
21	2	5.38	10.76
20	2	4.38	8.76
19	4	3.38	13.52
18	6	2.38	14.28
17	11	1.38	15.18
16	5	.38	1.90
15	4	−.62	−2.48
14	4	−1.62	−6.48
13	4	−2.62	−10.48
12	1	−3.62	−3.62
11	3	−4.62	−13.86
10	1	−5.62	−5.62
9	2	−6.62	−13.24
8	0	−7.62	0
7	1	−8.62	−8.62

$N = 50$
$M = 15.62$

$\Sigma fd = 128.80$
(when signs are ignored)

$$AD = \frac{\Sigma fd}{N}$$

$$= \frac{128.80}{50}$$

$$AD = 2.58$$

When the data are grouped, the identity of individual scores is lost, so the midpoints of the intervals are used in determining the deviations. The following is an example of computing AD from a grouped frequency distribution, using Data II:

X	$\overline{M}$	f	d	fd
135–139	137	2	35.6	71.2
130–134	132	1	30.6	30.6
125–129	127	5	25.6	128.0
120–124	122	4	20.6	82.4
115–119	117	3	15.6	46.8
110–114	112	9	10.6	95.4
105–109	107	6	5.6	33.6
100–104	102	12	.6	7.2
95–99	97	10	−4.4	−44.0
90–94	92	7	−9.4	−65.8
85–89	87	5	−14.4	−72.0
80–84	82	2	−19.4	−38.8
75–79	77	5	−24.4	−122.0
70–74	72	0	−29.4	0
65–69	67	1	−34.4	−34.3
60–64	62	3	−39.4	−118.2
		$N = 75$		$\Sigma fd = 990.3$
		$M = 101.40$		(when signs are ignored)

$$AD = \frac{\Sigma fd}{N}$$

$$= \frac{990.3}{75}$$

$$AD = 13.20$$

Computing Standard Deviation

Standard deviation (SD or σ) is the square root of the mean of the squared deviations. Most reliable of the measures of variability, standard deviation is used more than the other measures in research and other situations that require great accuracy. There are three formulas for calculating SD:

$$\text{Formula } A \quad \sigma = \sqrt{\frac{\Sigma d^2}{N}}$$

$$\text{Formula } B \quad \sigma = \sqrt{\frac{\Sigma fx^2}{N} - M^2}$$

$$\text{Formula } C \quad \sigma = SI \cdot \sqrt{\frac{\Sigma fd^2}{N} - \left(\frac{\Sigma fd}{N}\right)^2}$$

The following example uses formula A (with only a few scores):

X	M		d	d²
7	—	4	3	9
6	—	4	2	4
5	—	4	1	1
4	—	4	0	0
3	—	4	−1	1
2	—	4	−2	4
1	—	4	−3	9
$N = 7$				$\Sigma d^2 = 28$
$M = 4$				

$$\sigma = \sqrt{\frac{\Sigma d^2}{N}}$$

$$= \sqrt{\frac{28}{7}}$$

$$= \sqrt{4}$$

$$\sigma = 2$$

where

$$d = \text{deviation of the score from the } M$$

$$d = X - M$$

The following example uses formula B (with crude scores), and Data I.

X	f	x^2	fx^2
21	2	441	882
20	2	400	800
19	4	361	1444
18	6	324	1944
17	11	289	3179
16	5	256	1280
15	4	225	900
14	4	196	784
13	4	169	676
12	1	144	144
11	3	121	363
10	1	100	100
9	2	81	162
8	0	64	0
7	1	49	49
	$N = 50$		$\Sigma fx^2 = 12707$
	$M = 15.62$		

$$\sigma = \sqrt{\frac{\Sigma fx^2}{N} - M^2}$$

$$= \sqrt{\frac{12707}{50} - (15.62)^2}$$

$$= \sqrt{254.140 - 243.984}$$

$$= \sqrt{10.156}$$

$$\sigma = 3.19$$

The following example uses formula C (short form with grouped data) and Data II.

X	f	d	d^2	fd	fd^2
135–139	2	7	49	14	98
130–134	1	6	36	6	36
125–129	5	5	25	25	125
120–124	4	4	16	16	64
115–119	3	3	9	9	27
110–114	9	2	4	18	36
105–109	6	1	1	6	6
GA 100–104	12	0	0	0	0
95–99	10	−1	1	−10	10
90–94	7	−2	4	−14	28
85–89	5	−3	9	−15	45
80–84	2	−4	16	−8	32
75–79	5	−5	25	−25	125
70–74	0	−6	36	0	0
65–69	1	−7	49	−7	49
60–64	3	−8	64	−24	192
	$N = 75$			$\Sigma fd = -9$	$\Sigma fd^2 = 873$
	$SI = 5$				

$$\sigma = SI \cdot \sqrt{\frac{fd^2}{N} - \left(\frac{fd}{N}\right)^2}$$

$$= 5 \cdot \sqrt{\frac{873}{75} - \left(\frac{-9}{75}\right)^2}$$

$$= 5 \cdot \sqrt{11.640 - .014}$$

$$= 5 \cdot \sqrt{11.626}$$

$$= 5 \cdot 3.410$$

$$\sigma = 17.05$$

where $d =$ the number of step intervals each interval is from the GA (guessed average).

Formula *A* is the basic formula for computing standard deviation, but this formula is useful only if the data are limited.

Formula *B* is derived from formula *A* and is referred to as the crude score formula. This formula produces exact results with ungrouped data but slight error with grouped data. It should be used with extensive data only if a calculating machine is available for making the extensive mathematical computations.

Formula *C* is referred to as the short form formula. This formula is the most expedient with extensive data because it reduces the amount of mathematical computations. It may be used with either simple or grouped data, but again grouped data may cause slight error in the results.

The assumption used in calculating standard deviation from a grouped frequency distribution is the same as that used in calculating the mean (within each interval the mean of the scores is equal to the midpoint of the interval). If this assumption is not made, slight, although negligible, error may result; however, usually the convenience of using the grouped data process outweighs this disadvantage.

Assignment 6

1.   Using Data III and the means found under Assignment 4, find the *AD* for height. Use the formula

$$AD = \frac{\Sigma d}{N}$$

2.   Using Data III and the groupings suggested under Assignment 2, find the *AD* for height; for the high jump. Use the formula

$$AD = \frac{\Sigma fd}{N}$$

3.   Using the crude score formula *B*, find the *SD* for leg strength and the high jump.

4.   Using the short form formula *C* and the groupings suggested under Assignment 2, find the *SD* for height and weight.

5. You are a high school teacher and teach basketball to two tenth grade classes of students. You give each class a test which presumably measures their present basketball ability. The mean score for each class is 70, but the *SD* for one class is 6 and the other is 12. What is the significance of this difference from your point of view as a teacher? Which class would you rather teach? Why?

Percentiles

Percentiles and percentile rank are measures of relative status. They indicate the percent of scores below and above a given point along the scale of scores. For instance, the 30th percentile is the point where 30 percent of the scores are below and 70 percent are above. The 60th percentile is the point where 60 percent of the scores are below and 40 percent are above. The 50th percentile is the middle score and is equal to the median.

Percentiles may be found from a list of scores or from a simple or grouped frequency distribution. Finding percentiles from a simple frequency distribution is preferable because the procedure is convenient and produces no error. However, computing percentiles from grouped data may result in slight error.

Percentile rank gives approximately the same information as a percentile. If a score value is given, the percentile rank of that score may be found. For example, if, in a given distribution, a score of 56 has a percentile rank of 80, then this score is better than 80 percent of the other scores. If a percentile is given, then the score value which lies at the percentile may be determined.

To compute a percentile from a simple frequency distribution:

1. Add a cumulative frequency column to the distribution.

2. Multiplying N by the given percentile, determine the number of scores from the bottom that constitute the given percentile. (For example, $N = 50$. How many scores from the bottom is the 30th percentile? $30\% \times 50 = 15$. The 15th score is at the 30th percentile.)

3. Locate the position of that score (15th score) in the *cf* column. The score appearing opposite that number is at the given percentile.

The following are examples of how to compute a given percentile from a simple frequency distribution (data I).

X	f	cf
21	2	50
20	2	48
19	4	46
18	6	42
17	11	36
16	5	25
15	4	20
14	4	16
13	4	12
12	1	8
11	3	7
10	1	4
9	2	3
8	0	1
7	1	1
	$N = 50$	

To find the 20th percentile.

1. $20\% \times N (50) = $ 10th score.

2. The 10th score is in the 7th step from the bottom in the *cf* column.

3. The score in the X column opposite the 10th score has a value of 13. Therefore, a score of 13 is at the 20th percentile.

To find the 70th percentile.

1. $70\% \times N (50) = $ 35th score.

2. The 35th score is in the 11th step from the bottom in the *cf* column.

3. The score in the X column opposite the 35th score has a value of 17. Therefore, a score of 17 is at the 70th percentile.

To compute percentiles from a grouped frequency distribution, use the any-percentile formula and the procedure described in the section on computing the median.

To compute the percentile rank of a given score:

1.   Add a cumulative frequency column to the simple frequency distribution.

2.   Determine the number of scores below the given score by finding the score in the X column and adding half of the frequencies opposite that score to the cumulative frequencies in the interval just below that score.

3.   Divide the number of scores below the given score (answer from 2 above) by N and multiply by 100 to determine the percentile rank of the score.

The following is an example of how to compute a percentile rank from a simple frequency distribution.

X	f	cf
21	2	50
20	2	48
19	4	46
18	6	42
17	11	36
16	5	25
15	4	20
14	4	16
13	4	12
12	1	8
11	3	7
10	1	4
9	2	3
8	0	1
7	1	1
	$N = 50$	

Percentile rank (PR) of a score of 18 equals half of the frequencies opposite 18 plus the cf in the interval below 18 divided by N, then multiplied by 100. Therefore:

$$PR \text{ of } 18 = \frac{\frac{1}{2} \times 6 + 36}{50} \times 100$$

$$= \frac{3 + 36}{50} \times 100$$

$$PR \text{ of } 18 = 78$$

Deciles and Quartiles

Key percentiles in a distribution are called deciles and quartiles. They are useful as reference points along a percentile scale and as means for comparing two or more groups with each other. Deciles are indicated by D_1 (10th percentile), D_2 (20th percentile), and so on. Q_1, Q_2, Q_3 are the 25th, 50th, and 75th percentiles respectively. A table of deciles or quartiles consists of a title and three columns as shown in Tables 6-1 and 6-2.

Table 6-1
Deciles from a Simple Frequency Distribution of Scores of 75
High School Boys on the Right Grip Test (Data II)

Deciles	Scores	Interdecile Differences
d_{10}	139	
		14
d_9	125	
		11
d_8	114	
		4
d_7	110	
		6
d_6	104	
		3
d_5	101	
		3
d_4	98	
		4
d_3	94	
		5
d_2	89	
		10
d_1	79	
		19
d_0	60	

Table 6-1 provides various information. For instance, it shows that no boy gripped more than 139 pounds or less than 60 pounds. The middle 40 percent of the boys were between 94 and 110 pounds. Fifty percent of the boys did better and 50 percent did worse than 101 pounds. The interdecile differences show that the scores concentrated near the middle.

Table 6-2
Quartiles from a Simple Frequency Distribution of Scores of 75
High School Boys on the Right Grip Test (Data II)

Quartile	Grip Test Score	Interquartile Difference
Q_4	139	
		27
Q_3	112	
		11
Q_2	101	
		10
Q_1	91	
		31
Q_0	60	

The table of quartiles provides information similar to that provided by the table of deciles. It shows that no boy gripped more than 139 pounds or less than 60 pounds. Fifty percent of the boys gripped more, and 50 percent gripped less than 101 pounds.

Assignment 7

1.   Using Data I and the simple frequency distribution constructed in Assignment 5/1, compute the following percentiles: 10, 35, 70, 95.

2.   Using the same data, determine the percentile ranks of the scores 8, 11, 15, 19.

3.   Using Data II and the grouped frequency distribution constructed in Assignment 5/1, compute the following percentiles: 25, 50, 75.

Distribution Curves

A distribution is a line representing the frequencies along the scale of scores. The height of the curve at any point is proportional to the frequencies at that point. Therefore, the highest point of the curve is at the mode (most frequent score). For a clearer conception of a distribution curve, refer to the polygon in Figure 5-3. If that curve line were smoothed out, it would represent a distribution curve.

Probability is frequently stated as a ratio that always falls between the limits of 0 to 100 percent. If a coin is tossed once, the probability of its falling a head is 50 percent and a tail 50 percent. If two coins are tossed at the same time, the ratios are 2 heads 25 percent, one head and one tail 50 percent, and 2 tails 25 percent. If 20 pennies were tossed 1000 times and the results plotted, the curve line would approximate a normal curve. The chances that all the pennies would fall heads, or tails, would be extremely rare.

The normal curve is a unique bell-shaped curve, the exact definition of which is given only by its mathematical formula. Normal curves always have the same proportions; however, some normal curves may be higher or lower than others and still fit. the definition. Figure 6-1 illustrates the shape and characteristics of a normal distribution curve.

There are certain characteristics unique to the normal curve.

1. The mean, median, and mode fall at the same point and are, therefore, equal to one another.

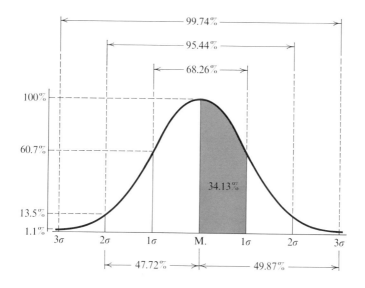

Figure 6-1. Normal curve with certain characteristics illustrated.

2.   At one *SD* (standard deviation) from the mean in either direction the height is always 60.7 percent of the height at the mean.

3.   At two *SD*s from the mean the height is 13.5 percent of the height at the mean.

4.   At three *SD*s from the mean the height is 1.1 percent of the height at the mean.

5.   The mean plus and minus one *SD* includes 68.26 percent of the scores (34.13 percent in one direction. See Appendix F.).

6.   The mean plus and minus two *SD*s includes 95.44 percent of the scores (47.72 percent in one direction).

7.   The mean plus and minus three *SD*s includes 99.74 percent of the scores (49.87 percent in one direction).

8.   The curve is bell-shaped, bilaterally symmetrical, unimodal, and the ends of the curve approach but never touch the baseline.

9.   A normal curve may be higher or lower than the one presented in Figure 6-1, but its proportions and characteristics must remain as described.

In addition the following points about the normal curve are of interest:

1.   The mean plus and minus *Q* (semi-interquartile range) includes the middle 50 percent of the scores.

2.   The mean plus and minus *AD* (average deviation) includes the middle 57.5 percent of the scores.

3.   The mean plus and minus *PE* (probable error) includes the middle 50 percent of the scores.

Skewed Curve

In a skewed distribution the mean, median, and mode are at different points, and the balance of the curve is thrown to the left or right (see Figure 6-2).

The degree of skewness of a distribution is measured by the formula:

$$\text{Skewness} = \frac{3(\text{mean} - \text{median})}{\sigma}$$

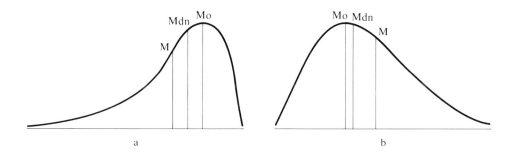

Figure 6-2.   Skewed curves: (a) extreme skew to the left (negative); (b) moderate skew
to the right (positive).

Skewness results from too few cases, from special selection, or from a true lack of normality in the data. When the mean and median are equal, skewness $= 0$.

Other Shapes of Distribution Curves

In addition to the normal curve and skewed curves a distribution may take other shapes, such as those illustrated in Figure 6-3.

Assignment 8

1.   Describe the following:
     a.   unimodal curve
     b.   bimodal curve
     c.   multimodal curve
     d.   bilaterally symmetrical curve
     e.   bell-shaped curve
     f.   normal curve

2.   You give a test of cardiovascular efficiency to a group of boys and find that $M = 72$ and $SD = 7$. If the distribution is near normal, give the score limits which will include approximately 68 percent, 95 percent, and 100 percent of the cases. What is the approximate range of the scores?

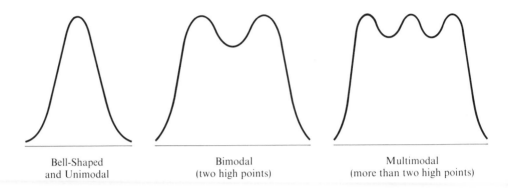

| Bell-Shaped and Unimodal | Bimodal (two high points) | Multimodal (more than two high points) |

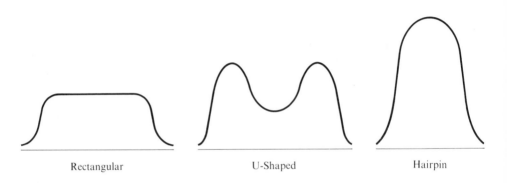

| Rectangular | U-Shaped | Hairpin |

Figure 6-3. Other shapes of curves.

3.   From the given measures of variability describe the probable shape of distribution A; of distribution B.

A   50th percentile = 80   B $Q_3 = 35$
      95th percentile = 100 $Q_2 = 25$
        5th percentile = 20 $Q_1 = 20$

Reliability Measures

When a test is administered to a group that represents a larger group, the smaller group is referred to as a *sample* and the larger group is referred to as the *population*. A sample will seldom truly represent the population from which it is taken; hence, a statistic derived from a sample will seldom equal the parameter (true statistic of the population). Therefore, we should usually not accept a statistic, such as the mean or standard deviation, computed from a sample for its face value but should consider it as only a statistic of a sample.

The usefulness of a statistic may depend on its proximity to the parameter. In other words the reliability or dependability of a statistic must be known to determine its significance. The amount of error in a sample statistic is estimated by sampling error procedures, which supply a description of the reliability of a statistic taken from a sample. Through these procedures the administrator can compute the standard error of the statistic and state its meaning.

Standard Error of the Mean

The standard error of the mean (σ_M) is the measure used to estimate the reliability of a mean computed from a sample of a population. If a large number of samples of the same size were drawn at random from a particular population, and if the means of the samples were formed into a distribution, then we would have a *sampling distribution of means*. If the means varied greatly from one another, then the distribution would have a large standard deviation. Conversely, if the means were near one another, the standard deviation of the sampling distribution of means would be small. If the means varied greatly, then we obviously could not place much confidence in any one of the means. Whereas, if the means were in close agreement, we could be more confident that any one mean was near the parameter. In other words the variability of the sampling distribution of means indicates the reliability of a mean taken from a sample.

The measure used to describe the reliability of a mean is the *SD* of the sampling distribution of means. The estimated *SD* of a sampling distribution of means is known as the *standard error of the mean*. Hence, the standard error of the mean is the standard deviation of the sampling distribution of means. The standard error is used to estimate the amount of error that may be present in the mean as a result of the chance factor in the process of random sampling. Although these errors cannot be controlled, they can be estimated; standard error formulas are designed for this purpose.

Because it is not practical to construct a sampling distribution of means for the purpose of computing the standard error of the mean, a formula has been derived which provides an estimate of the standard error. The derivation of the formula is relatively easy to follow and is explained in several books on statistics. The formula is:

$$\sigma_M = \frac{\sigma_{\text{sample}}}{\sqrt{N}}$$

where

$$\sigma_M = \text{standard error of the mean}$$
$$\sigma_{\text{sample}} = \text{standard deviation of the sample scores}$$
$$N = \text{number of cases in the sample}$$

Assume that the height measures found in Data III from Appendix A represent a sample from a larger group of students (a population). The mean of those scores is 65.92 inches, the *SD* is 3.23 inches, and *N* is 25. Place these figures in the formula:

$$\sigma_M = \frac{3.25}{\sqrt{25}} = \frac{3.25}{5} = .65$$

The σ_M of .65 indicates that if a sampling distribution of means were constructed, its *SD* would equal .65 inches. Normality of the sampling distribution can be assumed. Recall that in a normal distribution the mean plus and minus one *SD* includes approximately 68 percent of the scores; the mean plus and minus two *SD* includes approximately 95 percent of the scores; and the mean plus and minus three *SD* includes practically 100 percent of the scores. Since the σ_M is an estimate of the *SD* of the sampling distribution, there is a 68 percent chance that the mean obtained from the sample is within one σ_M of the parametric mean. In other words we can be 68 percent certain that the obtained mean deviates no more than .65 inches (1 σ_M) from the true (parametric) mean. Further, we can be 95 percent certain that the obtained mean deviates no more than 1.30 inches (2 σ_M) from the true mean. And we can be practically 100 percent certain that the obtained mean is no more than 1.95 inches (3 σ_M) away from the true mean.

A small σ_M indicates that the obtained mean is highly reliable; whereas a large σ_M indicates that the obtained mean has a low level of reliability.

Standard Errors of Measures Other Than the Mean

The reliability of statistics other than the mean may also be estimated. The following formulas are designed for that purpose:

$$\sigma_{SD} = \frac{\sigma_{\text{sample}}}{\sqrt{2N}}$$

$$\sigma_{SD} = .707 \text{ times } \sigma_M$$

$$\sigma_Q = .787 \text{ times } \sigma_M$$

$$\sigma_{Mdn} = 1.25 \text{ times } \sigma_M$$

The standard errors of measures other than the mean are interpreted the same as the σ_M, which was explained in the preceding section.

Standard Error of the Difference

Groups of scores are often compared according to their means or standard deviations. On the basis of these comparisons the groups are either alike or different.

The extent to which the obtained measures of difference are reliable and the degree to which the calculated measure of difference is dependable are determined by computing and interpreting the standard error of the difference (σ_{diff}) which is an estimate of the standard deviation of a sampling distribution of obtained differences.

The reliability of the difference between two means (M_1 and M_2) can be found by computing the standard error of the difference between means. The formula is:

$$\sigma_{\text{diff}} = \sqrt{\sigma_{M_1}{}^2 + \sigma_{M_2}{}^2}$$

remember that

$$\sigma_M = \frac{\sigma \text{ sample}}{\sqrt{N}}$$

Substituting:

$$\sigma_{\text{diff}} = \sqrt{\left(\frac{\sigma \text{ sample}^2}{\sqrt{N}}\right) + \left(\frac{\sigma \text{ sample}^2}{\sqrt{N}}\right)}$$

Suppose we have two means taken from two comparable random samples. For group 1, $M = 104$, $\sigma = 9$, and $N = 100$. For group 2, $M = 99$, $\sigma = 10$, and $N = 100$. The obtained difference in the means equals 5 ($104 - 99 = 5$). Is this difference real, or is it a result of chance error in sampling? In other words to what extent can we rely on this measure of difference? To determine reliability we compute the σ_{diff} between the two means. Substituting the correct numbers into the formula,

$$\sigma_{M_1} = \frac{9}{\sqrt{100}} = .9$$

$$\sigma_{M_2} = \frac{10}{\sqrt{100}} = 1.0$$

$$\sigma_{\text{diff}} = \sqrt{(.9)^2 + (1.0)^2} = \sqrt{.81 + 1.0} = \sqrt{1.81} = 1.34$$

What does this result mean? When the obtained difference (5) is divided by the σ_{diff} (1.34), the result is a critical ratio (CR). The CR parallels standard deviation units of the normal curve. Therefore, if the CR were 1.0, we could be approximately 68 percent certain that the obtained difference is real. If the CR were 2, we would be approximately 95 percent certain; and if the CR were 3, we could be practically 100 percent certain that the difference is real. In this problem, the obtained difference (5) divided by the σ_{diff} (1.34) equals 3.73 ($CR = 3.73$). Therefore, we are practically 100 percent certain that the obtained difference is real and not a result of chance alone. Hence, the difference is highly reliable.

Assignment 9

1.   Assume that the six sets of scores found in Data III from Appendix A represent samples from a population. Using the means and SDs already obtained, find the σ_M for each of the six factors. Interpret your answers.

2.   Find the σ_σ for height and high jump scores.

3.   Find the σ_{mdn} for height and high jump scores.

4.   Compute the σ_{diff} between the two means when the conditions are:

$$M_1 = 80, \ SD = 5, \ N = 100; \ M_2 = 83, \ SD = 3, \ N = 100.$$

Correlation

The statistical technique known as correlation results in a coefficient (number) which expresses the relationship between two variables. The coefficient of correlation is designated by the symbol r. The r can range from 0 to $+1$ and from 0 to -1; hence, from -1 to $+1$. (If r is greater than 1, the computation is incorrect.) A positive correlation indicates positive relationship. A zero correlation indicates absence of relationship. A negative correlation indicates inverse relationship.

If $r = +1$, the relationship is perfect and positive; that is, if the first variable (trait) were increased, the second variable would increase a proportional amount. For instance, the relationship of the diameter to the circumference of a circle is perfect and positive. If we were to change the diameter, we would always change the circumference by 3.1416 times that amount.

If $r = -1$, the relationship is perfect and negative; that is, as the first variable increases, the second variable decreases a proportional amount. For example, a perfect negative relationship exists between velocity and time in the 100-yard run. As velocity increases, time decreases proportionately.

When $r = 0$, there is no relationship between the variables; that is, if the first variable were changed, the second variable would not be affected in any way.

Although the coefficient of correlation is a convenient index of relationship, the degree of relationship between two variables should be interpreted with caution. A coefficient of correlation of .60, for example, does not represent exactly twice as much relationship as one of .30. The correlation should be interpreted in relation to the character and extent of the problem under investigation. In one instance an r of .50 might be considered to be quite high as a significant value, while in another instance an r of .50 might be considered to be too low. Generally a correlation of .80 is considered to be substantial, and below .40 is usually considered to be low.

Correlation is a frequently used statistical technique to determine validity, reliability, and objectivity of tests. It also serves as a basis for construction of standard tests and for prediction of results. If a high relationship exists between two traits and one trait is measured, then the other trait can be predicted with a relatively high degree of accuracy. Measures of correlation help us to understand people and the relationships that exist among them. Correlation theory is important in some of the more advanced statistical techniques.

Two sets of corresponding scores are necessary. The raw score method is a convenient approach to compute correlation when the number of cases is relatively small, a computing machine is available, and a scattergram is not needed. The formula for the raw score method is:

$$r_{xy} = \frac{\dfrac{\Sigma XY}{N} - M_x\, M_y}{\sqrt{\dfrac{\Sigma X^2}{N} - M_x^{\,2}} \cdot \sqrt{\dfrac{\Sigma Y^2}{N} - M_y^{\,2}}}$$

The formula may also be written:

$$r_{xy} = \frac{\dfrac{\Sigma XY}{N} - (M_x \cdot M_y)}{\sigma_x \cdot \sigma_y}$$

To obtain the coefficient of correlation from an unordered list of paired scores, with the use of this formula:

1. Compute the mean and standard deviation of each set of scores.

2. Multiply the two raw scores for each individual, add the products, and divide by N.

3. Multiply the mean of the X scores and the mean of the Y scores and subtract the result from the answer in step 2.

4. Divide the answer from step 3 by the product of the two standard deviations.

Table 6-3 uses the raw score formula:

Table 6-3
Scores for 10 High School Boys in the High Jump
(X Scores) and Standing Long Jump (Y Scores)

Subject	X*	Y*	XY	X²	Y²
1	60	72	4320	3600	5184
2	62	70	4340	3844	4900
3	64	68	4352	4096	4624
4	58	68	3944	3364	4624
5	48	52	2496	2304	2704
6	56	66	3696	3136	4356
7	44	50	2200	1936	2500
8	52	60	3120	2704	3600
9	48	56	2688	2304	3136
10	58	68	3944	3364	4624
$N = 10$	$M = 55.0$	$M = 63.0$	$\Sigma XY = 35100$	$\Sigma X^2 = 30652$	$\Sigma Y^2 = 40252$

* Scores given in inches.

$$r_{xy} = \frac{\frac{\Sigma XY}{N} - M_x M_y}{\sigma_x \cdot \sigma_y}$$

$$= \frac{\frac{35100}{10} - (55)(63)}{(6.34)(7.50)}$$

$$= \frac{3510 - 3465}{47.55} = \frac{45.00}{47.55} = .95$$

where: $\sigma_x = \sqrt{\frac{\Sigma x^2}{N} - (M_x)^2}$

$\sigma_x = 6.34$

$\sigma_x = \sqrt{\frac{\Sigma y^2}{N} - (M_y)^2}$

$\sigma_y = 7.50$

Assignment 10

1.   Using the following data, complete the columns in the table and compute
     r with the raw score formula.

Subject	X	Y	XY	X²	Y²
1	65	56			
2	66	51			
3	68	55			
4	67	47			
5	69	54			
6	66	48			
7	62	49			
8	69	52			
9	68	47			
10	60	46			

2.   Using the raw score means and standard deviations already obtained
     from Data III in Appendix A, compute the correlations between height
     and weight, and height and high jump.

Computing
Correlation by the Short Method

When many scores are to be correlated without a computing machine, an
economical procedure is to compute *r* from a scatter diagram by the *short method*
(also called Pearson Product Moment Method), in which each score is expressed as
a deviation from the guessed average of the distribution. When deviations are taken
from the guessed average, correction factors are necessary and the formula then
becomes:

$$r_{xy} = \frac{\dfrac{\Sigma XY}{N} - (C_x)(C_y)}{(\sigma_x)(\sigma_y)}$$

substituting when

$$C_x = \frac{\Sigma fd_x}{N} \text{ and } C_y = \frac{\Sigma fd_y}{N}$$

$$r_{xy} = \frac{\dfrac{\Sigma XY}{N} - \left(\dfrac{\Sigma fd_x}{N}\right)\left(\dfrac{\Sigma fd_y}{N}\right)}{\sqrt{\dfrac{\Sigma fd_x{}^2}{N} - \left(\dfrac{\Sigma fd_x}{N}\right)^2}\sqrt{\dfrac{\Sigma fd_y{}^2}{N} - \left(\dfrac{\Sigma fd}{N}\right)^2}}$$

The application of this formula requires a specially prepared chart (scattergram) as shown in Figure 6-4. Printed copies of the chart may usually be purchased in college bookstores.

To compute r with the use of the scattergram and the short method formula:

1. Establish step intervals for the data as in a frequency distribution. Then record the interval limits for the X variable across the top and for the Y variable along the left hand column. The data may be grouped or simple, depending on the range.

2. Label the extra columns and rows with f_y, f_x, and so on as illustrated in Figure 6-4.

3. Plot a tally mark in the appropriate square for each pair of scores. The mark must be placed in the square below the correct interval for the X variable and opposite the correct interval for the Y variable. For example, in Figure 6-4 four boys, 68 inches tall, high-jumped 58 inches or 59 inches, so they were tallied in that square.

4. Add the frequencies in each row and record the sums in the f_y column. Add the frequencies in each column and record those sums in the f_x row.

5. In the d_y column record plus and minus deviations from the GA and do the same in the d_x row (see Figure 6-4).

6. By multiplying the numbers in f_y by those in d_y fill in the fd_y column. Do the same for the fd_x row.

7. Fill in the numbers in the $fd_y{}^2$ column by squaring each d_y number and multiplying the result by the corresponding f_y. Do the same for the $fd_x{}^2$ row.

8. Compute *moments* for each square in which tally marks appear, by multiplying the number of intervals the square is from the GA column by the number of steps it is from the GA row. Then multiply that product by the number of tallies in the square. Circle the answer. The moments

X Variable (Height in Inches)

Y Variable (High Jump in Inches)	58	59	60	61	62	63	64	65	66	67	68	69	70	fy	dy	fdy	fdy^2	*XY* −	*XY* +	
														0	5	0	0			
60–61											I (20)		I (28)	2	4	8	32		48	
58–59									I (9)		IIII (60)	I (18)	I (21)	7	3	21	63		108	
56–57										I (8)	I (10)	I (12)		3	2	6	12		30	
54–55						I		II (4)		I (4)				4	1	4	4		8	
52–53							I		I	I				3	0	0	0			GA
50–51			I (3)											1	−1	−1	1		3	
48–49					I (2)									1	−2	−2	4		2	
46–47														0	−3	0	0			
44–45	I (20)		I (12)											2	−4	−8	32		32	
42–43												I (30)		1	−5	−5	25	30		
40–41						I								1	−6	−6	36			
fx	1	0	2	0	1	2	1	2	2	3	6	3	2	N=25		Σ=17	Σ=209	Σ=201		
dx	−5	−4	−3	−2	−1	0	1	2	3	4	5	6	7							
fdx	−5	0	−6	0	−1	0	1	4	6	12	30	18	14	Σ=73						
fdx^2	25	0	18	0	1	0	1	8	18	48	150	108	98	Σ=475						
						GA														

Figure 6-4. Scatter diagram (scattergram) for computing coefficient of correlation between body height and high-jump achievement (Data III, Appendix A).

in the plus quadrants (upper right and lower left) of the scattergram are recorded in the XY plus column, while the moments in the minus quadrants are recorded in the XY minus column. The ΣXY is the difference between the plus column and the minus column. Using the information from Figure 6-4,

$$r_{xy} = \frac{\dfrac{201}{25} - \left(\dfrac{73}{25}\right)\left(\dfrac{17}{25}\right)}{\sqrt{\dfrac{475}{25} - \left(\dfrac{73}{25}\right)^2}\sqrt{\dfrac{209}{25} - \left(\dfrac{17}{25}\right)^2}}$$

$$= \frac{8.004 - (2.920)(.680)}{\sqrt{19 - 8.526}\sqrt{8.360 - .462}}$$

$$= \frac{8.004 - 1.986}{\sqrt{10.474}\sqrt{7.898}}$$

$$= \frac{6.018}{(3.236)(2.810)}$$

$$= \frac{6.018}{9.093}$$

$$r_{xy} = .66$$

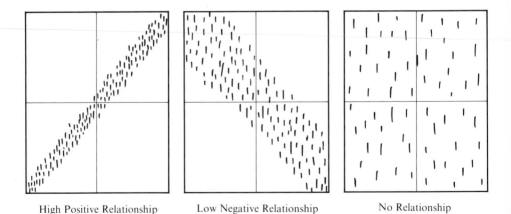

High Positive Relationship	Low Negative Relationship	No Relationship

Figure 6-5. Tally-mark patterns on scattergrams illustrating amount and type of relationship.

When the scores represented by tally marks tend to cluster along a line running diagonally from the lower left to the upper right on the scattergram the relationship is positive, because these quadrants are positive. The closer the tallies cluster along the diagonal line the higher is the correlation. If all the tallies fell exactly on the diagonal line, the relationship would be perfect positive. Different degrees of relationship in both positive and negative directions are shown in Figure 6-5.

Assignment 11

Following the example given in Figure 6-4, make an appropriate scattergram and compute the coefficient of correlation between height and the long jump scores in Data III from Appendix A.

7

Interpreting Scores

To obtain a raw score is sometimes a simple matter, but to interpret the meaning and significance of the score is more difficult. For instance, if a 16-year-old boy were to do 10 dips on the parallel bars and 12 chins (pull-ups) on the high bar, a suitable standard of comparison would be necessary to determine the degree of excellence of his performance. A standard scale is often developed for a specific test to assist in the interpretation of scores and to serve as a standard against which to compare any raw score from the particular test.

In general a standard scale provides a technique for converting a distribution of raw scores into standard scores. Specifically a standard scale provides a measure of relative status for a raw score and thus permits a more adequate interpretation of the score. It also provides a technique for computing the averages of several different kinds of scores. Any standard scale developed from a large sample of raw scores can serve as a standard against which to compare any raw score of the same type. Thus a standard scale is used to develop norms.

One widely used standard scale is the percentile scale discussed in Chapter 6. Although the information from this scale is easy to understand and interpret, it is relatively unstable and unreliable because the scale is nonarithmetic and may be influenced by the irregularities in the distribution of scores. While percentiles are frequently averaged to secure composite measures for administrative convenience, this practice is not strictly valid.

In view of the limitations of the percentile scale, it is important to know that there are three types of arithmetic standard scales: the z-scale, the T-scale, and the 6 sigma-scale. These scales are more reliable than percentiles, but they are often less convenient and more difficult to interpret.

z-Scores

The z-scale normally extends from -3 to $+3$. The mean of the scale $= 0$, and the standard deviation $= 1$. When plotted on the normal distribution curve, the z-scale appears as Figure 7-1. Thus, if a raw score were equal to the mean of the distribution, it would have a z value of 0. A score of 2 SDs above the mean would have a z value of $+2$, and a score of 1 SD below the mean would have a z value of -1. The z score tells how many SDs above or below the mean a raw score lies. A score equal to $+3$ on the z-scale would be at or near the top of the scale (excellent), whereas one equal to a z of -3 would be at or near the bottom of the scale (very poor). A score equal to a z of 0 would be average (at the mean).

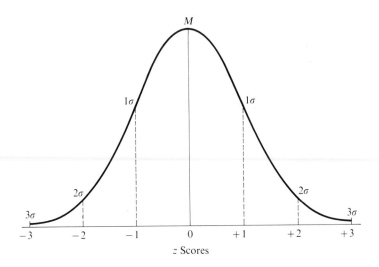

Figure 7-1.   z-scale plotted on a normal curve.

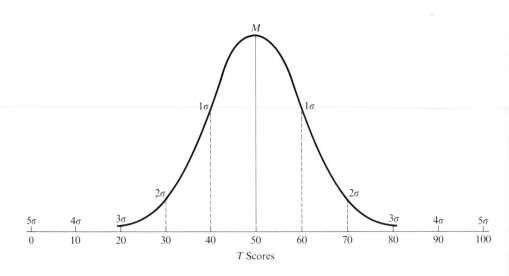

Figure 7-2.   T-scale plotted on a normal curve.

T-Scores

On the *T*-scale $M = 50$ and $SD = 10$. When plotted on a normal distribution curve, the *T*-scale appears as Figure 7-2. If a raw score is equal to the mean of the distribution, then it has a *T* value of 50. A score at 2 *SD*s above the, mean would have a *T* value of 70, and a score at 1 *SD* below the mean would have a *T* value of 40. A score with a *T* value of 80 would be equal to a *z* value of $+3$ and would be considered excellent in relation to others within the sample. A score with a *T* value of 20 would be equal to a *z* value of -3 and would be considered very poor.

6 σ-Scores

The 6 σ-scale extends from 0 to 100 and covers 6 *SD*s as its name implies. On the 6 σ-scale $M = 50$ and $SD = 16.66$. When plotted on a normal distribution curve, the scale appears as Figure 7-3.

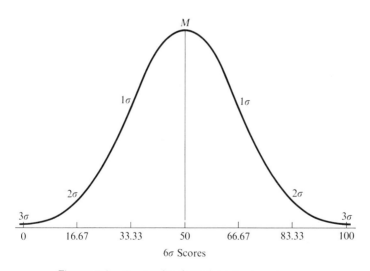

Figure 7-3.   6 σ-scale plotted on a normal curve.

If a raw score is equal to the mean of the distribution, it has a 6 σ value of 50. A score at 2 *SD*s above the mean has a 6 σ value of 83.33, while a score at 1 *SD* below the mean has a 6 σ value of 33.33. The 6 σ standard scale simply divides a 100-point range into 6 equal segments representing 6 *SD*s which include approximately 100 percent of the scores in a normal distribution.

Table 7-1 presents a comparison of the three types of standard scales and gives their percentile equivalent.

Table 7-1
A Comparison of the Standard Scales:
Standard Score Values at 1, 2, and 3 SDs from the Mean

	-3σ	-2σ	-1σ	M	$+1\sigma$	$+2\sigma$	$+3\sigma$
z-Scale	−3	−2	−1	0	+1	+2	+3
T-Scale	20	30	40	50	60	70	80
6 σ-Scale	0	16.66	33.33	50	66.66	83.33	100
Percentile equivalent	.13	2.18	15.87	50	84.13	97.22	99.87

Computing Standard Scores

The formula for computing any standard score from a raw score is:

$$\text{standard score} = \frac{\sigma_s (X - M)}{\sigma_X} + M_s$$

where

σ_s = SD of the standard scale; for example, 1 for z-scale, 10 for T-scale, and 16.67 for 6 σ-scale

X = Raw score under consideration

M = Mean of the scores

σX = SD of the scores

M_s = Mean of the standard scale; for example, 0 for z-scale, 50 for T-scale, and 50 for 6 σ-scale.

X

24
23
22
21
20
19
18
17
16
―――
180
$M = 20$
$\sigma X = 2.6$

Example:

a.   Find the z score for a raw score of 21.

$$z = \frac{1\ (21 - 20)}{2.6} + 0 = .385$$

b.   Find the T score for a raw score of 21.

$$T = \frac{10\ (21 - 20)}{2.6} + 50 = 53.85$$

c.   Find the 6 σ score for a raw score of 21.

$$6\ \sigma = \frac{16.67\ (21 - 20)}{2.6} + 50 = 56.41$$

To develop a standard scale from a distribution of raw scores:

1.   Arrange all raw score values in a column from high to low, as in a simple frequency distribution.

2.   Place the mean of the standard scale opposite the mean of the raw scores.

3.   Using the standard score formula, compute the standard score value of the raw score immediately above the mean and record that standard score opposite the corresponding raw score.

4.   Determine the reciprocal (R) by the formula $R = \dfrac{\sigma_s}{\sigma_X}$.

5.   Add this reciprocal value to the result of step 3 to get the standard score for the next higher raw score value. Continue the process for all raw scores above the mean.

6.   Repeat steps 3, 4, and 5 for the score values below the mean. (For scores below the mean the reciprocal is successively added in the case of the z-scale and successively subtracted in the case of the T- and 6 σ-scales.)

Table 7-2
The z, T, and 6 σ Equivalents for the Scores Made by 50
High School Girls on the Sit-Up Test (Data I)

X	z	T	6σ
21	1.67	66.85	78.15
20	1.36	63.72	72.92
19	1.05	60.59	67.69
18	.74	57.46	62.46
17	.43	54.33	57.23
16	.12	51.20	52.00
M = 15.62	0	50.00	50.00
15	−.19	48.10	46.83
14	−.50	44.97	41.60
13	−.81	41.84	36.37
12	−1.12	38.71	31.14
11	−1.43	35.58	25.91
10	−1.74	32.45	20.08
9	−2.05	29.32	15.45
8	−2.36	26.19	10.22
7	−2.67	23.06	4.99

$$M \ = \ 15.62$$

$$SD = \ \ 3.19$$

$$N \ = 50$$

Since the mean of the distribution equals 15.62, this value is 0 on the z-scale, 50 on the T-scale, and 50 on the 6 σ-scale. As stated in step 2 we place those values opposite the mean of the distribution. In accordance with step 3, we compute the standard score value of the raw score immediately above the mean. That score is 16. Therefore,

$$z \ = \frac{1 \ (16 - 15.62)}{3.19} + 0 = .12$$

$$T \ = \frac{10 \ (16 - 15.62)}{3.19} + 50 = 51.20$$

$$6 \, \sigma = \frac{16.67 \ (16 - 15.62)}{3.19} + 50 = 52.00$$

According to step 4 the reciprocal $(R) = \dfrac{\sigma_s}{\sigma_x}$. Hence,

$$R_z = \frac{1}{3.19} \text{ which } = .31$$

$$R_T = \frac{10}{3.19} \text{ which } = 3.13$$

$$R_{6\,\sigma} = \frac{16.67}{3.19} \text{ which } = 5.23$$

As stated in step 5 we add the R value successively to the obtained standard score. After this step the portion of the standard scale above the mean is complete. The raw score 16 has a z value of .12, a T value of 51.20, and a $6\,\sigma$ value of 52.00. Likewise the raw score 17 has a z-value of .43, a T value of 54.33 and a $6\,\sigma$ value of .57.23. To complete the scales below the mean follow the instructions in step 6. For scores below the mean in the T-scale and the $6\,\sigma$-scale remember to successively subtract instead of add the R value.

We can now read the z, T, or $6\,\sigma$ score corresponding to any raw score in Table 7-2. For example, the z value of the score 10 is -1.74. This figure tells us that 10 is 1.74 SD below the mean.

In a practical situation only one of the standard scales would be established, not all three of them as done on this example. Therefore, one problem is to choose which standard scale is best for the particular situation. If a large number of students were tested on a strength test and if these scores were converted to standard scores, then the scale of standard scores could serve as a norm against which to compare the raw scores of like students on the same test.

Advantages of Each Type of Standard Scale

The z-scale is the simplest to calculate and the easiest to interpret if the reader understands the meaning of standard deviation. The z value identifies position in the distribution in terms of standard deviation units above or below the mean. This scale is most meaningful when the distribution approaches normality. Since it involves decimals and both negative and positive values, a z-scale may be confusing to some people.

The T-scale involves no decimals or negative values, is plotted on a 100-point scale, and is thus easy to interpret. However, it covers ten standard deviations when only six standard deviations include almost 100 percent of the cases in a normal distribution.

The 6 σ-scale involves no negative values, covers a 100-point scale in 6 *SD*, and is thus also easy to interpret. However, it does involve decimals and the values at the *SD* points are awkward to work with.

Increased Increment Scale

The increased increment scale is an attempt to devise a method by which performers are awarded scores proportional to the excellence of the performance. It has been recognized that as an individual approaches the limit of his present capacity in a given activity in which he is being tested, improvement becomes more difficult. The man who reduces his time in the 100-yard run from 10 seconds to 9.5 seconds has accomplished more than the man who reduces his time from 13 seconds to 12.5 seconds. The graphical representation of such a scale is a parabolic curve that moves slowly upward from the baseline and increases more rapidly as the distance between the baseline and the curve widens. An example of an increased increment scale is the one used for scoring the decathlon in track and field. Valid increase increment scales are difficult to devise and therefore seldom used.

Rating Scales

Rating scales are useful mainly for adding accuracy to subjective judgments. Frequently rating systems are set up on 5-point scales. However, they sometimes appear on 3-, 7-, or even 10-point scales; and in some cases it may be desirable to use a scale even more refined than 10 points, such as a 100-point scale. Note these examples of rating scales.

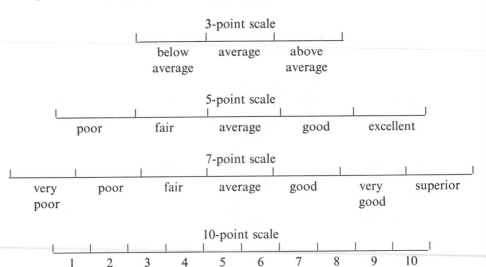

Assignment 12

Problems

1. Using the high jump scores in Data III, construct a z-scale.

2. Using the long jump scores in Data III, construct a T-scale.

3. Using the height measures in Data III, construct a 6 σ-scale.

4. If $M = 17$ and $SD = 15$, find the z score, T score, and 6 σ score for each of the following raw scores: 81, 100, 57.

Questions

1. A student earned a z score of 1.6. What does this score mean?

2. A student made a z score of zero. Interpret his score.

3. A student had a z score of zero and yet his score is higher than the 50th percentile. Interpret this result.

4. In a large and representative sample of weights of 15-year-old boys, one boy had a z score of 3.3. Characterize him in terms of very heavy, medium, light, very light. Another boy had a z score of $-.7$. Characterize him in the same terms.

THREE
Measurements
of Body Structure

This section includes descriptions of growth and nutrition measures, body type measures, posture evaluation, and plans for classifying students for instruction and competition.

8

Measurements of
Body Structure and Type

Sculptors in ancient India, Egypt, Athens, and Rome measured individuals in various ways in attempts to find the ideal structure and proportions of man. Throughout history great athletic performers have been studied to determine the unique features of their structures. In the United States Edward Hitchcock at Amherst College in the 1860s, and Dudley A. Sargent, first at Yale and later at Harvard, made many structural measurements of college students and prepared profile charts. Since then numerous other studies have been completed. At present, with our knowledge about body structure and with the aid of measurements, we can recognize individual differences and appraise individual potential with more insight.

Growth and Nutrition Measurements

In combination growth (change in size) and development (change in function) are a process of maturation. In some cases development may affect growth since growth changes are largely a result of maturation rate. The teacher has more influence over and more concern with development than with growth and therefore may only indirectly affect growth.

Growth tends to be continuous, but its rate is not constant; it follows a pattern of spurts and plateaus. Variations in growth rate occur among different individuals and also in the same individual from time to time. Many variations in growth rate are simply normal irregularities, but some variations may result from illness, body defects, nutrition changes, and environmental changes. Glandular malfunctions may produce excessive growth or retarded growth. Because of irregularities in growth rate, a child's present growth status and rate are best compared with his own record of the past rather than with the growth rate of other persons.

Wetzel Grid

Norman C. Wetzel (1948) developed a chart known as the Wetzel Grid based on age, height, and weight and used to show the growth rate of children.

Wetzel classified physique into nine categories on the grid so that the plottings of a child's age, height, and weight determine his position on the chart. Plottings at reasonable age intervals (at least once a year) show the child's growth status in relation to the normal growth expectation. The child who proceeds normally tends to remain in his channel on the chart. If he deviates from his channel, he should be given special attention to determine the cause of his deviation and the means for correction. Its primary purpose is to identify children who need special attention because of abnormal growth patterns. The chart is especially useful for early identification of malnourishment.

In his original study Wetzel compared the grid ratings of 2093 children, in kindergarten through grade twelve, with physicians' appraisals. There was an 87.5 percent agreement between the physicians' ratings and the grid ratings. When one of the categories (fair) was omitted from the comparison of results, the percentage of agreement between the physicians and the grid increased to 94.5 percent.

Since Wetzel's original study, several other studies involving the Wetzel Grid have been completed.[1] The evidence indicates that this technique is useful for identifying abnormal growth patterns, provided the child is located in the correct channel in the beginning.

Pryor Weight–Width Tables

Because of the inadequacy of age–height–weight standards for evaluating nutritional status, Helen Pryor (1940) developed a set of weight–width tables for persons between the ages of one and 41 years. The tables are designed to serve as a basis for screening individuals with nutritional deficiencies. This useful system for measuring nutritional status takes into account the bony framework and body structure in addition to age, height, weight, and sex.

To use these tables the teacher records the child's age to the nearest year, height to the nearest one-quarter inch, and weight to the nearest pound. With calipers he measures hip width (bi-illiac diameter) to the nearest one-tenth centimeter. With calipers he also measures chest width to the nearest one-tenth centimeter. Then he selects the appropriate table according to the child's age, sex, and chest width, and opposite the child's height and under his bi-illiac diameter the teacher finds the appropriate weight in pounds. Finally he compares the child's actual weight with the appropriate weight. On the basis of such a comparison the teacher can identify students who show signs of malnutrition.[2] Students identified as malnourished should be placed under the direction of the school medical staff.

Meredith Height–Weight Chart

Howard Meredith (1949) constructed a useful zone classification system for height and weight of boys and girls ages four through 18 years. His chart contains

---

[1] Copies of the Wetzel Grid chart along with specific instructions for its use may be obtained from the NEA Service, Inc., 1200 West 3rd St., Cleveland, Ohio.
[2] Pryor's Weight–Width Tables may be obtained from the Stanford University Press, Stanford, California. The tables are accompanied by specific instructions for measuring and scoring.

curved zones for height and weight upon which the child's growth progress can be plotted. There are five zones for height: *tall, moderately tall, average, moderately short*, and *short*. Similarly there are five zones for weight: *heavy, moderately heavy, average, moderately light*, and *light*. The height zones are at the top of the chart and the weight zones at the bottom.

After the child's height and weight are plotted at the appropriate age column, an immediate check is available to see whether the child's height and weight are in similar zones; a moderately short child is expected to be light; a tall child, heavy; and so on. If the zones are dissimilar, the child's physique may account for the dissimilarity, for example, a child may be naturally tall and slender, or short and stocky. If this is not the case, then further examination should be made for possible health problems such as malnutrition, obesity, and illness. Moreover, as successive plottings are made, growth patterns can be observed. A child's height and weight will essentially parallel each other in that they will proceed along the same zones. Any marked deviation from one zone to another is usually cause for referral.[3]

Body Type Measurements

Amount of body fat, extent of muscular development, and dimensions of body structure are factors generally used in evaluating physique or body type. Within certain limits diet and exercise may affect the development of musculature and amount of fatty tissue but not basic body type (morphology) which results from heredity.

Observation of individual athletes and research both indicate that body build relates considerably to one's ability to perform. A certain body build may be an advantage or a disadvantage in performance, depending upon the nature of the activity. For example, height is clearly an advantage in basketball and volleyball. Generally it is less advantageous in skating, ice hockey, and football and still less advantageous in soccer, gymnastics, and wrestling. A tall and heavy stature is an advantage in the shot put, discus throw, and hammer throw but a distinct disadvantage in the two-mile run and in several gymnastic activities. Obese and very stocky people tend to be nonathletic; however there are some exceptions to this generalization. People of medium structure with well developed muscles are generally good performers in such sports as swimming, gymnastics, and wrestling; and people with slight builds tend to do reasonably well in track events, especially distance running, and in some individual and dual sports.

A study of the physiques and ages of the champions in the 1964 Olympic Games

[3] Copies of Meredith's chart along with specific instruction may be obtained from the American Medical Association, 535 N. Dearborn St., Chicago, Illinois or from the National Education Association, 1201 Sixteenth St., N.W., Washington, D.C.

furnishes evidence of the relationship of body build to performance. The Olympic basketball players and the volleyball net players were lean and tall, did not have excessive weight, and did not have a great deal of muscularity. The hockey and soccer players were rather small but stout. The gymnasts were generally small but strong. The weight lifters had short arms and were heavy and strong. The shot, discus, and hammer throwers were large and strong; the high jumpers, tall and lean. The pole vaulters were shorter and heavier because of the strength needed in the arms and shoulder girdle muscles. The distance runners, requiring much endurance, tended to be lean and small, more so as the distances increased, and the short-distance runners were heavier because of the demand for strength and speed. In addition to the Olympic players described, football linemen tend to be large and heavy; ends, tall and lighter; and backs, lighter than the linemen. Of course there are exceptions to these generalizations.

Knowledge that body build and size influence performance in certain ways can be useful to physical education teachers, especially those who coach athletic teams. But a student should not be deprived of opportunities to excel simply because his body build tends to deviate from those who usually excel in the activity.

Sheldon's Somatotype System

Of the various methods used to classify people by physique or body build the somatotype classification (Sheldon 1954) designed by William H. Sheldon, Stevens, and Tucker is generally the most useful in physical education. Somatotyping may be applied to boys, girls, men, and women. With Sheldon's system individuals may be classified according to endomorphic, mesomorphic, or ectomorphic characteristics (see Figure 8-1).

The endomorph tends to be thickset, and his body has a large amount of viscera and fatty tissue. He has a large round head; relatively short, thick neck; short, thick arms; thick chest with fatty breasts; thick, fatty abdomen, heavy buttocks, and thick legs. In general he has a pear-shaped structure and tends toward obesity.

The mesomorph, often referred to as the athletic type, has heavy, well-defined muscles throughout, large bones, broad shoulders, relatively narrow hips, large hands and arms. In general he has a V-shaped structure.

The ectomorph has small bones; light, fairly undefined musculature; long, slender arms; small chest; flat, slender abdomen; narrow hips, and slender legs. He may be described as the bean pole type.

Nearly all persons possess a mixture of the traits of the three primary body types. Therefore, three ratings are used to identify a person's body type, one rating for each component. Each rating is signified by a number between one and seven, with the higher numbers indicating dominance of that particular component. The first number refers to endomorphy, the second to mesomorphy, and the third to ectomorphy. Thus a person rated 7–1–1 would have dominant endomorphic characteristics and would lack mesomorphic and ectomorphic characteristics. A person with prominent mesomorphic characteristics might be rated 1–7–1, and one with

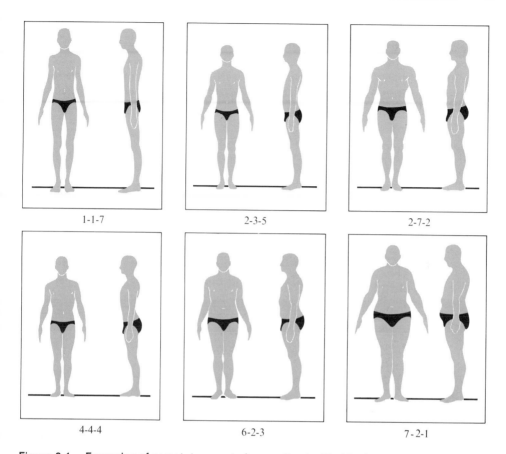

1-1-7   2-3-5   2-7-2

4-4-4   6-2-3   7-2-1

Figure 8-1. Examples of somatotypes rated according to Sheldon's somatotype system.

prominent ectomorphic traits might receive a 1–1–7 rating. Most people would not receive a one or seven rating. More typical would be ratings of 2–6–4 or 5–3–2.[4]

Except for research purposes somatotyping in the schools will probably continue to be done by judgment based on observation, rather than detailed objective measurements.

Cureton's Simplified Somatotype Method

Thomas Cureton (1947) devised a simplified method for somatotyping which gives the same results as Sheldon's system and is quite satisfactory for use other

---

[4] For greater detail about somatotyping refer to Sheldon's *Atlas of Man* in which he describes the entire somatotyping process and uses a large number of photographs to identify different body types.

than research. However, the body-type numbers of Cureton's simplified system do not have the same meaning as those of Sheldon's system. The method rates three aspects of the body—external fat, muscular development and condition, and skeletal development—from one to seven. The ratings (numbers) are given in accordance with the information in rating scales A, B, and C:

A. Scale for Rating External Fat

1	2	3	4	5	6	7

Extremely low in adipose tissue and relatively small anteroposterior dimensions of the lower trunk	Average in tissue and physical build of lower trunk	Extremely obese with large quantities of adipose tissue and unproportionately thick abdominal region

B. Scale for Rating Muscular Development and Condition

1	2	3	4	5	6	7

Extremely underdeveloped and poorly conditioned muscles squeezed or pushed in the contracted state (biceps, abdominals, thighs, calves)	Average in skeletal muscular development and condition	Extremely developed with large and hard muscles in the contracted state; firm under forceful squeezing

C. Scale for Rating Skeletal Development

1	2	3	4	5	6	7

Extremely thick and heavy bones, short and ponderous skeleton with relatively great cross-section of ankle, knee, and elbow joints	Average size bones and joints in cross-section and length	Extremely thin, frail bones, tall linear skeleton with relatively small cross-section of ankle, knee, and elbow joints

Thus a student rated 6–4–4 would be obese, average in muscle development, and average in skeletal development.

Posture and Body Mechanics

Posture refers to the relative positions of the different body segments. Posture is both static (body position while sitting and standing) and dynamic (body position during movement). Because dynamic posture is difficult to judge, there is a tendency to evaluate posture in only the standing and the sitting position. Silhouettes, photographs, posture charts, and posture rating scales have been used in evaluating the posture of students.

Correct posture is important because it enhances the functioning of the organic systems; reduces the strain on muscles, ligaments, and tendons and thereby retards the onset of muscle fatigue; increases the attractiveness of the person; and may influence the self-concept of the person and the view of others toward him.

Individual differences in structure and function result in part from heredity, so no precise standard of posture can be applied to all persons, although there are postural guides that apply in general. Logically posture must be evaluated from the physiological, anatomical, and aesthetic points of view.

Physiological Correctness

Posture is physiologically correct when it allows the body systems to function efficiently. Posture which restricts circulation, respiration, digestion, and elimination is less than correct. Research indicates that changes in posture influence heart rate in static positions and also required cardiac output during exercise.

Anatomical Correctness

Posture is anatomically correct when the body is in good balance and alignment for the least amount of muscle strain. Posture with each weight-bearing segment balanced upon the segment beneath demands less muscular effort than posture with segments formed in a zigzag alignment. Anatomically the best posture has body structure in good alignment and muscles as relaxed as possible.

Aesthetic Correctness

Posture is aesthetically correct when it contributes most to the attractiveness of the person. Aesthetically correct posture also tends to be anatomically and physiologically correct (see Figure 8-2). The concept of aesthetic posture may change slightly from time to time and from one segment of society to another: What is

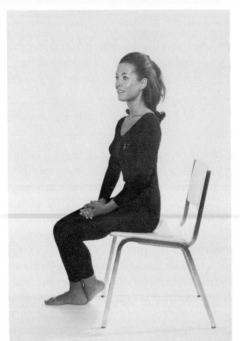 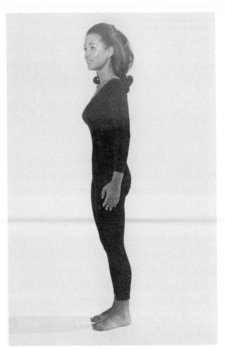

Figure 8-2. Illustrations of good posture, sitting and standing.

aesthetically correct for fashion models and for military personnel is indeed different.

Posture has strong psychological implications. A shy person may display a withdrawn type of posture to be less obvious, while a highly aggressive person may display a straight and outgoing type of posture to be more obvious.

Causes of Poor Posture

Posture characteristics may be inherited or developed. Children are inclined to have postures similar to their parents because of heredity and imitation. Height may influence posture; for example, short people tend to extend their height by standing straight, and tall people tend to reduce their height by settling at the joints and hunching at the upper back and neck.

Different physical education activities influence posture in different ways. Dance, gymnastics, diving, and fencing contribute to a straight and somewhat rigid posture and precision in movement. Wrestling and boxing seem to contribute to a slightly hunched posture. Long-distance running and swimming may contribute to a relaxed and often slouchy posture. Work conditions may also cause certain habitual postures. For instance, excessive study over a desk tends to develop rounded shoulders and forward head tilt.

Poor posture may be caused by body defects, disease, malnutrition, lack of muscle tone and strength, emotional states, attitudes, and lack of knowledge about the importance of good posture. In many cases the well-informed physical educator can help a student correct poor posture by motivating him to want to correct his posture and by specifying a program of exercise that will increase the strength and tone of the muscles to be used in correcting the particular deviation. Increased strength must be accompanied by increased flexibility of the opposing muscles.

Evaluation of Posture

Postural evaluation considers both the lateral and anteroposterior alignments of the different body segments. Spinal deviations include kyphosis (hunchbacked curvature), lordosis (exaggerated forward curvature in the lower part of the back), scoliosis (lateral curvature), and forward tilt of the head. Other deviations are rounded shoulders and sunken chest, lateral or medial rotation of the legs and feet, and abdominal ptosis (sagging). The following guides should be considered in the evaluation of posture:

1. The weight-bearing body segments should be correctly aligned.

2. The extension of the weight-bearing joints should be an easy extension, not rigid and tense.

3. The feet should point straight forward and be placed far enough apart to form a base of support so that the body can be easily balanced.

4. Excessive forward or lateral tilt of the pelvis should be avoided.

5. The spinal column, viewed from the rear, should be straight and the natural curves of the spine, viewed laterally, should not be excessive.

6. The abdominal wall should have good tone and should be kept flat.

7. The chest should not be sunken and the shoulders should not rotate forward.

8. The neck should be held straight so that the neck muscles are not under unnecessary strain.

Postural Screening Tests

Even though most postural deviations are apparent to one who knows correct posture, there are some postural screening tests that may be helpful to teachers who have had little or no instruction on posture deviation and correction. The Kraus–Weber Refined Posture Test (Kraus and Weber 1945), the Massey Posture Test (Massey 1943), the Wellesley Posture Test (MacEwan and Howe 1932), and the

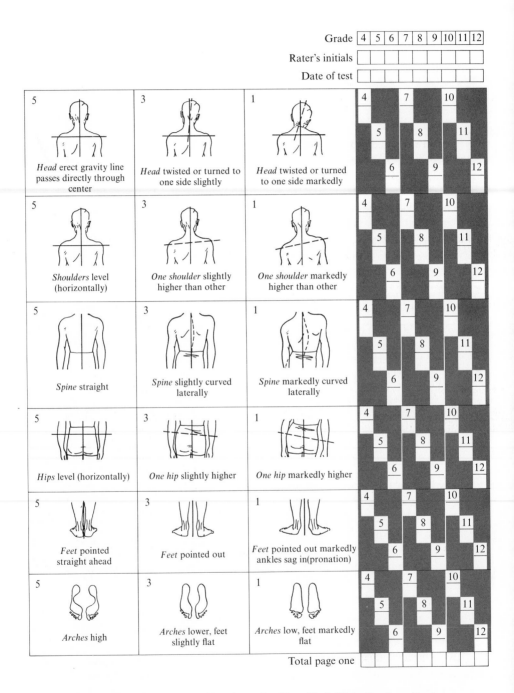

Figure 8-3.   Posture profiles from the New York State Posture Test.

Grade | 4 | 5 | 6 | 7 | 8 | 9 | 10 | 11 | 12

Total page one

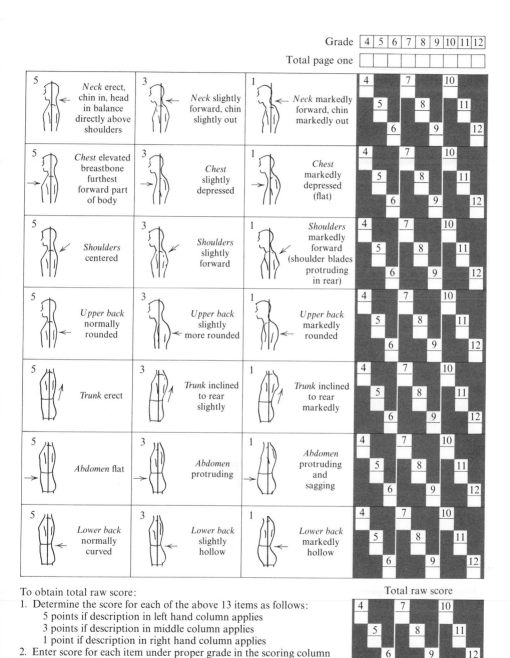

| 5 | *Neck* erect, chin in, head in balance directly above shoulders | 3 | *Neck* slightly forward, chin slightly out | 1 | *Neck* markedly forward, chin markedly out |

| 5 | *Chest* elevated breastbone furthest forward part of body | 3 | *Chest* slightly depressed | 1 | *Chest* markedly depressed (flat) |

| 5 | *Shoulders* centered | 3 | *Shoulders* slightly forward | 1 | *Shoulders* markedly forward (shoulder blades protruding in rear) |

| 5 | *Upper back* normally rounded | 3 | *Upper back* slightly more rounded | 1 | *Upper back* markedly rounded |

| 5 | *Trunk* erect | 3 | *Trunk* inclined to rear slightly | 1 | *Trunk* inclined to rear markedly |

| 5 | *Abdomen* flat | 3 | *Abdomen* protruding | 1 | *Abdomen* protruding and sagging |

| 5 | *Lower back* normally curved | 3 | *Lower back* slightly hollow | 1 | *Lower back* markedly hollow |

To obtain total raw score:

1. Determine the score for each of the above 13 items as follows:
   - 5 points if description in left hand column applies
   - 3 points if description in middle column applies
   - 1 point if description in right hand column applies
2. Enter score for each item under proper grade in the scoring column
3. Add all 13 scores and place total in appropriate space

Total raw score

Wickens and Kiphuth Posture Test (Wickens and Kiphuth 1937) are useful measures of posture.

The manual for the New York State Fitness Test (1958) includes a convenient posture rating system. The system includes a series of profiles (see Figure 8-3) against which any student's posture may be compared.

Procedure: The examiner hangs a plumb line from a stationary support about four feet in front of a screen or other suitable background against which to view the student. Then at a right angle from the screen he passes a line of masking tape directly under the plumb line and extends it ten feet toward him (see Figure 8-4). In the first part of the examination the student stands between the screen and the plumb line facing the screen, directly over the line of masking tape so the plumb line passes directly up the middle of the back. The examiner then rates the student's posture from the rear view by comparing the student with the rear view profiles (see Figure 8-4). In a similar fashion the student assumes a side position and the examiner completes the examination.

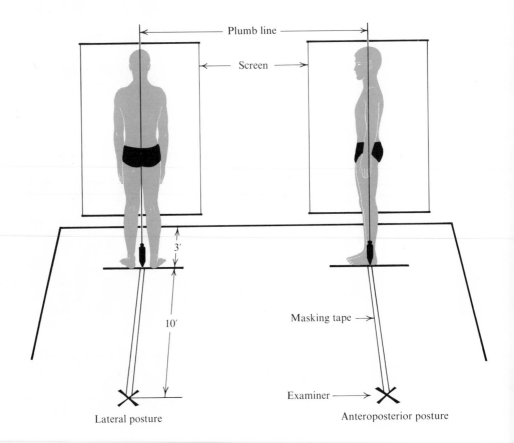

Figure 8-4. New York state posture testing station.

Scoring: The examiner assigns a score of five, three, or one for each body area, according to the profile that best matches the student and records the score in the square corresponding to the student's grade level. He then totals the 13 scores to obtain a final score and compares the final score to the norm based on a percentile scale (see Table 8-1).

Table 8-1
Norms for the New York State Posture Test

Final Score	Percentile
65	98
63	93
61	84
59	69
55–57	50
49–53	31
39–43	7
35–37	2
0–33	1

How To Correct Posture

In most cases the well-informed physical educator can help a student correct poor posture by motivating him to correct his posture and by leading him through a corrective program, consisting of selected exercises to add strength and tone to muscles which need to apply more tension and to add flexibility to opposing muscle groups.

The following is considered a successful postural corrective procedure:

1. Correctly identify the postural deviation and inform the individual of its nature and the importance of correction.

2. Attempt to identify the basic causes of the deviation and control the causes.

3. Motivate the individual to correct the deviation. (In the absence of such motivation, postural corrective exercises will probably fail.)

4. Prescribe an exercise program designed to correct the condition.

5. Periodically evaluate the effects of the program.

A well-prepared physical educator should be able to tell which muscles must be strengthened and which must have increased flexibility to bring about the desired postural changes. He should also be able to select effective exercises.

Selected References

Cureton, Thomas K., "Physical Fitness Appraisal and Guidance." St. Louis: C. V. Mosby Company, 1947, p. 120.

Kraus, Hans, and Weber, S., "Evaluation of Posture Based on Structural and Functional Measurements," *Physiotherapy Review*, 1945, *26* (6).

MacEwan, Charlotte G., and Howe, Eugene C., "An Objective Method of Grading Posture," *Research Quarterly*, 1932, *3* (3).

Massey, Wayne W., "A Critical Study of Objective Methods for Measuring Anterior-Posterior Posture with a Simplified Technique," *Research Quarterly*, 1943, *14* (1).

Meredith, Howard V., "A Physical Growth Record for Use in Elementary and High Schools," *American Journal of Public Health*, 1949, *39*, 878–885.

The New York State Physical Fitness Test: A Manual for Teachers of Physical Education. Albany, N.Y.: Division of Health, Physical Education and Recreation, New York State Education Department, 1958.

Pryor, Helen B., *Weight–Width Tables.* Stanford, Calif.: Stanford University Press, 1940.

Sheldon, William H., *Atlas of Men.* New York: Harper & Brothers, 1954.

Wetzel, Norman C., "The Treatment of Growth Failure in Children." Cleveland: NEA Service, 1948.

Wickens, J. Stuart, and Kiphuth, Oscar, "Body Mechanics Analysis of Yale University Freshmen," *Research Quarterly*, 1937, *3* (4).

9

Student
Classification Plans

Sometimes students are classified for competition and instruction by some method other than age or grade. Experience and research have led to the conclusion that age, height, and weight measures form a sound basis for the classification of elementary and junior high school boys and girls and for high school boys. Height and weight may be used for the classification of college men. (Age contributes little in classifications of this group.) Age, height, and weight measures are not satisfactory for classifying high school girls or college women. For students other than high school girls and college women age–height–weight classification plans have been used extensively to establish achievement scales that evaluate a student's performance, measure his improvement in skills, stimulate his interest in total development, and help the teacher select activities to meet individual needs.

The examiner can determine height with a stadiometer and weight with a balanced scale. He can compute age conveniently and accurately by the following method:

First he finds the difference between the year during which the age is being

Month Age Is Being Computed

Birth Month	Jan.	Feb.	Mar.	Apr.	May	June	July	Aug.	Sept.	Oct.	Nov.	Dec.
Jan.	0	1	2	3	4	5	6	7	8	9	10	11
Feb.	1	0	1	2	3	4	5	6	7	8	9	10
March	2	1	0	1	2	3	4	5	6	7	8	9
April	3	2	1	0	1	2	3	4	5	6	7	8
May	4	3	2	1	0	1	2	3	4	5	6	7
June	5	4	3	2	1	0	1	2	3	4	5	6
July	6	5	4	3	2	1	0	1	2	3	4	5
Aug.	7	6	5	4	3	2	1	0	1	2	3	4
Sept.	8	7	6	5	4	3	2	1	0	1	2	3
Oct.	9	8	7	6	5	4	3	2	1	0	1	2
Nov.	10	9	8	7	6	5	4	3	2	1	0	1
Dec.	11	10	9	8	7	6	5	4	3	2	1	0

Add

Subtract

Figure 9-1

computed and the year the student was born. This number will be the base years. Since the teacher will usually be working with similar age groups, the base years for a given group will not vary widely. Then he uses a classification chart (see Figure 9-1) to determine the month difference to be added to, or subtracted from, the base years to produce an accurate age in years and months. For example, if the difference between the present year and the year the student was born is 14, this number will be the base years. If the computation is made in February and the student was born in September, then using the classification chart, the examiner looks down the February column and across the September row to find that the month difference is 7. He then subtracts this number from the base years, 14. The result is 13 years 5 months. The chart, of course, can be used with any base years.

Neilson and Cozens
Classification Plan for Elementary
and Junior High School Students

The Neilson and Cozens age–height–weight classification plan has been used extensively for elementary and junior high school students. It was first developed in the Oakland, California, public schools as an adaptation of the classification scheme used in connection with the California Decathlon Charts, which were outgrowths of Frederick Reilly's plan of rational athletics. Through research Frederick W. Cozens clearly established the validity of the Neilson and Cozens plan. Use of the plan for the classification of students is illustrated by the following example:

Age–Height–Weight	Exponent*
Height = 59 inches	8
Age = 13 years and 7 months	8
Weight = 119 pounds	12
Sum of exponents	28
Class of student	E

* Derived from Table 9-1.

The following 6 σ achievement scales (Neilson, Van Hagen, and Comer 1966) are based on the Neilson and Cozens classification plan.

For Girls

Agility Run (Shuttle Run)	Run—60 yards
Basketball Throw for Goal	Soccer Dribble
Jump and Reach (Vertical Jump)	Softball Throw for Accuracy
Run and Catch	Standing Long Hop
Run—50 yards	Standing Three Hops

For Boys

Agility Run (Shuttle Run)	Run—75 yards
Basketball Throw for Goal	Running High Jump
Jump and Reach (Vertical Jump)	Soccer Dribble
Pull-up	Softball Throw for Accuracy
Push-up	Standing Hop, Step, Jump
Run—50 yards	Standing Long Jump

Table 9-1
Neilson and Cozens Classification Chart for Elementary
and Junior High School Boys and Girls

Exponent	Height in inches	Age in years	Weight in pounds
1	50 to 51	10 to 10-5	60 to 65
2	52 to 53	10-6 to 10-11	66 to 70
3		11 to 11-5	71 to 75
4	54 to 55	11-6 to 11-11	76 to 80
5		12 to 12-5	81 to 85
6	56 to 57	12-6 to 12-11	86 to 90
7		13 to 13-5	91 to 95
8	58 to 59	13-6 to 13-11	96 to 100
9		14 to 14-5	101 to 105
10	60 to 61	14-6 to 14-11	106 to 110
11		15 to 15-5	111 to 115
12	62 to 63	15-6 to 15-11	116 to 120
13		16 to 16-5	121 to 125
14	64 to 65	16-6 to 16-11	126 to 130
15	66 to 67	17 to 17-5	131 to 133
16	68	17-6 to 17-11	134 to 136
17	69 and over	18 and over	137 and over

Sum of exponents	Class	Sum of exponents	Class
9 and below	A	25 to 29	E
10 to 14	B	30 to 34	F
15 to 19	C	35 to 38	G
20 to 24	D	39 and above	H

Neilson and Cozens Classification Plan for Secondary School Boys

Using 20,000 performance records of boys in a wide variety of individual athletic events, Cozens arrived at the Best-Fit Index of $2A + .475H + .16W$, where A refers to age in years, H to height in inches, and W to weight in pounds. Table 9-2 was produced from the Best-Fit Index. In this classification plan junior high school boys predominate in classes F, E, D, and C, while senior high school boys fall mainly in classes C, B, and A.

The following example uses Table 9-2 for the classification of a boy who is 12 years old, 54 inches tall, and weighs 160 pounds.

Age–Height–Weight	Exponent
Height = 54 inches	26
Age = 12.0 years	24
Weight = 160 pounds	26
Sum of exponents	76
Class of student	D

Table 9-2
Neilson and Cozens Classification Plan for Secondary School Boys
Grades 7 to 12 inclusive*

Exponent	Age	Height	Weight	Exponent	Age	Height	Weight
9			53– 59	24	11:9–12:2	49.5–51.5	147–153
10			60– 65	25	12:3–12:8	52 –53.5	154–159
11			66– 71	26	12:9–13:2	54 –55.5	160–165
12			72– 78	27	13:3–13:8	56 –57.5	166–171
13			79– 84	28	13:9–14:2	58 –59.5	172–178
14			85– 90	29	14:3–14:8	60 –62	179–184
15			91– 96	30	14:9–15:2	62.5–64	185–190
16			97–103	31	15:3–15:8	64.5–66	191–up
17			104–109	32	15:9–16:2	66.5–68	
18			110–115	33	16:3–16:8	68.5–70.5	
19			116–121	34	16:9–17:2	71 –72.5	
20			122–128	35	17:3–17:8	73 –74.5	
21			129–134	36	17:9–18:2	75 –up	
22	10:9–11:2	47–down	135–140	37	18:3–18:8		
23	11:3–11:8	47.5–49	141–146	38	18:9–19:2		

Sum of exponents	Class	Sum of exponents	Class
88 and over	A	75–78	D
83–87	B	70–74	E
79–82	C	69 and below	F

* For purposes of competition in interschool athletics and in individual events—derived from the formula 2A (years) +.475H (inches) +.16W (pounds)

Appendix C has numerous achievement scales for secondary school boys that are based on this classification plan.

Cozens Classification
Plan for College Men

In studying the problem of classification of college men for competition in individual athletic events, Cozens found a negligible correlation between age and height and between age and weight. He also found that with college men age has little or no bearing on performance. Although height and weight have some influence on performance, the correlations are not large enough to use in the prediction of performance. On the basis of these findings, Cozens formed nine stature groups: tall slender, tall medium, tall heavy, medium slender, medium medium, medium heavy, short slender, short medium, and short heavy, as shown in Table 9-3. (All heights and weights are to be taken without clothing.)

According to the information in Table 9-3 a student five feet eight inches in height and 138 pounds in weight would be classified as medium medium in stature. A student six feet three inches in height and 153 pounds in weight would be classified as tall slender in stature.

Table 9-3
Cozens Height–Weight Class Division
of College Men

	Height	Slender	Medium	Heavy
			Weight	
Short	4–11	up to 92	93–108	109 up
	5-0	up to 97	98–112	113 up
	5-1	up to 101	102–117	118 up
	5-2	up to 106	107–121	122 up
	5-3	up to 110	111–126	127 up
	5-4	up to 114	115–131	132 up
	5-5	up to 118	119–135	136 up
	5-6	up to 121	122–139	140 up
Medium	5-7	up to 124	125–143	144 up
	5-8	up to 128	129–147	148 up
	5-9	up to 131	132–150	151 up
	5-10	up to 134	135–153	154 up
Tall	5-11	up to 138	139–157	158 up
	6-0	up to 142	143–162	163 up
	6-1	up to 146	147–166	167 up
	6-2	up to 150	151–171	172 up
	6-3	up to 154	155–175	176 up
	6-4	up to 158	159–179	180 up

Appendix D has numerous achievement scales for college men that are based on this classification plan.

Classification Plan for
High School Girls and College Women

The relationships of age, height, and weight of high school girls and college women to their performance records is low. However, research is needed to determine, whether the classification plan used for college men would be desirable in some of the activities. Appendix B has several achievement scales for secondary school girls that are based on the Cozens and Neilson Classification Index. The scales were prepared by the American Association of Health, Physical Education, and Recreation (AAHPER).

McCloy Classification Indexes

On the basis of extensive study Charles H. McCloy established three age–height–weight indexes:

For high school:	Classification Index I	20 (age in years) + 6 (height in inches) + weight in pounds
For college:	Classification Index II	6 (height in inches) + weight in pounds
For elementary school:	Classification Index III	10 (age in years) + weight in pounds

McCloy (McCloy and Young 1954), in recommending the indexes for different age levels, found that age ceased to make a contribution at 17 years and that height was not an important factor at the elementary school level.

Selected References

Barrow, Harold M., "Classification in Physical Education." *The Physical Educator*, 1960, *17*, 101.

Clarke, H. Harrison, and Degutis, Ernest W., "Comparison of Skeletal Age and Various Physical and Motor Factors with the Pubescent Development of 10, 13, and 16 Year Old Boys." *Research Quarterly*, 1962, *33*, 356–68.

Clarke, H. Harrison, and Harrison, James C. E., "Differences in Physical and Motor Traits Between Boys of Advanced, Normal, and Retarded Maturity." *Research Quarterly*, 1962, *33*, 13–25.

Cozens, Frederick W., Cubberley, Hazel J., and Neilson, N. P., *Achievement Scales in Physical Education Activities for Secondary School Girls and College Women*. New York: A. S. Barnes, 1937.

Cozens, Frederick W., Trieb, Martin H., and Neilson, N. P., *Physical Education Achievement Scales for Boys in Secondary Schools*. New York: A. S. Barnes, 1936.

Cozens, Frederick W., Trieb, Martin H., and Neilson, N. P., "The Classification of Secondary School Boys for Purposes of Competition." *Research Quarterly*, 1939, *7*, 36.

Espenschade, Anna S., "Restudy of Relationships Between Physical Performances of School Children and Age, Height, and Weight." *Research Quarterly*, 1963, *34*, 144–53.

Lockhart, Aileene, and Mott, Jane A., "An Experiment in Homogeneous Grouping and Its Effect on Achievement in Sports Fundamentals." *Research Quarterly*, 1951, *22*, 58–62.

Gross, Elmer A., and Casciani, Jerome A., "Value of Age, Height, and Weight as a Classification Device for Secondary School Students in the Seven AAHPER Youth Fitness Tests." *Research Quarterly*, 1962, *33*, 51–58.

McCloy, Charles H., *The Measurement of Athletic Power*. New York: A. S. Barnes, 1932.

McCloy, Charles H., and Young, Norma D., *Tests and Measurements in Health and Physical Education*, 3rd ed. New York: Appleton-Century-Crofts, 1954, p. 59.

Miller, Kenneth D. "A Critique on the Use of Height–Weight Factors in the Performance Classification of College Men." *Research Quarterly*, *23*, 402–16, December 1952.

Neilson, N. P., *An Elementary Course in Statistics, Tests and Measurements in Physical Education*. Palo Alto, Calif.: National Press Publications, 1960.

Neilson, N. P., and Cozens, Frederick W., *Achievement Scales in Physical Education Activities for Boys and Girls in Elementary and Junior High Schools*. New York: A. S. Barnes, 1934.

Neilson, N. P., Van Hagen, Winifred, and Comer, James L., *Physical Education for Elementary Schools*, 3rd ed. New York: The Ronald Press, 1966.

Pierson, William R., and O'Connell, Eugene R., "Age, Height, Weight, and Grip Strength." *Research Quarterly*, 1962, *33*, 439–43.

Reilly, Frederick J., *New Rational Athletics for Boys and Girls*. Boston: D. C. Heath, 1917.

FOUR
Measurements of
Interpretive and Impulsive Traits

Physical educators have made considerable progress in the area of anthropometric measurements and in tests of such functional traits as strength, skill, and endurance. A few standardized tests of knowledge about physical education activities have been constructed. Much less progress has been made in accurate measurements of student interests, attitudes, emotions, and ideals which determine to a large extent choices in behavior.

Tests and ratings of interpretive and impulsive traits are difficult to construct and use, yet they are valuable and should be as valid, reliable, and objective as possible. This section includes the more useful tests of interpretive and impulsive traits.

10

Tests of
Interpretive Traits

Measurements of interpretive traits include tests dealing with ideas, concepts, facts, and the ability to make judgments, and they determine the extent to which the student has attained knowledge in these areas. Comparison of a student's level of knowledge at the beginning of a physical education course with that at the end of the course indicates the amount of progress made. Such tests should motivate the student to learn as well as help the teacher to improve the quality of instruction.

Tests of knowledge in physical education may vary in length and content and be specific or comprehensive in nature. They may be individual tests or a battery of tests designed to cover a number of areas. The tests may refer to the history of physical education; the history of a given activity; the organization and rules of the activity; the techniques of performance; and the strategies, facilities, or terminology used in the activity. A participant or spectator who is ignorant of the rules and procedures in physical education activities often displays undesirable behavior during these events. However, despite the importance of knowledge of rules and procedures, the time involved in giving such tests should not be excessive since the student's primary interest is to participate in the activities, not to talk or read about them.

Standardized Knowledge Tests

The development of standardized knowledge tests in physical education began in 1929 when J. G. Bliss devised his knowledge test on basketball. Recognition of the importance of knowledge about physical education activities and efforts to establish physical education as an academic discipline influenced the construction and use of such tests.

A large number of physical education activities have standardized tests of knowledge constructed for boys and girls on the secondary school level and for men and women on the college level. Various issues of the *Research Quarterly* and the *Journal of Health, Physical Education and Recreation* have reported these tests.

When a well-informed person has carefully constructed a knowledge test about some phase of physical education and has given evidence that the test is highly valid and reliable, then physical educators may accept the test as standardized and use its established norms. A standardized test should cover an adequate amount of important information about the subject. Those who use the test must include in their instruction the content covered by the test. The purpose of the test is to discover the degree to which the students in the class have learned the subjects covered in the test. Under these conditions standardized knowledge tests are difficult to adapt to a local situation—that is, to a particular group of students in a particular situation—and are therefore used infrequently. However, teachers often find such tests useful as sources of good questions which may be selected to fit the teacher's particular needs.

Teacher-Made Tests

Most tests of interpretive traits used by physical educators are in the form of local, teacher-made tests constructed for specific situations. For example, following a unit of instruction on tennis a teacher may construct a test to measure the students' knowledge about tennis. He may follow the same procedure in connection with units of instruction on other activities.

Teacher-made knowledge tests are closely related to the teacher's conception of what the students should have learned and are highly local in nature. The teacher administers such tests to discover what the students have and have not learned. This information is then available to the teacher and the student. The tests become guides for future instruction and learning.

When he constructs a knowledge test for a given course, the teacher should select test items that are important in relation to the objectives of the course and should state the items clearly. He should take an adequate sample of ideas from the course content in balance with their emphasis in the course. He should avoid long, involved statements that are poorly worded or poorly substantiated by facts. He should also avoid use of such words as *all*, *never, always,* and *none* because they tend to make the answer apparent. Refer to *Chapter 22* for specific information on test construction.

Knowledge Tests
in Relation to Objectives

Teachers who instruct students in an activity course or in a physical education lecture course must be aware of certain important objectives. As far as the expected results of activities are concerned, the teacher and the students should have the same objectives; if they do not, teaching and learning become inefficient. Knowledge tests in the activities should be related to the expected results.

Let us consider the examples of archery and girls basketball. In archery it is expected that the student will know how to:

1.   Choose a bow.

2.   Nock a bow.

3.   Stand in relation to the target.

4.   Pick up and hold an arrow.

5.   Nock an arrow.

6.   Judge the shooting range.

7.   Allow for the direction and intensity of the wind.

8.   Hold the bow before loosing an arrow.

9.   Establish the point of aim.

10.   Draw the bow.

11.   Release an arrow.

12.   Pull an arrow from the target.

13.   Pull an arrow from the grass.

14.   Score in archery using the various methods.

15.   Practice courtesy and etiquette.

16.   Unnock the bow.

17.   Care for a bow.

18.   Care for arrows.

19.   Care for the target.

In girls basketball it is expected that the student will know:

1.   The rules of the game.

2.   The terms used in basketball.

3.   The importance of developing a variety of skills.

4.   How to start a movement quickly.

5.   How to stop a movement quickly.

6.   How to jump for a tie ball.

7.   How to catch the ball.

8.   The various techniques to be used in passing.

9.   How to dribble the ball.

10.   How to pivot.

11.   How to feint and dodge.

12.   How to guard an opponent.

13.   How to avoid making fouls.

14.   Game strategy and play patterns.

15.   The techniques of foul shooting.

16.   The various techniques to be used in shooting from the field.

17.   The courtesies that should be extended to teammates.

18.   The courtesies that should be extended to opponents.

19.   The courtesies that should be extended to officials.

20.   The personal health practices that influence performance.

Available Sports Knowledge Tests

Even though the teacher usually wants to design knowledge tests to fit his particular situation, prepared tests are often helpful for ideas. There are numerous sources for test items that will fit a local situation.

Wadsworth Sports Series

Wadsworth Publishing Company in Belmont, California has published individual booklets on a number of sports. Each booklet, prepared by an expert in the particular sport, contains a short, written knowledge test. Booklets on the following activities are available:

Archery
Badminton
Basketball for men
Bowling
Conditioning
Field hockey
Folk dancing
Golf
Handball
Paddleball
Skiing
Skin and scuba diving
Soccer

Social dance
Softball
Square dance
Swimming
Tennis
Track and field
Trampolining
Tumbling and floor exercise
Volleyball
Weight training
Wrestling
Personal defense for women

William C. Brown Activity Series

Subsequent to the Wadsworth series William C. Brown Company in Dubuque, Iowa published a series of booklets on sports. There are written knowledge tests for the following activities included in the series:

Archery
Badminton
Basketball for men
Basketball for women
Biophysical values of muscular activity
Bowling
Canoeing
Circuit training
Conditioning
Contemporary square dance
Fencing
Field hockey
Figure skating
Folk dance
Golf
Gymnastics
Handball
Judo

Lacrosse
Modern dance
Physical and physiological
   conditioning for men
Skiing
Skin and scuba diving
Soccer
Social dance
Softball
Squash racquets
Swimming
Table tennis
Tap dance
Tennis
Track and field
Trampolining
Volleyball
Weight training

Other Sports Knowledge Tests

A large number of carefully prepared knowledge tests have resulted from research studies. Some of these tests have been standardized. The following sources are good references for a variety of sports knowledge tests:

Archery

> Ley, Katherine L., Constructing Objective Test Items to Measure High School Levels of Achievement in Selected Physical Education Activities. Microcarded doctoral dissertation, University of Iowa, 1960. Includes archery, badminton, basketball, golf, soccer, softball, and volleyball.
>
> Snell, Catherine, "Physical Education Knowledge Tests." *Research Quarterly*, 1935, *6*. Includes baseball, basketball, golf, soccer, tennis, and volleyball.

Badminton

> Fox, Katherine, "Beginning Badminton Written Examinations." *Research Quarterly*, 1953, *24*.
>
> French, Esther, "The Construction of Knowledge Tests in Selected Professional Courses in Physical Education." *Research Quarterly*, 1943, *14*. Includes basketball, dance, golf, soccer, softball, swimming, tennis, and volleyball.
>
> Goll, Lillian M., Construction of Badminton and Swimming Knowledge Tests for High School Girls. Microcarded master's thesis, Illinois State Normal University, 1956.
>
> Hennis, Gail M., "Construction of Knowledge Tests in Selected Physical Education Activities for College Women." *Research Quarterly*, 1956, *27*. Includes basketball, softball, tennis, and volleyball. (Also see Physical Education Microcards.)
>
> Ley, Katherine L. (see Archery).
>
> Phillips, Marjorie, "Standardization of a Badminton Knowledge Test for College Women." *Research Quarterly*, 1946, *17*.
>
> Scott, Gladys M., "Achievement Examination in Badminton." *Research Quarterly*, 1941, *12*.

Baseball

> Goldberg, Isidor H., The Development of Achievement Standards in Knowledge of Physical Education Activities. Microcarded doctoral dissertation, New York University, 1953.
>
> Hemphill, Fay, "Information Tests in Health and Physical Education for High School Boys." *Research Quarterly*, 1932, *3*.

Basketball

> French, Esther (see Badminton).
>
> Hennis, Gail M. (see Badminton).
>
> Ley, Katherine L. (see Archery).

Dance

French, Esther (see Badminton).

Murry, Josephine K., An Appreciation Test in Dance. Unpublished master's thesis, University of California, 1943.

Field Hockey

Deita, Dorothea, and Frech, Beryl, "Hockey Knowledge Test for Girls." *Journal of Health, Physical Education and Recreation*, 1940, *11* (6).

Kelly, Elen D., and Brown, J. E., "The Construction of a Field Hockey Test for Women Physical Education Majors." *Research Quarterly*, 1952, *23* (3).

Golf

French, Esther (see Badminton).

Ley, Katherine L. (see Archery).

Snell, Catherine (see Archery).

Waglow, I. F., and Rehling, C. H., "A Golf Knowledge Test." *Research Quarterly*, 1953, *24.*

Soccer

French, Esther (see Badminton).

Heath, Marjorie L., and Rodgers, E. G., "A Study in the Use of Knowledge and Skill Tests in Soccer." *Research Quarterly*, 1932, *3.*

Knighton, Marion, "Soccer Questions." *Journal of Health and Physical Education*, 1930 (1).

Ley, Katherine L. (see Archery).

Snell, Catherine (see Archery).

Softball

French, Esther (see Badminton).

Hennis, Gail M. (see Badminton).

Ley, Katherine L. (see Archery).

Waglow, I. F., and Stephens, Foy, "A Softball Knowledge Test." *Research Quarterly*, 1955, *26* (2).

Swimming

French, Esther (see Badminton).

Goll, Lillian M. (see Badminton).

Scott, M. Gladys, "Achievement Examinations for Elementary and Intermediate Swimming Classes." *Research Quarterly*, 1939, *11.*

Tennis

Broer, Marion R., and Miller, Donna M., "Achievement Tests for Beginning and Intermediate Tennis." *Research Quarterly*. 1950, *21*.

French, Esther (see Badminton).

Hennis, Gail M. (see Badminton).

Hewitt, Jack E., "Comprehensive Tennis Knowledge Test." *Research Quarterly*, 1937, *8*.

Hewitt, Jack E. "Hewitt's Comprehensive Tennis Knowledge Test." *Research Quarterly*, 1964, *35*.

Miller, Wilma K., "Achievement Levels in Tennis Knowledge and Skill for Women Physical Education Major Students." *Research Quarterly*, 1953, *24*.

Scott, M. Gladys, "Achievement Examination for Elementary and Intermediate Tennis Classes." *Research Quarterly*, 1941, *12*.

Snell, Catherine (see Archery).

Volleyball

French, Esther (see Badminton).

Hennis, Gail M. (see Badminton).

Langston, Dewey F., "Standardization of a Volleyball Knowledge Test for College Men Physical Education Majors." *Research Quarterly*, 1955, *26*.

Ley, Katherine L. (see Archery).

Snell, Catherine (see Archery).

Selected References

Barrow, Harold M., "The Construction and Evaluation of Objective Knowledge Tests," *A Practical Approach to Measurement in Physical Education*. Philadelphia: Lea & Febiger, 1966.

Bliss, J. G., *Basketball*. Philadelphia: Lea & Febiger, 1929.

Clarke, Harrison H., "Knowledge Tests," *Application of Measurement*. Englewood Cliffs, N.J.: Prentice-Hall, 1967.

Colvill, Frances, The Learning of Motor Skills as Influenced by a Knowledge of General Principles of Mechanics. Unpublished doctoral dissertation, University of Southern California, 1956.

Johnson, Barry L., "The Measurement of Knowledge," *Practical Measurements for Evaluation in Physical Education*. Minneapolis: Burgess Publishing Company, 1969.

Mohr, Dorothy R., and Barrett, Mildred E., "Effect of Knowledge of Mechanical Principles in Learning to Perform Intermediate Swimming Skills." *Research Quarterly*, 1962, *33*.

11

Measurements
of Impulsive Traits

There are only a few noteworthy instruments in physical education that measure impulsive traits (interests, attitudes, emotional behavior, and character). Much additional work needs to be done in this area of measurement.

Ratings of Interests

People involved in physical education are interested in participating in physical activities as well as in learning about their organization, techniques, and environment. In addition, rather than participate, other people may enjoy watching the active participants or reading in newspapers and magazines about such participation. This widespread interest on the part of participants and observers helps to maintain the interscholastic, intercollegiate, and professional sports.

When making studies of human interests physical educators frequently formulate a list of items and then have the student rate himself as to his degree of interest in each item. The rating scale generally provides for several degrees of interest: high, above average, average, below average, and little interest. Teachers often find profitable the use of interest rating scales related to physical education activities or to the expected outcomes from participation in the activities.

Ratings of Attitudes

An attitude is a predisposition to feel favorably or unfavorably toward something. A person's attitudes strongly influence his thinking and behavior and have an important influence on the learning process. Attitudes may relate to activities, people, leadership, and the environment. Since attitudes impel one to act, they may be inferred from observed behavior.

To be effective, teachers of physical education must be concerned with the appraisal of student attitudes and with the development of desirable attitudes. However, since objective tests of attitudes are impossible, teachers must rely on careful observation of behavior, student reactions to attitude inventories, anecdotal records, and the information from rating scales.

Ratings of Emotional Behavior

Emotional behavior is involved in most motor performances. The emotional elements inherent in swimming (fear of water, for example) are different from the emotional elements in gymnastics, wrestling, basketball, football, or golf. Each activity has its own type and level of emotional involvement. Active participation offers unusual opportunities for evaluation of emotional behavior and for the development of desirable behavior patterns.

Ratings of Character

Character is a complex of one's behavior traits; hence ratings of behavior are essentially ratings of character traits. Behavior rating scales are the result of efforts to evaluate character as a whole or some aspect of character as exhibited in physical education activities. The following examples are desirable behavior traits: friendly attitude toward teammates and opponents; accuracy in keeping score; loyalty to the team, coach, and school; modesty in winning; courage in contact sports; refinement in manners; control of emotions; sense of humor in appropriate situations; tact at necessary times.

Construction and Use of Rating Scales

Several factors must be considered in the construction of rating scales for the evaluation of impulsive traits: How should the traits be selected? How many traits should be selected? How should the traits be defined? Should general or specific traits be listed? Should both desirable and undesirable traits be listed? Should different degrees of a trait be measured? To what degree is the trait desirable or undesirable? Who is to do the rating? How frequently does the person exhibit the trait?

A teacher should attempt ratings of character traits only after intentional and accurate observation over a reasonable period of time. He should use these ratings as an aid in changing undesirable forms of student conduct, not for the purpose of grading.

The teacher might make the process of rating a class project and allow students with some training to assist in the evaluation process by rating themselves or their classmates. In this way students may learn the importance of good behavior and become interested in improving their own ways of behaving.

Useful Measures of Impulsive Traits

The following selected measuring instruments have proved to be useful in school programs:

Neilson Character Rating Scale

This scale was prepared by N. P. Neilson to measure how well a student of junior high school, high school, or college age demonstrates desirable character traits. The evaluator, usually the teacher, rates the student on each of the 24 items and records the appropriate score (listed at the top of each column) opposite the item. Five is the highest possible score on each item. There are 120 points possible.

Neilson Character Rating Scale

Name_____ Age_____ Grade_____

Date_____ Evaluator_____

CHARACTER TRAITS	poor 1	fair 2	average 3	good 4	excellent 5
1. *Accuracy:* precise, correct					
2. *Alertness:* watchful; ready to act.					
3. *Cheerfulness:* joyous; in good spirit.					
4. *Confidence:* reliant; sure; free from doubt.					
5. *Cooperation:* ability to work harmoniously with other persons.					
6. *Courage:* meets difficulties with firmness or valor.					
7. *Dependability:* trustworthy; reliable.					
8. *Enthusiasm:* inspired; ardent; interested.					
9. *Honesty:* truthful; having integrity.					
10. *Industry:* diligent; not slothful or idle.					
11. *Initiative:* to begin action in new fields.					

Neilson Character Rating Scale *continued*

CHARACTER TRAITS	poor 1	fair 2	average 3	good 4	excellent 5
12. *Judgment:* making intelligent decisions.					
13. *Language:* good choice of words; avoids profanity.					
14. *Leadership:* directing action; being followed by others.					
15. *Loyalty:* giving active support to a cause.					
16. *Modesty:* not boastful or egotistical; absence of arrogance.					
17. *Neatness of dress:* being clean and appropriately dressed.					
18. *Obedient:* compliance with requests of one in authority.					
19. *Refinement in manners:* actions are pleasing and in good taste.					
20. *Self-control:* control over emotions; self-direction.					
21. *Sense of humor:* ability to appreciate amusing situations.					
22. *Social adaptability:* friendly with people and at ease in their presence.					
23. *Sportsmanship:* fairness; respect for rights of others; a good loser and graceful winner.					
24. *Tact:* ability to deal with others without giving offense.					

Cowell's Social Adjustment Index

This index (Cowell 1958) was developed to measure how well students of junior high school through college age are adjusted to their social environment. The index has a reported validity coefficient of .63 and a reliability coefficient of .82.

Procedure: The teacher rates each student on both Form A and Form B.

Scoring: He then computes the score (listed at the top of the columns) in the appropriate column opposite each item and computes the raw score by subtracting the total score on Form B from the total score on Form A. The higher scores are indications of good social adjustment.

Cowell's Social Adjustment Index (Form A)

Name_____ Age_____ Grade_____

Date_____ Describer's name_____

Behavior Trends	Descriptive of the Student			
	Markedly (+3)	Somewhat (+2)	Only Slightly (+1)	Not at All (+0)
1. Enters heartily and with enjoyment into the spirit of social intercourse.				
2. Frank; talkative and sociable, does not stand on ceremony.				
3. Self-confident and self-reliant, tends to take success for granted, strong initiative, prefers to lead.				
4. Quick and decisive in movement, pronounced or excessive energy output.				
5. Prefers group activities, work or play; not easily satisfied with individual projects.				
6. Adaptable to new situations, makes adjustments readily, welcomes change.				
7. Is self-composed, seldom shows signs of embarrassment.				
8. Tends to elation of spirits, seldom gloomy or moody.				
9. Seeks a broad range of friendships, not selective or exclusive in games and the like.				
10. Hearty and cordial, even to strangers, forms acquaintanceships very easily.				

Cowell's Social Adjustment Index (Form B)

Name_____ Age_____ Grade_____

Date_____ Describer's name_____

Behavior Trends	Descriptive of the Student			
	Markedly (−3)	Somewhat (−2)	Only Slightly (−1)	Not at All (−0)
1. Somewhat prudish, awkward, easily embarrassed in his social contacts.				

Cowell's Social Adjustment Index (Form B) *continued*

Behavior Trends	Descriptive of the Student			
	Markedly (−3)	Somewhat (−2)	Only Slightly (−1)	Not at All (−0)
2. Secretive, seclusive, not inclined to talk unless spoken to.				
3. Lacking in self-confidence and initiative, a follower.				
4. Slow in movement, deliberative or perhaps indecisive. Energy output moderate or deficient.				
5. Prefers to work and play alone, tends to avoid group activities.				
6. Shrinks from making new adjustments, prefers the habitual to the stress of reorganization required by the new.				
7. Is self-conscious, easily embarrassed, timid or "bashful".				
8. Tends to depression, frequently gloomy or moody.				
9. Shows preference for a narrow range of intimate friends and tends to exclude others from his association.				
10. Reserved and distant except to intimate friends, does not form acquaintanceships readily.				

Mercer Attitude Inventory

The Mercer Attitude Inventory (Mercer 1961) was constructed to evaluate the attitudes of high school girls toward the psychological, sociological, moral, and spiritual values of their physical education experience. The inventory has a reported validity coefficient of .72 and a reliability coefficient of .92.

Procedure: The student responds to each of the statements by placing a check mark on the answer sheet to indicate the appropriate answer from the following choices:

strongly disagree	disagree	neutral– undecided	agree	strongly agree
( )	( )	( )	( )	( )

Scoring: The statements included on the inventory are both positive and negative as marked on the answer sheet. The best answer on positive statements would be five, indicating strong agreement. The best answer on negative statements would also be five, indicating strong disagreement. The final score is the total of all the score values for the 40 items. There are 200 points possible. Achievement scales are not available.

Mercer Attitude Inventory

Name_____ Age_____

Date_____ Grade _____

1. Physical education activities are likely to be emotionally upsetting to many girls.
2. The saying, "Rules are made to be broken," is true in highly competitive sports.
3. It would be better to study than to spend time in physical education classes.
4. Physical education contributes nothing toward character development.
5. Girls who are skilled in active games and sports are not popular with boys.
6. Social dancing helps one to improve in grace and poise.
7. Competitive activities break down emotional self-controls.
8. Physical education classes are not looked forward to with enthusiasm.
9. Learning to accept situations as they are rather than as they should be is learned through participation in competitive sports.
10. An appreciation for art and beauty can be learned from physical education.
11. Archery is an activity in which one learns to score honestly.
12. Opportunities for making friends are provided more in other classes than in physical education.
13. Feelings of joy and happiness may be expressed through physical activities.
14. Girls who excel in sports are not as intellectual as other girls.
15. A good team is composed of individuals each working for her own particular good.
16. The spending of money for "exercise" and "play" is unnecessary and wasteful.
17. There is no apparent spiritual basis for physical education.
18. Working together as a team does not reduce the value of human relationships.
19. Being dishonest in calling balls good or bad in tennis is not related to personal integrity and honesty.
20. Physical education is not related to any other subject in the school program.
21. Learning to play by the rules of the game is not related to learning good moral and spiritual conduct.
22. Participation in competitive games and sports gives an opportunity for self-control.
23. Girls who enjoy physical activities are "unfeminine."
24. Individual student interests are not considered in physical education classes.
25. Accepting defeat graciously is not learned from participation in games and sports.
26. Physical education activities offer many opportunities for emotional expression.
27. Accepting your own capabilities is learned from participation in physical education.
28. Physical education activities do not provide opportunities for learning moral and spiritual values of living.
29. Physical education should be required in grades 1–2, and in college.
30. Just playing is not as important as having instruction in physical education.
31. A team should play according to the rules regardless of how unfairly the opposing team plays.
32. Associating with others in physical education activities is fun.
33. Physical education should be concerned with the learning of physical skills.
34. Physical activities are embarrassing for girls who are not skilled.
35. Each player on a team should play in every game regardless of her skill.
36. Physical education makes important contributions to the mental health of an individual.
37. Physical education offers little of importance to the general education of high school girls.
38. No opportunities are offered for students to become leaders in the physical education classes.
39. Physical education activities provide no opportunity for learning emotional control.
40. Physical education activities develop socially desirable standards of conduct.

Scoring Key

	Code	Strongly Disagree	Disagree	Negative	Agree	Strongly Agree		Code	Strongly Disagree	Disagree	Negative	Agree	Strongly Agree		Code	Strongly Disagree	Disagree	Negative	Agree	Strongly Agree

```
        5 4 3 2 1              5 4 3 2 1                1 2 3 4 5
— 1. ( )( )( )( )( )    —14. ( )( )( )( )( )    +27. ( )( )( )( )( )
        5 4 3 2 1              5 4 3 2 1                5 4 3 2 1
— 2. ( )( )( )( )( )    —15. ( )( )( )( )( )    —28. ( )( )( )( )( )
        5 4 3 2 1              5 4 3 2 1                1 2 3 4 5
— 3. ( )( )( )( )( )    —16. ( )( )( )( )( )    +29. ( )( )( )( )( )
        5 4 3 2 1              5 4 3 2 1                1 2 3 4 5
— 4. ( )( )( )( )( )    —17. ( )( )( )( )( )    +30. ( )( )( )( )( )
        5 4 3 2 1              1 2 3 4 5                1 2 3 4 5
— 5. ( )( )( )( )( )    +18. ( )( )( )( )( )    +31. ( )( )( )( )( )
        1 2 3 4 5              5 4 3 2 1                1 2 3 4 5
+ 6. ( )( )( )( )( )    —19. ( )( )( )( )( )    +32. ( )( )( )( )( )
        5 4 3 2 1              5 4 3 2 1                5 4 3 2 1
— 7. ( )( )( )( )( )    —20. ( )( )( )( )( )    —33. ( )( )( )( )( )
        5 4 3 2 1              5 4 3 2 1                5 4 3 2 1
— 8. ( )( )( )( )( )    —21. ( )( )( )( )( )    —34. ( )( )( )( )( )
        1 2 3 4 5              1 2 3 4 5                1 2 3 4 5
+ 9. ( )( )( )( )( )    +22. ( )( )( )( )( )    +35. ( )( )( )( )( )
        1 2 3 4 5              5 4 3 2 1                1 2 3 4 5
+10. ( )( )( )( )( )    —23. ( )( )( )( )( )    +36. ( )( )( )( )( )
        1 2 3 4 5              5 4 3 2 1                5 4 3 2 1
+11. ( )( )( )( )( )    —24. ( )( )( )( )( )    —37. ( )( )( )( )( )
        5 4 3 2 1              5 4 3 2 1                5 4 3 2 1
—12. ( )( )( )( )( )    —25. ( )( )( )( )( )    —38. ( )( )( )( )( )
        1 2 3 4 5              1 2 3 4 5                5 4 3 2 1
+13. ( )( )( )( )( )    +26. ( )( )( )( )( )    —39. ( )( )( )( )( )
                                                        1 2 3 4 5
                                                +40. ( )( )( )( )( )
```

Behavior Attitude Checklist

This checklist (Dexter 1957) was constructed to provide junior and senior high school students with a self-appraisal of behavior in physical education classes. The objective is to motivate the students to develop good behavior and to make them aware of poor behavioral traits.

Procedure: Each student rates himself on each item by placing a check mark in the column opposite the appropriate item. The test may be given periodically during the year to determine whether the physical education course has motivated the students toward better behavior.

Scoring: There are no numerical score values involved. The examiner simply evaluates the responses to determine which behavioral traits need to be improved.

Behavior Attitude Checklist

Name_____ Age_____

Date_____ Grade_____

Always	Often	Seldom	Never	
				Self-Direction
				1. I work diligently even though I am not supervised.
				2. I practice to improve the skills I use with least success.
				3. I follow carefully directions that have been given me.
				4. I willingly accept constructive criticism and try to correct faults.
				5. I play games as cheerfully as I can.
				6. I appraise my progress in each of my endeavors to learn.
				Social Adjustment
				1. I am considerate of the rights of others.
				2. I am courteous.
				3. I am cooperative in group activities.
				4. I accept gladly responsibility assigned me by a squad leader.
				5. I accept disappointment without being unnecessarily disturbed.
				6. I expect from the members of my group only the consideration to which I am entitled.
				Participation
				1. I am prompt in reporting for each class.
				2. I dislike being absent from class.
				3. I ask to be excused from an activity only when it is necessary.
				4. I do the best I can regardless of the activity in which I am participating.
				5. I give full attention to all instructions that are given in class.
				6. I encourage others with whom I am participating in an activity.
				Care of Equipment and Facilities
				1. I use equipment as I am supposed to use it.
				2. I return each piece of equipment to its proper place after using it.
				3. I avoid making my dressing area untidy.
				4. I arrange my clothes neatly in my locker.
				Personal Attractiveness
				1. I am particular about my personal appearance.
				2. I take a shower after I have participated in any vigorous activity.
				3. I wear clean clothes in physical education.
				4. I dress appropriately for each activity.
				5. I bathe regularly even during my menstrual period.

Blanchard Behavior Rating Scale

Name_____ Age_____ Grade_____

Date_____ Name of rater_____

	No Opportunity to Observe	Never	Seldom	Fairly Often	Frequently	Extremely Often	Score
Leadership							
1. He is popular with classmates.		1	2	3	4	5	
2. He seeks responsibility in the classroom.		1	2	3	4	5	
3. He shows intellectual leadership in the classroom.		1	2	3	4	5	
Positive Active Qualities							
4. He quits on tasks requiring perseverance.		5	4	3	2	1	
5. He exhibits aggressiveness in his relationship with others.		1	2	3	4	5	
6. He shows initiative in assuming responsibility in unfamiliar situations.		1	2	3	4	5	
7. He is alert to new opportunities.		1	2	3	4	5	
Positive Mental Qualities							
8. He shows keenness of mind.		1	2	3	4	5	
9. He volunteers ideas.		1	2	3	4	5	
Self-Control							
10. He grumbles over decisions of classmates.		5	4	3	2	1	
11. He takes a justified criticism by teacher or classmate without showing anger or pouting.		1	2	3	4	5	
Cooperation							
12. He is loyal to his group.		1	2	3	4	5	
13. He discharges his group responsibilities well.		1	2	3	4	5	
14. He is cooperative in his attitude toward the teacher.		1	2	3	4	5	
Social Action Standards							
15. He makes loud-mouthed criticisms and comments.		5	4	3	2	1	
16. He respects the rights of others.		1	2	3	4	5	
Ethical Social Qualities							
17. He cheats.		5	4	3	2	1	
18. He is truthful.		1	2	3	4	5	
Qualities of Efficiency							
19. He seems satisfied to "get by" with tasks assigned.		5	4	3	2	1	
20. He is dependable and trustworthy.		1	2	3	4	5	
21. He has good study habits.		1	2	3	4	5	
Sociability							
22. He is liked by others.		1	2	3	4	5	
23. He makes a friendly approach to others in the group.		1	2	3	4	5	
24. He is friendly.		1	2	3	4	5	

This rating scale (Blanchard 1936) was constructed to measure behavior characteristics of students. The scale has a reported validity coefficient of .93 and a reliability coefficient of .71.

Procedure: The teacher rates each student on the scale by circling the appropriate number opposite each of the 24 items.

Scoring: The score for each item is the circled number. The higher scores are indications of better behavior. There are 120 points possible.

Evaluation of
Accomplishment of Objectives

This evaluation form was prepared by Neilson to help students of junior high school through college age evaluate how well they accomplished certain important objectives.

Procedure: The form should be completed at the end of a unit instruction or at the end of a semester. Usually the student completes the form but the teacher can fill in the information if he so desires.

Scoring: The student or teacher records the score in the appropriate column opposite each of the 20 items. The highest score for each item is 5. There are 100 points possible.

Evaluation of Accomplishment of Objectives

Name_____ Age_____ Grade_____

Date _____ Evaluator_____

To what extent did you:	1	2	3	4	5
1. Make new friends?					
2. Develop a sense of humor?					
3. Learn to know your own limitations?					
4. Work hard in order to succeed?					
5. Do your best under difficult situations?					
6. Respect the ability of opponents?					

Evaluation of Accomplishment of Objectives *continued*

To what extent did you:	1	2	3	4	5
7. Respect the ability of teammates?					
8. Become tolerant of the success of others?					
9. Share with teammates in the struggle to accomplish a goal?					
10. Sacrifice your own desires, when necessary, for the good of the group?					
11. Exhibit loyalty to the leader and the school?					
12. Strive for an ideal?					
13. Learn to make decisions quickly when necessary?					
14. Understand the strategy in the activities?					
15. Learn to be a leader?					
16. Keep your body clean?					
17. Abide by training rules (eating, sleeping, and avoiding tobacco, alcoholic drinks, and drugs)?					
18. Develop strength?					
19. Develop skill?					
20. Develop endurance?					

How Is Your Physical
Education Coming Along?

This checklist (National Education Association 1955) was established to assess a student's progress in achieving the objectives of physical education. Students may use it as a periodical appraisal of themselves or as a goal toward achievement of various items. Boys and girls of junior and senior high school age may use the checklist.

Procedure: The student answers yes or no to each of the questions listed under A, B, C, and D according to his best judgment.

Scoring: A student should achieve the indicated score on each set of questions to pass the evaluation in good standing. He records his total score at the end of the checklist.

Checklist

Name_____ Age_____

Date_____ Grade_____

A. Developing Good Living Habits   (6 out of 6)
  1. I get enough sleep (8–10 hours each night) so that I am rested and refreshed in the morning.
  2. I drink milk every day and eat three good meals that include plenty of fruit and vegetables. _____
  3. I take a bath or shower frequently. _____
  4. I am concerned about my personal appearance and try to be neat and clean at all times.
  5. I always take reasonable precautions for the safety of myself and others. _____
  6. I have regular dental and medical examinations and seek correction of any defects that are found. _____

B. Acquiring Skills in Sports and Other Recreational Activities   (6 out of 7)
  1. I swim well enough to feel safe in, on, or about the water. _____
  2. I can play well one or more individual sports like archery, bowling, golf, or tennis. I am a good player in one or more team sports (softball, soccer, volleyball, and the like) and can take part in several others. _____
  3. I am a member of an intramural or a varsity team. _____
  4. I have a hobby that I hope to enjoy the rest of my life. _____
  5. I participate regularly throughout the year in some vigorous activity outside school hours.
  6. I enjoy a vigorous activity (modern dancing, gymnastics, tumbling, wrestling, track and field, and the like) that helps to develop my strength, endurance, agility, coordination, and balance. _____
  7. I dance well enough to enjoy school dances and similar social functions. _____

C. Learning Facts about Sports   (4 out of 6)
  1. I enjoy watching and discussing sports because I understand the rules, vocabulary, and basic strategy of the popular sports.
  2. I know the rules of one or more sports well enough to officiate in class or intramural contests. _____
  3. In each sport I play, I know the proper safety precautions to take in order to avoid injuring myself and others. _____
  4. I have learned to recognize and appreciate good sports equipment and know how to care for it to obtain maximum service. _____
  5. I know the origin of many popular sports and how they have affected the life of my community. _____
  6. I know about several outstanding sports personalities and their achievements. _____

D. Learning and Living the Good-Sportsman's Code   (10 out of 10)
  1. I consider athletic opponents and officials to be guests of my school and treat them accordingly.
  2. I respect the rights and feelings of those who cheer the rival team. _____
  3. I respect the authority and judgment of the coach. _____
  4. I respect the property of the school and the authority of school officials. _____
  5. I cheer good plays and good sportsmanship whether displayed by my school's team or its opponents.
  6. I appreciate the responsibility of sports officials and accept their decisions. _____
  7. I maintain self-control at all times during and after the game. _____
  8. I try to be modest in victory and gracious in defeat. _____
  9. I do what I can to encourage both players and spectators to act in the spirit of fair play and sportsmanship. _____
  10. I try to observe the code of the good sportsman not only on the playing field but wherever I go. _____

Yes: _____   No: _____

Other Measurements
of Impulsive Traits

In addition to the aforementioned measurements of impulsive traits the following are also useful: Action-Choice Tests for Competitive Sports Situations (Haskins and Hartman 1960), Cowell Personal Distance Scale (Cowell 1958), Outcomes of Sports: An Evaluation Checksheet (Cowell 1957), Social Evaluation Score Card (Barrow 1956), A Subjective Rating Scale for Social, Personal, and Emotional Development (*Physical Education* 1960), Carr Attitude Inventory (Carr 1945), Kneer Attitude Inventory and Diagnostic Statements (Kneer 1956), Scale to Measure Attitudes Toward Intensive Competition for High School Girls (McGee 1956), Wear Attitude Inventory (Wear 1951).

Selected References

Barrow, Harold M., *A Practical Approach to Measurement in Physical Education*. Philadelphia: Lea & Febiger, 1966.

Barrow, Harold M., Unpublished Study, Winston-Salem, N.C.: Wake Forest College, 1956.

Blanchard, B. E., Jr., "A Behavior Frequency Rating Scale for the Measurement of Character and Personality in Physical Education Classroom Situation." *Research Quarterly*, 1936, 7, 56–66. The Blanchard Behavior Rating Scale is reprinted by permission of the American Association for Health, Physical Education, and Recreation.

Carr, Martha G., "The Relationship Between Success in Physical Education and Selected Attitudes Expressed in High School Freshmen Girls." *Research Quarterly*, 1945, 16, 176–91.

Cowell, Charles C., "Our Function Is Still Education!" *The Physical Educator*, 1957, 14, 6–7.

Cowell, Charles C., "Validating an Index of Social Adjustment for High School Use." *Research Quarterly*, 1958, 29, 7–18. Form A and B of the Index are reprinted by permission of the American Association for Health, Physical Education, and Recreation.

Dexter, Genevie (Ed.), *Teachers' Guide to Physical Education for Girls in High School*. Sacramento: California State Department of Education, 1957, p. 318.

Haskins, Mary Jane, and Hartman, Betty Grant, Unpublished Study. (Copies may be obtained by writing to Mary Jane Haskins, Department of Physical Education, Ohio State University, Columbus, Ohio, or to Betty Grant Hartman, School of Physical Education, University of Connecticut, Storrs, Connecticut.)

National Education Association, "How Is Your Physical Education Coming Along?" *NEA Journal*. 1955, 44, 353.

Kneer, Marian E., The Adaptation of Wear's Physical Education Attitude Inventory for Use with High School Girls. Unpublished master's thesis, Illinois State Normal University, 1956.

McGee, Rosemary, "Comparison of Attitudes Toward Intensive Competition for High School Girls." *Research Quarterly*, 1956, 27, 60–73.

Mercer, Emily-Louise, An Adaptation and Revision of the Galloway Attitude Inventory for Evaluating the Attitudes of High School Girls Toward Psychological, Moral–Spiritual, and Sociological Values in Physical Education Experiences. Unpublished master's thesis, The Woman's College of the University of North Carolina, 1961.

Physical Education—Guide for North Dakota Elementary Schools, Grades 1–6. Bismarck, N.D.: Department of Public Instruction, 1960, p. 17.

Wear, Carlos L., "The Evaluation of Attitudes Toward Physical Education as an Activity Course." *Research Quarterly*, 1951, *22*, 114–26.

FIVE
Measurements
of Neuromuscular Traits

Performance tests that measure primarily the efficiency of the nervous and muscular systems fall into the category of neuromuscular tests of strength, power, agility, flexibility, speed, reaction time, balance, perception, and specific skills. This section includes descriptions and other pertinent information about the more useful neuromuscular tests.

12

Muscular
Strength Tests

Strength is defined as the ability of the body, or a segment of it, to apply force. Strength has often been considered as the contractile force of a muscle or group of muscles. But the definition of strength and the methods used to measure it indicate that strength is a combination of the combined contractile forces of the muscles causing the movement, the mechanical ratio of the particular body levers involved, and the ability to coordinate the agonistic muscles into one unified force working with the antagonistic and stabilizer muscles.

Strength is dependent upon the force with which each contributing muscle can contract. As the contractile forces of the contributing muscles increase, strength increases. In addition strength depends upon the relative length of the body levers and the positions of muscle attachments to these levers. Mechanical ratio changes as a body segment moves through its range of motion, causing strength to differ at various positions through the range of motion.

Relationship of
Strength to Performance

The definition of strength implies its importance in athletic performance. Even though nearly all movements are performed against some resistance, athletes perform movements against greater resistance than usual. For example, in the shot put, discus throw, pole vault, various gymnastic movements, jumping, running, swimming, and leaping, the body segments exert maximum force. If all else remains equal, greater strength often results in better performances; in fact some prominent physical educators have claimed that strength is the most important single contributor.

In addition to being an important trait by itself strength is a factor in several other traits which influence athletic performance. Strength is an element in power. Expressed in a simple formula, power = force × velocity. Increased strength results in the ability to apply more force; hence strength contributes to power.

Strength is also a factor in muscular endurance, the ability of the muscles to resist fatigue while doing work. Suppose a man were to move a given resistance through a particular range of motion 100 times. If his strength were increased 50 percent, he would then be able to move (provided resistance is constant) through the range of motion with greater ease; hence he would be able to repeat the movement considerably more than 100 times. This example illustrates how strength, within limits, contributes to muscular endurance.

143

Strength is an important contributor to agility because adequate strength is required to control the weight of the body against the force of inertia and to maneuver the body and its parts rapidly. Strength is also a factor in running speed since great force is required to accelerate the body and to propel it at a fast speed.

Types of Strength

There are two types of strength: static (isometric) and dynamic (isotonic). Static strength is the ability to apply force at a particular position without moving through the range of motion. It involves the isometric muscle contractions involved in pulling against a fixed object, a cable tensiometer, or a back and leg lift dynamometer. Dynamic strength is the ability to apply force through the range of motion. It involves the isotonic muscle contractions demonstrated in pull-ups or dips on the parallel bars. Dynamic strength is used more in athletics, but the two types of strength are closely correlated. Static strength can be measured more accurately than dynamic strength.

Since strength is so necessary in vigorous performance, it is important to identify the lack of strength and to attempt to correct the condition. For this reason strength tests have been devised.

Instruments for Measuring Strength

The back and leg lift dynamometer, the hand dynamometer, and the cable tensiometer are instruments designed specifically to measure strength.

The back and leg lift dynamometer is a meter with a chain and bar attached, mounted on a platform. A performer, holding the bar, stands on the platform and applies force upward. The meter indicates in pounds amount of force exerted. This instrument measures the strength of the leg muscles or back muscles, depending on how the force is applied.

The hand dynamometer tests right- and left-hand grip strength. With attachments it is useful for measuring strength of the arm and shoulder abductor and adductor muscles.

The cable tensiometer tests the strength of numerous muscle groups. With the use of a well-designed testing table this instrument, attached to almost any segment of the body, measures the strength of that segment (see Figure 12-1).

Static Strength Tests

Static strength tests, the most accurate measures of strength, are useful in school programs. However they have two limitations: static tests measure strength at only

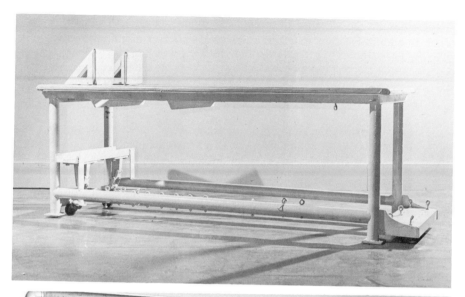

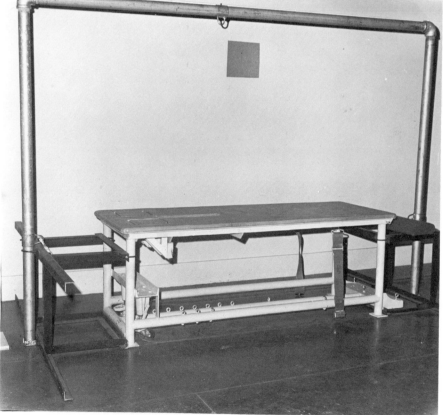

Figure 12-1.   Strength testing tables.

one angle despite the variance of strength at different angles through the range of motion. In addition static strength is a less valid indicator of ability to perform than is dynamic strength.

Leg Lift Test

This test measures the strength of the leg extensor muscles; the results indicate total leg strength. A leg lift dynamometer with a belt attachment is the only equipment necessary. About 25 students can be tested in a 40-minute period.

Procedure: The student holds the bar with both hands (palms down) so that the bar rests at the juncture of his thighs and trunk. He maintains this position while the belt is fastened to the handle and adjusted to his body. He then takes his position on the dynamometer platform so that the pull will be directly upward. Bending his knees slightly, he holds this position while the chain length is adjusted (see Figure 12-2). At a signal from the leader the student exerts a maximum force upward by extending his legs, at the same time keeping his arms and back straight, his head erect, and his chest high.

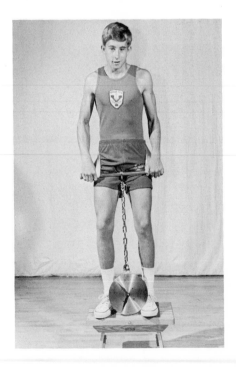 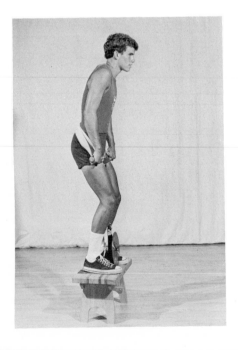

Figure 12-2. Leg lift strength test.

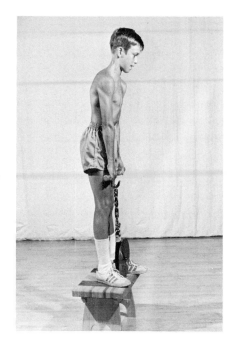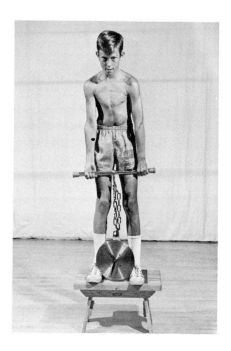

Figure 12-3. Back lift strength test.

Scoring: Each student takes two trials: the better of the lifts is recorded to the nearest pound. Achievement scales (norms) are not available for this test; therefore the examiner must interpret scores by comparing the scores of the different students or by comparing the scores of the same student taken at different times.

Back Lift Test

This test measures the strength of the back extensor muscles. It requires the same amount of time and the same equipment as the leg lift test, without the use of the belt.

Procedure: The student stands in position on the dynamometer platform. When the chain length has been properly adjusted, he bends forward and grasps the bar firmly with one palm upward and one palm downward, keeping his legs straight, his feet flat on the platform, his head up, and his eyes straight forward (see Figure 12-3). At a signal from the leader he lifts steadily with maximum force.

Scoring: The same method is used as for the leg lift test.

Hand Grip Test

This test measures the grip strength of the right and left hands. The only equipment needed is a hand grip dynamometer. About 30 students can be tested in a 40-minute period.

Procedure: The student places the grip dynamometer in the palm of his right hand (with the dial toward the palm) so that the convex edge is between the first and second joints of the fingers and the rounded edge is against the base of the hand. He bends his elbow slightly and raises his arm upward; he then moves his arm forward and downward, gripping with maximum force. At the same time he is careful not to touch his body or any object. He then repeats the test using his left hand.

Scoring: Each student has two trials with each hand. The better of the grips is recorded.

Arm Abduction Test

This test measures the strength of the arm abductor and shoulder girdle protractor muscles. It requires a hand grip dynamometer with push and pull attachments. Thirty students can be tested in a 40-minute period.

Procedure: With the dynamometer in front of his chest and with the dial facing outward, the student grasps the handles with his two hands. On a signal from the leader he pulls steadily outward with both hands, applying maximum force.

Scoring: The same method is used as for the leg lift test.

Arm Adduction Test

This test measures the strength of the arm adductor and shoulder girdle retractor muscles. It requires the same equipment and the same amount of time as the arm abduction test.

Procedure: The student, in the same position as in the arm abduction test, grasps the handles of the dynamometer with both hands and pushes them toward each other with maximum force.

Scoring: The method is the same as for the leg lift test.

Cable Tensiometer Tests

The cable tensiometer accurately measures the static strength of almost any body segment, provided the tests are administered correctly.

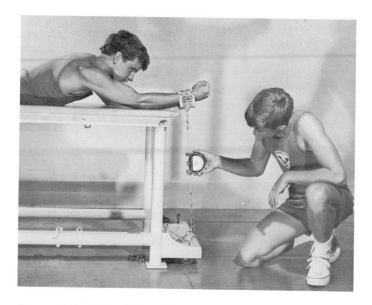

Figure 12-4. Test of elbow flexion strength, using tensiometer.

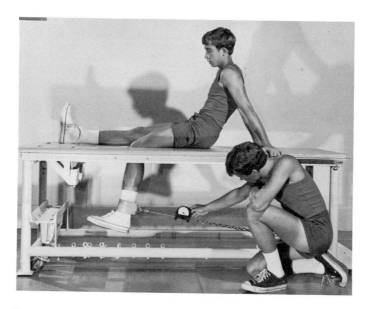

Figure 12-5. Test of knee extension strength, using tensiometer.

After experimenting for several years, H. Harrison Clarke (1953) identified 38 different muscle groups that can be tested by use of the cable tensiometer. Physical educators with the necessary background and insight into muscular actions can identify the muscle groups they want to test and the angle at which to apply the test.

Procedure: The student is placed in the desired testing position. Then one end of the tensiometer cable is attached to the body segment to be tested and the other end to a fixed object. The tensiometer is placed on the cable and the amount of force applied by the segment is then measured. For measures of this type to be accurate the body must be in a stable position to allow for the application of maximum force by the body segment (see Figures 12-4 and 12-5).

Scoring: Test scores that are to be compared must be obtained at the same angle of pull. For example, a comparison of the scores of two students on the elbow flexion test would not be valid if one student were tested with his elbow at a 90 degree angle and the other student with his elbow at a 120 degree angle.

Dynamic Strength Tests

Pure dynamic strength is difficult to measure. Maximum lifts with weight training equipment probably give the best results. This approach is not totally satisfactory because a certain amount of experimentation is necessary to determine the maximum weight that can be lifted at once. When it is determined, the maximum weight represents the dynamic strength score for that particular movement. Figures 12-6 through 12-10 are some of the more standard lifts useful for testing dynamic strength of major muscle groups.

Dynamic Strength–Endurance Tests

Often movements against one's body weight, such as pull-ups, have been used as measures of dynamic strength. Such tests do not measure pure strength but rather a combination of strength and endurance. Any test calling for repetitions of a movement (such as a maximum number of pull-ups) combines strength with endurance. A pure strength test involves only a single maximum muscle contraction; a second maximum contraction in succession will likely be less intense than the first one, and a third contraction will be even less than the second.

The extent to which strength or endurance is the primary factor in a particular strength–endurance test depends on the number of times a person can execute the movement. If a student is able to perform only one pull-up, then his strength rather than his endurance is measured. A failure to do even one pull-up results from

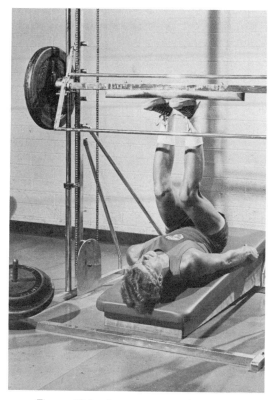

Figure 12-6.   Leg press test (dynamic).

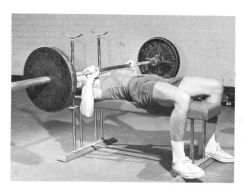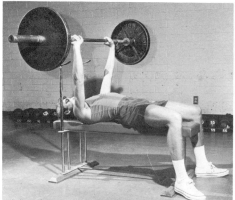

Figure 12-7.   Bench press test (dynamic).

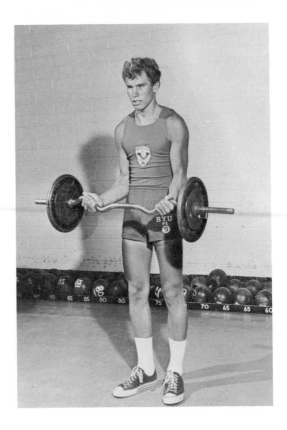

Figure 12-8. Two Arm Curl test (dynamic).

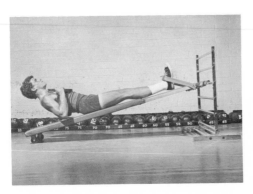 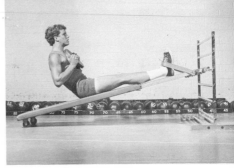

Figure 12-9. Sit-up test with weight.

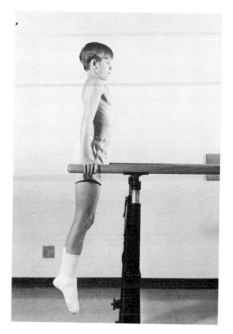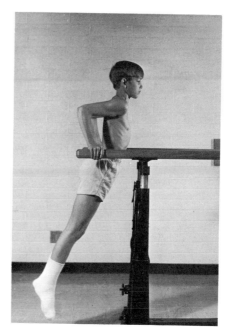

Figure 12-10.   Parallel bar dips.

insufficient strength, not from a lack of endurance. On the other hand, if a student performs 25 pull-ups, then the test measures endurance primarily rather than pure strength. Although a student must be strong to do 25 pull-ups, his great strength contributes to his endurance.

Many muscular strength–endurance tests are simple to administer and require limited space and little or no special test equipment. These tests are reasonably good indicators of general ability to perform in athletics. They also provide an immediate sense of achievement for students as they see themselves accomplish work.

Dips on Parallel Bars

This test measures strength and endurance of the elbow extensor, shoulder flexor, and shoulder girdle depressor muscles. With the use of a testing station at each end of the apparatus about 60 students can be tested in 40 minutes.

Procedure: The student stands at the end of the parallel bars (adjusted to the proper height and width), grasps one bar in each hand, and jumps to the front support position, keeping his arms straight. Lowering his body until the angle at the elbows is a right angle (90 degrees) or less (see Figure 12-10), he executes the bar dip as many times as possible without jerking or kicking.

Scoring: The jump to the support position counts one and each additional dip properly executed counts one. Improperly executed dips count one-half. Achievement scales with which each student's score can be evaluated appear in Appendixes C and D.

Floor Push-Ups

This test measures strength and endurance of the elbow extensor and shoulder flexor muscles. Because the trunk must be held straight throughout the exercise, extreme weakness of the hip flexor and abdominal muscles may also be detected with this test. The test can be administered to several students at one time, with a counter for each student.

Procedure: The student lies down facing the floor, with his body straight, his arms bent, and his hands flat on the floor beneath his shoulders (see Figure 12-11). From this position he pushes upward to a straight arm position and then lowers his body to touch the counter's hand which is placed palm down under the chest. The student should keep his body rigid throughout, touching only his hands and toes to the floor. He repeats the action as many times as possible.

Scoring: The total number of push-ups correctly done in succession is counted. Achievement scales for this test appear in Appendixes C and D.

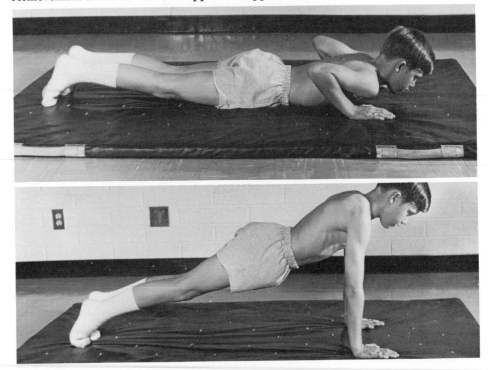

Figure 12-11.   Push-ups.

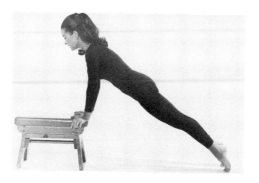

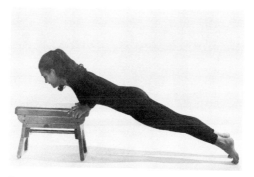

Figure 12-12. Modified push-ups (bench).

Modified Push-Ups

This test is the same as the floor push-up test, with modifications to suit the needs of girls.

Procedure: The student grasps the outer edges of a bench (15 inches high and 15 inches long) at the nearest corners (see Figure 12-12). In the front leaning rest position she performs push-ups as described in the floor push-up test. The knee push-up (see Figure 12-13) is another version of a modified push-up used by girls.

Scoring: The method is the same as for the floor push-up test. However, achievement scales are not available.

Pull-Ups

This test measures the strength and endurance of the elbow, wrist, and finger flexors; the shoulder extensors; and the shoulder girdle depressor muscles. A high horizontal bar is the only equipment required. About 40 students can be tested in 40 minutes at each station.

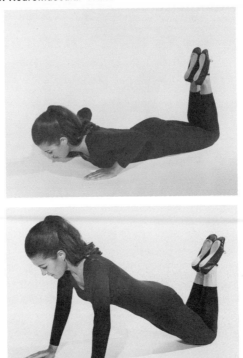

Figure 12-13.   Modified push-ups (knee).

Procedure: The student takes a straight-arm hang position (hands directly above shoulders) on the horizontal bar with his body fully extended. Using the forward grip (palm forward), he raises his body until he can place his chin over the bar without kicking or swinging. He then lowers his body to the original position. He repeats the procedure as many times as possible.

Scoring: The score is the total number of pull-ups correctly performed in succession. Pull-ups done incorrectly count half. Achievement scales appear in Appendixes C and D.

Modified Pull-Ups

This test is the same as the pull-up test, with modifications to suit the needs of girls. The bar is adjusted to a height equal to the base of the student's sternum, when she is standing erect.

Procedure: The student grasps the bar with a forward grip (palms forward) and slides her feet under the bar until her arms are straight and the angle between arms and trunk is 90 degrees (see Figure 12-14). Keeping her body straight and rigid, she executes as many pull-ups as possible, bringing her chin over the bar each time.

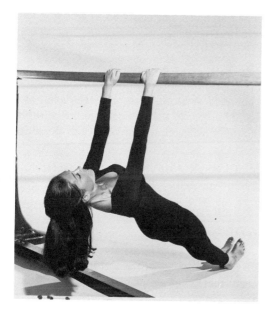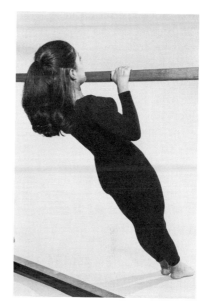

Figure 12-14. Modified pull-ups (low bar).

Scoring: The method is the same as for the boys' pull-up test. However, achievement scales are not available.

This test measures the strength and endurance of the fingers, wrist, and elbow flexors; the shoulder extensors; and the shoulder girdle depressor muscles. A stopwatch and a suspended rope not less than one and one half inches or more than two inches in diameter are necessary. About 40 students can be tested in 40 minutes at one station.

Procedure: From a standing position the student grasps the rope. At the signal he climbs the rope, using both his hands and feet, until one hand reaches the 20 foot mark.

Scoring: The student is allowed two trials; the examiner records the better time to the nearest tenth of a second. Achievement scales appear in Appendixes C and D.

This test measures the strength and endurance of the trunk and hip flexor muscles. If the students are arranged into pairs to count for each other and to check each other's performance, a large number of students can be tested in a short time. The counter sits on the performer's legs midway between the knees and ankles and holds the feet down by applying force at the ankles.

Procedure: The student lies in a supine position with his hands clasped behind his head. Keeping his knees straight, he comes to a sitting position and touches one elbow to the opposite knee and then the other elbow to the alternate side. Returning to the supine position, the student repeats the movement as many times as possible.

Scoring: The score is the number of complete sit-ups the student performs correctly. Achievement scales are available in Appendixes B, C, and D.

Body Curl

This test is used to measure strength and endurance of the abdominal muscles. The body curl is the same as the sit-up except that the performer's knees are elevated, the feet are placed flat on the floor, and the hands are clasped behind his head (see Figure 12-15). Achievement scales are not available.

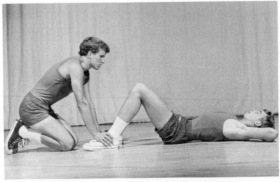

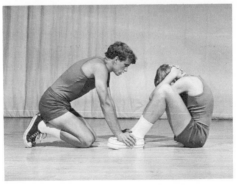

Figure 12-15.   Body curl.

This test measures strength and endurance of the leg and foot extensor muscles. It requires no special equipment. If students are arranged into pairs to serve as counters and checkers for each other, a large number can be tested in a short time.

Procedure: The student takes a standing position with one foot 12 to 15 inches forward of the other foot and his hands clasped behind his head. He jumps upward just high enough to exchange positions of his feet and, upon landing, dips to a half squat position. Resuming the standing position, he repeats the jump, exchanging positions of the feet, and continues this procedure as many times as possible.

Scoring: The score is the number of jumps the student correctly executes in succession. Achievement scales are not available.

Static Strength–Endurance Tests

If certain muscles are contracted against the body weight and held in position as long as possible, their endurance can be tested. The following simple tests measure the strength–endurance of the major muscle groups. Except for the flexed arm hang test achievement scales are not available.

Flexed Arm Hang

The height of the horizontal bar should be adjusted so that it is approximately equal to the student's standing height. The student should use an overhand (forward) grasp. With the assistance of two spotters, one in front and one in back, the student raises off the floor to a position where the chin is above the bar, the elbows are flexed, and the chest is close to the bar. He holds this position as long as possible.

The stopwatch is started as soon as the student takes the correct hanging position. The watch is stopped at three points: when the student touches his chin to the bar, when the student tilts his head backward to keep his chin above the bar, and when the student lets his chin fall below the level of the bar. The length of time the student holds the hanging position is recorded in seconds to the nearest second. Achievement scales for girls and women appear in Appendix B.

Half-Flexed Arm Hang

This test measures the strength–endurance of arm and shoulder muscles. The student grasps a horizontal bar as if he were going to perform a pull-up. He pulls himself upward until the angle at the elbows is 90 degrees and holds this position as long as possible. The longer he holds the position, the greater is the ability of his arm and shoulder muscles to resist fatigue when contracted against the weight of his body. The score is the length of time the student can hold the position, measured to the nearest second.

Straight Arm Hang

This test is performed the same as the half-flexed arm hang test, except that the student's arms are fully extended.

Leg Raise and Hold

This test measures the ability of the abdominal and hip flexor muscles to hold against the weight of the legs and feet. Lying on his back with hands clasped behind his head, feet together, and legs straight, the student raises both feet 4 inches above the floor and holds this position as long as possible.

Chest Raise and Hold

This test measures the ability of the back and neck extensors to hold against the weight of the upper body. The student assumes a prone position with hands clasped behind his head and elbows held horizontally. Another student sits on the performing student's lower legs. By contracting the back and neck extensor muscles, the performer raises his chest from the floor and holds this position as long as possible.

Sit and Hold

This test measures the ability of the knee extensor (thigh) muscles to hold against the body weight. With the back and head flat against a wall the student lowers his body and moves his feet away from the wall until right angles form at the hip and knee joints (sitting position). He holds this position as long as possible.

Strength Test Batteries

Each test measures the strength of only one body region. A battery of tests consists of several test items and may, therefore, be a much better indicator of total body strength. Usually the scores of the several items are combined to give the total score for the battery.

Larson Muscular Strength Test

Leonard Larson (1940) designed this test to measure dynamic strength of high school boys and college men. The test consists of pull-ups and dips, which measure a combination of strength and endurance, and the vertical jump, which mainly measures explosive power. All three test items depend heavily on strength, but none measures pure strength. With a chinning bar, parallel bars, and a vertical jump board, about 30 students can be tested in a 40-minute period.

Procedure: All students should perform the tests in the following sequence:

1.   Pull-ups: See description on page 155.

2.   Vertical jump: See description on page 172.

3.   Dips: See description on page 153.

Scoring: The number of pull-ups, the height of the vertical jump to the nearest half inch, and the number of dips are the raw scores. Achievement scales for high school boys and college men were printed in *The Physical Educator* (Bookwalter 1942).

Rogers Strength Test

This test of total body strength consists of seven items, some of which measure pure strength while others test strength and endurance (Rogers 1926). Necessary equipment are an adjustable horizontal bar, parallel bars, back and leg lift dynamometer, hand grip dynamometer, girl's push-up bench, height and weight measuring equipment, and a wet spirometer. With all testing stations operating simultaneously, about 20 students can be tested in a 40-minute period.

Procedure: All students should perform the items of the test in the sequence in which they are listed. Age, height, and weight should be measured and recorded to the nearest month, half inch, and pound respectively.

1.   Hand grips (right and left): See description on page 148. Record the scores for both the right and left hands.

2.   Back lift: See description on page 147.

3.   Leg lift: See description on page 146.

4.   Pull-ups: See description on page 155.

5.   Push-ups: See description on page 154.

6.   Lung capacity: There is no evidence that this item relates to strength in any significant way. But since lung capacity was included in the original test, the item must be retained if the established norms are to be useful. This aspect of the test measures the amount of air that can be expelled from the lungs in one breath. The student inhales as much air as possible; then he places his mouth over the sterilized mouthpiece and expels as much air into the spirometer as possible. The score is recorded in cubic inches.

Scoring: There are two steps in scoring this test: computing arm strength and determining the strength index (*SI*).

$$\text{arm strength} = \text{pull-ups} + \text{push-ups} \times \left(\frac{\text{weight}}{10} + \text{height} - 60\right)$$

The student's weight is recorded in pounds and his height in inches. If the student is 60 inches or less in height, the minus 60 phase of the formula is eliminated.

Strength index (*SI*)
    = arm strength + right grip + left grip + back lift + leg lift + lung capacity

The student's strength index may be compared to *SI* norms (Rogers 1926).

Frederick Rogers proposed that a person's physical fitness could be measured by the following formula:

$$\text{physical fitness index } (PFI) = \frac{\text{achieved } SI}{\text{normal } SI} \times 100$$

The physical fitness index is discussed in more detail in Chapter 21.

Kraus–Weber Test of Minimal Strength

The Kraus–Weber tests (Kraus and Hirschland 1954a, 1954b) were constructed from clinical experience over a period of 18 years. The six test items included in the battery are considered the most valid of a large number of tests administered under clinical situations. These diagnostic tests are designed to identify students age 6 through 18, whose strength is below minimal level. However they are only screening tests to detect cases of subnormal strength and are not valid measures of maximum strength. To pass each item the student must make the maximum score, without having done warm-up exercises prior to the test.

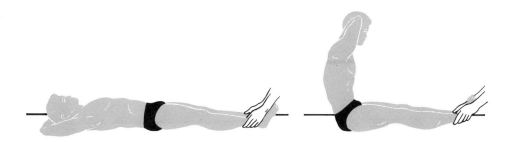

Figure 12-16. Kraus–Weber Test 1.

Test 1 measures minimal strength of the abdominal and hip flexor muscles. The student lies on his back with his legs straight and together and his hands clasped behind his neck (see Figure 12-16.) With a partner holding down his feet he tries to roll up to a sitting position. Twisting of the trunk or absence of the rolling action indicates weak abdominal muscles. If he cannot raise his shoulders, the student scores zero. If the examiner must help him half way to the sitting position, the student scores five. If he performs the sit-up correctly and unaided, the student scores 10.

Test 2 measures minimal strength of the abdominal muscles. From a supine position with knees elevated to release the hip flexor muscles from action, feet held down, and hands behind the neck, the student rolls up to a sitting position (see Figure 12-17). He is scored the same as for Test 1.

Test 3 measures minimal strength of the hip flexor and lower abdominal muscles. From a supine position with legs straight and hands behind his neck, the student lifts his feet 10 inches above the surface and holds this position for 10 seconds (see Figure 12-18). The student scores one point for each second he holds the position; the maximum he can score is 10.

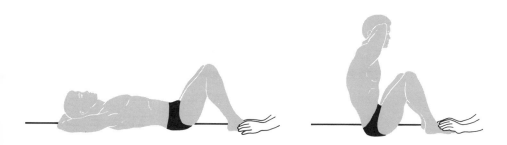

Figure 12-17. Kraus–Weber Test 2.

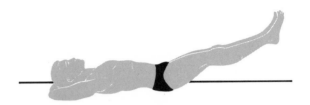

Figure 12-18.   Kraus–Weber Test 3.

Test 4 measures minimal strength of the upper back muscles. The student lies in a prone position with a pillow under his hips and lower abdomen. With a partner holding his feet the student raises his chest, shoulders, and head from the surface and holds this position for 10 seconds (see Figure 12-19). He is scored the same as for Test 3.

Test 5 measures minimal strength of the lower back. The student takes the same position as in Test 4, except that he places his forearms on the surface with his hands under his face. With a partner holding down his trunk the student raises his legs and feet above the surface, keeping his knees straight, and holds this position for 10 seconds (see Figure 12-20). He is scored the same as for Test 3.

Test 6 measures the flexibility of the hamstring and lower back muscles. The student removes his shoes and stands erect with feet together. Keeping his knees

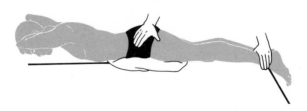

Figure 12-19.   Kraus–Weber Test 4.

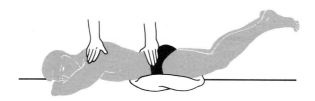

Figure 12-20.   Kraus–Weber Test 5.

straight he bends slowly forward until he touches the floor with his fingertips. He
holds this position without bobbing for three seconds (see Figure 12-21). If he touches
the floor he passes the test. If he does not touch the floor he receives a minus score of
one for each inch between the floor and his fingertips.

The Kraus–Weber test has caused much excitement and controversy because
it has been used as the testing instrument in a number of studies in which school
children of the United States have been compared with children of other countries.
The United States children have fared poorly in the comparisons, as illustrated in
Table 12-1. As a result this test has been effective in stimulating greater efforts toward
physical fitness of our young people.

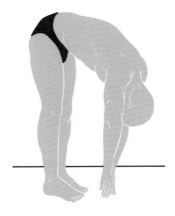

Figure 12-21.   Kraus–Weber Test 6.

Table 12-1
Results of the Kraus–Weber Test Administered to Children of the
United States and European Countries*

	Austrian	Italian	Swiss	American
		percent		
Number tested	678	1036	1156	4264
Failure	9.5	8.0	8.8	57.9
Incidence of failure	9.7	8.5	8.9	80.0

* H. Kraus and R. P. Hirschland, "Minimum Muscular Fitness Tests in School Children." *Research Quarterly*, 1954, *25*, 177–88. Reprinted by permission of the American Association for Health, Physical Education, and Recreation.

Precautions in the Interpretation of Strength Test Results

A strength score is not usually meaningful unless it is interpreted in view of the following facts: Larger people must be stronger than smaller people to perform at the same level; hence raw scores by people of different sizes cannot logically be compared. For people of the same size men are normally stronger than women. When body size is equal, young adults (ages 20–25) are normally stronger than youth or older people. Mesomorphs (with heavy musculature) are normally stronger for their size than ectomorphs or endomorphs, and ectomorphs are usually stronger for their size than endomorphs. Thus, to be meaningful, strength tests must be interpreted relative to age, sex, size, and body type.

How to Increase Strength

Through experimentation we have learned that strength can best be increased by applying the basic principles of strength overload and progressive resistance. The principle of strength overload simply means that if muscles are contracted regularly against resistance heavier than they are accustomed to, they will respond by increasing in strength. If they are not loaded beyond their usual levels, muscles will gain only the strength resulting from normal growth. The principle of progressive resistance means that as the muscles become stronger the loads against which they contract must progressively be increased in order to continue to apply overload.

Any form of exercise which applies heavier than usual resistance to muscle contractions will stimulate an increase in strength. For example, hard manual labor or vigorous athletic performance; specific exercises against body weight, as in pull-ups or dips; exercises against external movable resistance, such as weight-training equipment and wall pulleys; and muscle tensions against a fixed object or another body part are all strength-building stimuli.

The first three stimuli examples result in isotonic contractions: The muscles change in length, and movement of body segments occurs. The fourth stimuli example results in isometric contractions: The muscles apply tension but do not shorten, and little or no movement of body segments occurs.

Isotonic Strength-Building Methods

Thomas DeLorme and A. L. Watkins (1848) declared that strength can rapidly be increased with the use of heavy resistance for 10 repetitions and three sets. They specifically recommended that every other day the person should do one set of 10 repetitions with 1/2 10 RMs,[1] one set of 10 repetitions with 3/4 10 RMs, and one set of 10 repetitions with 10 RMs.

Currently many experts disagree on the best program for building strength, but most people accept the following points:

1.   Exercises must be selected to work the specific muscles in which strength is to be developed.

2.   Muscles should be contracted regularly (every other day) against heavy resistance.

3.   Near-maximum weight for 10 repetitions or less should be used.

4.   The weight must progressively be increased as strength increases, to provide continual overload to the muscles. (This is progressive resistance.)

Isometric Strength-Building Methods

In 1963 E. A. Muller and W. Rohmert of Germany established evidence that strength will increase more rapidly by use of isometrics when near-maximum muscle contractions are used and when five to 10 repetitions are used. They also established the theory that strength will increase more evenly throughout the range of motion if the contractions are executed at various positions.

[1] R means repetition maximum. Ten RMs is 10 repetitions of an exercise using the maximum weight that can be lifted successively 10 times.

On the basis of evidence available at present, the following points serve as guides in the design of isometric strength-building programs:

1.   The best results can be obtained by use of near-maximum contractions of five to six seconds in length and repetitions of five or more times, with a few seconds of rest between contractions.

2.   The exercises should be performed daily.

3.   The contractions should be applied at varying points throughout the range of motion if maximum strength is desired throughout the full range. Where strength is needed only at the beginning of the motion, as in ballistic movements, the exercises should be designed accordingly.

Other Strength-Building Methods

In addition to pure isometric and isotonic methods some programs combining the two methods have received limited attention. Reasonable success has been experienced with the following procedure:

1.   The muscles are contracted isometrically against a rope or cable arrangement. After tension has been held for five or six seconds, the resistance which holds the rope is reduced so as to allow slow-motion isotonic contractions to occur.

2.   Each exercise is repeated five to six times daily.

Selected References

Berger, Richard A., "Optimum Repetitions for the Development of Strength." *Research Quarterly*, 1962, *33*, 334–38.

Berger, Richard A., "Comparison of Static and Dynamic Strength Increases." *Research Quarterly*, 1962, *33*, 329–33.

Bookwalter, Karl W., "Achievement Scales in Strength Tests for Secondary School Boys and College Men." *The Physical Educator*, 1942, *11*, 130–41.

Capen, Edward K., "Study of Four Programs of Heavy Resistance Exercises for Development of Muscular Strength." *Research Quarterly*, 1965, *27*, 132–42.

Clark, H. Harrison, *A Manual: Cable-Tension Strength Tests*. Chicopee, Mass., Brown-Murphy Company, 1953.

DeLorme, Thomas L., and Watkins, A. L., "Techniques of Progressive Resistance Exercise," *Arch. Phys. Med. Rehabil.*, 1948, *29*, 262–73.

Jensen, Clayne R., "Facts on Weight Training for Athletics." *Coach and Athlete*, 1963.

Jensen, Clayne R., "The Significance of Strength in Athletic Performance." *Coach and Athlete*, 1966.

Kraus, Hans, and Hirschland, Ruth P., "Minimum Muscular Fitness Tests in School Children." *Research Quarterly*, 1954a, *25*, 177–88.

Kraus, Hans, and Hirschland, Ruth P., "Muscular Fitness and Orthopedic Disability." *New York State Journal of Medicine*, 1954b, *54*, 212–15.

Larson, Leonard A., "A Factor and Validity Analysis of Strength Variables and Tests with a Test Combination of Chinning, Dipping, and Vertical Jump." *Research Quarterly*, 1940, *11* (4).

McCloy, Charles H., and Young, Norma D., *Tests and Measurements in Health and Physical Education*, 3rd ed. New York: Appleton-Century-Crofts, 1954.

Rogers, Frederick Rand, *Physical Capacity Tests in the Administration of Physical Education*. New York: Bureau of Publications, Teacher's College, Columbia University, 1926.

13

Measures of Power

Muscular power, often referred to as explosive power, is a combination of speed and strength. Such power is the ability to apply force at a rapid rate and is typically demonstrated in the long jump or the shot put. The individual uses his muscles to apply strong force at a rapid rate to give the body or the object the momentum necessary to carry it the desired distance through space. In formula form, power = force × velocity.

A person can be extremely strong and still not be extremely powerful. He may also be able to move with great speed but may lack the strength to move rapidly against resistance. However, if he has great strength combined with great speed of movement, then he is powerful.

Relationship of Power to Performance

Muscular power is important to vigorous performance because it determines how hard a person can hit, how far he can throw, how high he can jump, and to some extent how fast he can run or swim. Certain performers are described as power athletes: the player who kicks the football into the end zone; hits the home run in baseball; makes a long golf drive; tosses the shot, discus, or javelin a long distance; outjumps his opponent in basketball or volleyball; or drives through the line in football.

In addition, in running, which involves a series of body projections, power affects an individual's running speed, which is basic to many athletic performances.

Tests of Power

Tests of power ordinarily take three forms: ability to project one's body, ability to project an object, and ability to strike and kick. Power tests involve skills in which some people are more proficient than others. For the measure of power to be accurate, those being tested should be taught the particular skill and should then be given adequate practice. For example, with some basic instruction in throwing and a limited amount of practice most people can improve considerably in throwing events.

Vertical Jump (Jump and Reach)

The vertical jump test was first reported by Dudley A. Sargent in 1921 and is therefore often referred to as the Sargent jump test. It is also known as the jump and reach test.

This test measures explosive power of the extensor muscles of the legs and feet and the toe flexors. A validity coefficient of .78 has been reported when the test was correlated with four power events in track and field. A reliability coefficient of .93 has been reported. With a vertical jump board and a yardstick, about 30 students can be tested in 40 minutes at each station.

Procedure: The student faces the wall with both feet flat on the floor, toes touching the wall. He then reaches as high as possible with either hand and makes a chalk mark on the jump board (chalkboard). From the desired jump position, with the preferred side to the wall, he jumps as high as possible and at the peak of the jumping makes another chalk mark above the first one (see Figure 13-1). After each test the chalk marks should be erased.

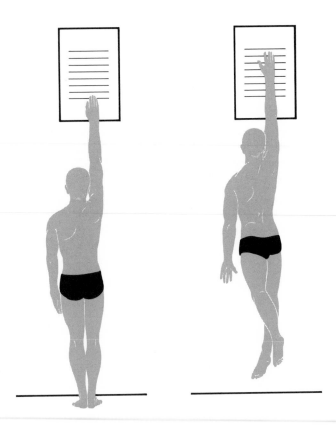

Figure 13-1. Vertical jumping test.

Scoring: The final score is the best of three jumps measured to the nearest half inch. The measurement is the distance between the two marks. Achievement scales for boys and men appear in Appendixes C and D. Achievement scales for girls and women are in Appendix B.

Standing Long Jump

This test measures about the same qualities as the vertical jump test and requires about the same amount of time. A validity coefficient of .61 was obtained when the test was compared to pure power. A reliability coefficient of .96 has been established. Each testing station requires a yardstick, a take-off mark on the floor, and for measurement purposes additional marks at six and nine feet in front of the take-off mark. The marks may be made with masking tape. About 30 students can be tested in 40 minutes at each station.

Procedure: The student stands with his feet a comfortable distance apart and his toes just behind the take-off mark. He crouches, leans forward, swings his arms backward, and then jumps horizontally as far as possible, jumping from both feet and landing on both feet (see Figure 13-2).

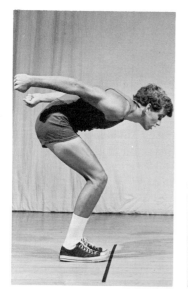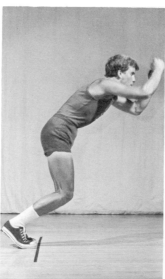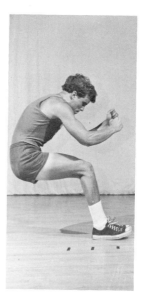

Figure 13-2. Standing long jump.

Scoring: The best of three jumps is measured to the nearest inch. The measurement is taken from the back of the take-off mark to the nearest point where the student touches the floor at the completion of the jump. Achievement scales appear in Appendixes B, C, and D.

Softball Throw for Distance

This throwing test measures power of the total body with emphasis on the upper extremities. Its validity and reliability are accepted at face value. Each testing station needs two or more softballs, 12 inches in circumference, and a steel measuring tape. On the field should be a restraining line, behind which the throw is made, and additional lines, placed 100 feet and 150 feet beyond the restraining line, for measurement purposes. About 25 students can be tested at each station in a 40-minute period.

Procedure: The student stands the desired distance behind the restraining line, up to a maximum of 15 feet. Using the typical baseball throwing approach, he moves up to the line and throws the ball as far as possible with the overarm throwing technique, being careful not to cross over the restraining line.

Scoring: The student is allowed three trials; the best throw is recorded to the nearest foot. Measurement is taken from the back of the restraining line to the spot where the ball first strikes the ground. Achievement scales appear in Appendixes B, C, and D.

Shot Put

This test for boys and men measures total body power. Its validity and reliability are accepted at face value. The test requires a shot (8 pounds for junior high school students, 12 pounds for high school students, and 16 pounds for college students), a shot-put ring 7 feet in diameter, and a steel measuring tape 50 feet long. About 20 students can be tested at each station in a 40-minute period.

Procedure: The student holds the shot on his four fingers and thumb, with his hand near the top and front portion of his shoulder. He starts near the back edge of the ring with his back toward the direction of the put. Using the typical shot-putting technique, he moves across the ring and thrusts the shot as far as possible.

Scoring: The student is allowed three trials; the best put is recorded to the nearest inch. Measurement is taken from inside the front of the ring to the nearest mark made by the fall of the shot. Achievement scales appear in Appendixes C and D.

Football Punt

This test for boys and men measures kicking power. Its validity and reliability are accepted at face value. Two regulation footballs and a steel measuring tape are needed at each testing station. On the field should be a restraining line, behind which the punt is performed, and additional lines, placed 50 feet and 100 feet beyond the restraining line, for measurement purposes. About 25 students can be tested at each station in 40 minutes.

Procedure: The student stands the desired distance behind the restraining line. He approaches the line and punts the ball as far as possible, being careful not to cross over the restraining line (see Figure 13-3).

Scoring: The student is allowed three trials; the best punt is recorded to the nearest foot. Measurement is taken from the back of the restraining line to the spot where the ball first strikes the ground. Achievement scales are not available.

Bar Snap

This test measures the power of the arms and shoulders. Its validity and reliability are accepted at face value. With a chinning bar set at a height of 4 feet 6 inches about 30 students can be tested in 40 minutes at each station.

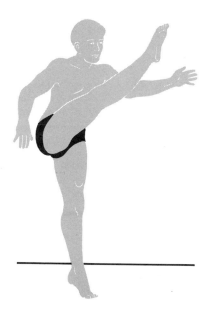

Figure 13-3.   Football punt.

Procedure: The student stands close to the bar and grasps it with both hands using the forward grip (palms forward). His body and arms should be straight with feet closer than the shoulders to the vertical plane of the bar. Taking off from both feet, he jumps upward slightly and then flexes his hips so that the insteps of his feet come close to the bar. As his flexed body swings under the bar, he shoots his feet upward, arches his back, and with his arms thrusts his body as far as possible in the horizontal direction, landing on his feet (see Figure 13-4).

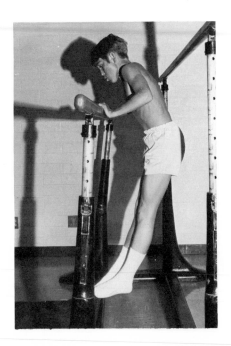
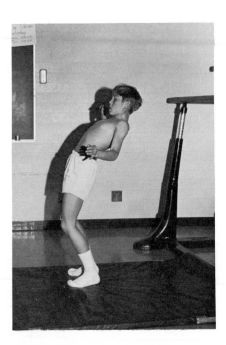

Figure 13-4. Bar snap.

Scoring: The distance is measured along the floor from directly below the bar to the place where the feet contact the floor nearest the bar. The student is allowed three trials; the best jump is recorded. Achievement scales are not available.

Other Muscular Power Tests

In addition to the aforementioned tests there are the basketball throw for distance, the football pass for distance, and the running long jump. Achievement scales for these events are not available.

How to Increase Power

There are various ways to increase power: by increasing strength without sacrificing speed, by increasing speed of movement without sacrificing strength, and by increasing both speed and strength. The best approach to increase power is to increase strength (see Chapter 12). Weight lifting against heavy resistance is the most expedient method. Speed can also be increased a limited amount as a result of training (see p. 202). Both speed and force can be stressed by applying strong force through rapid, explosive motion.

Selected References

Berger, Richard A., and Henderson, Joe M., "Relationship of Power to Static and Dynamic Strength." *Research Quarterly*, 1966, *37*, 9.

Burley, Lloyd R., and Anderson, Roy, "Relation of Jump and Reach Measures of Power to Intelligence Scores and Athletic Performances." *Research Quarterly*, 1955, *28*, 28–34.

Capen, Edward K., "The Effect of Systematic Weight Training On Power, Strength, and Endurance." *Research Quarterly*, 1950, *21*, 83–93.

Chui, Edward F., "Effects of Isometric and Dynamic Weight-Training Exercises Upon Strength and Speed of Movement." *Research Quarterly*, 1964, *35*, 246–57.

Chui, Edward F., "The Effect of Systematic Weight Training on Athletic Power." *Research Quarterly*, 1950, *21*, 188–94.

Gray, R. K., Start, K. B., and Glencross, D. J., "A Test of Leg Power." *Research Quarterly*, 1962, *33*, 44–50.

Gray, R. K., and others, "A Useful Modification of the Vertical Power Jump." *Research Quarterly*, 1962, *33*, 230–35.

Gray, R. K., Start, K. B., and Walsh, A. "Relationship Between Leg Speed and Leg Power." *Research Quarterly*, 1963, *33*, 395–400.

Meadows, P. E., The Effect of Isotonic and Isometric Muscle Contraction Training on Speed, Force, and Strength. Microcarded doctoral dissertation, University of Illinois, 1959, pp. 93–95.

14

Measures
of Agility

Agility is the ability to change the direction of the body or its parts rapidly. It is dependent primarily on strength, reaction time, speed of movement, and specific muscle coordinations. People with great agility have been said to be less accident prone because of their ability to make quick adjustments in body position and direction of movement.

Relationship of Agility to Performance

Agility is important in activities involving quick changes in positions of the body and its parts. In court games such as basketball, tennis, badminton, and volleyball and in field games such as soccer, football, speedball, and baseball, fast starts and stops and quick changes in direction are fundamental to good performances. Gymnastics and diving depend largely upon rapid body movements and quick changes in body positions. Skiing, skating, and certain forms of dance require rapid adjustments in position and quick changes in direction. However, such activities as track events and swimming do not depend on agility to any large degree.

Agility Tests

Agility tests are especially useful for classifying students into homogeneous groups for instruction in field and court games, skating, skiing, and other types of performance requiring quick changes in direction. Most agility tests involve running.

Squat Thrust (10 Seconds)

This test was first reported by Royal H. Burpee and is often referred to as the Burpee Test. The test measures agility of the total body. Validity and reliability coefficients of .55 and .92 respectively have been established. The only equipment needed is a stopwatch. A large number of students can be tested in a short time if they are arranged into pairs to count for each other and to check each other's performance.

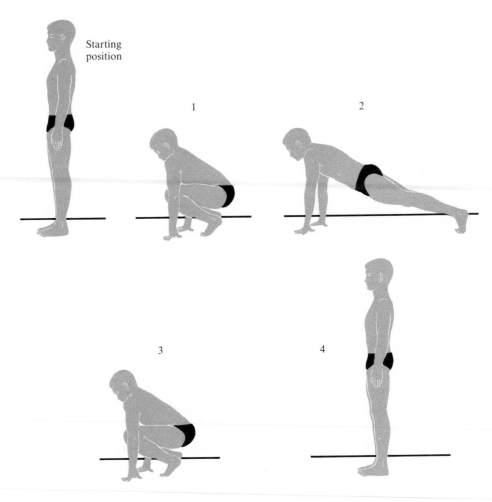

Figure 14-1.   Squat thrust test.

Procedure: The student takes a standing position. On the signal he moves to a squatting position, then to a front leaning rest position, back to a squatting position, and finally to the erect standing position. In the standing and front leaning rest positions his body should be straight (see Figure 14-1). In the squatting position his hands should touch the floor. He repeats the movement as rapidly as possible for 10 seconds.

Scoring: Each completed squat thrust counts one point and every quarter movement counts one-quarter point. For example, if a student finished four complete squat thrusts and started the fifth but reached only the squat position on the way down, his score would be four and one-quarter points. If he reached the front leaning rest position, his score would be four and one-half points. If he returned to the squatting position from the front leaning rest position, his score would be four and three-quarters points. The best of three trials is recorded as the final score. Achievement scales are not available.

Dodging Run

The dodging run (McCloy and Young 1954) is a running test of total body agility which has proved to be among the better agility tests. Validity and reliability coefficients of .82 and .93 respectively have been established. Four hurdles and a stopwatch are necessary at each station; about 30 students can be tested at one station in 40 minutes.

Procedure: The instructor places a starting line three feet long on the floor. He then places a hurdle 15 feet in front of the starting line, a second hurdle six feet beyond the first hurdle, a third hurdle six feet beyond the second hurdle, and a fourth hurdle six feet beyond the third hurdle. He should stagger the hurdles as shown in Figure 14-2. On the signal the student starts running and follows the course indicated by arrows on the dotted lines. He runs the course two complete times before stopping.

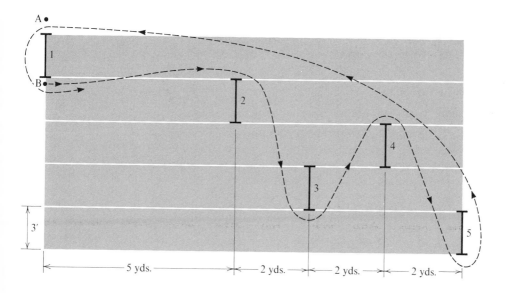

Scoring: The score is the time required to run the course two times, measured to the nearest tenth of a second. Achievement scales are not available.

Shuttle Run
(Agility Run or Potato Race)

The shuttle run (AAHPER 1961) measures total body agility. Validity and reliability are accepted at face value. Equipment required at each testing station includes two small wooden blocks or suitable substitutes and a stopwatch. About 30 students can be tested in a 40-minute period.

Procedure: The instructor places two small blocks of wood 30 feet from the starting point. At the signal the student starts from behind the starting line, retrieves one of the blocks, and places it behind the starting line. He then retrieves the second block and sprints back across the starting line. If two stopwatches are available, two students can compete against each other.

Scoring: The student is allowed two trials, with a short rest between trials. If the student commits an error, he should stop immediately and start again at the beginning. The score is the time required to complete the course correctly, recorded to the nearest tenth of a second. The time for the better run is recorded. Achievement scales appear in Appendixes B, C, and D.

Right-Boomerang Test

This test (McCloy and Young 1954) measures running agility. Validity coefficients of .82 for boys and .72 for girls and reliability coefficients of .93 for boys and .92 for girls have been established. The equipment needed is a jumping standard or similar object placed at the center point, four Indian clubs or other such object for the outside points, and a stopwatch. About 25 students can be tested at each station in 40 minutes.

Procedure: The student stands at the starting line. At the signal he runs to the center point, turns 90 degrees to the left, and continues through the remainder of the course as rapidly as possible (see Figure 14-3).

Scoring: The time for the better run is recorded to the nearest tenth of a second. Achievement scales are not available.

Sidestep Test

This test is a modification of H. D. Edgren's test (1932); it measures the speed with which the person can change direction moving sideward. A stopwatch is the only equipment needed. Forty students can be tested in 40 minutes.

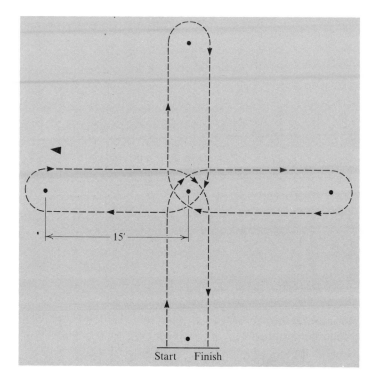

Figure 14-3.   Right-boomerang course.

Procedure: The instructor places three parallel lines five feet apart on the floor. The student straddles the middle line. On the signal he sidesteps to the right until his right foot crosses over the line to the right; then he sidesteps to the left until his left foot crosses over the line to the left (see Figure 14-4). He repeats these movements as rapidly as possible for 20 seconds.

Scoring: Each time the performer crosses over the center line he scores one point. Current achievement scales are not available.

Other Agility Tests

In addition to the tests described in this chapter the following are also useful tests of agility: forty-yard maze run (McCloy and Young 1954), loop-the-loop run (McCloy and Young 1954), zigzag run (McCloy and Young 1954), quadrant jump (Johnson and Nelson 1969), and LSU agility test (Johnson and Nelson 1969).

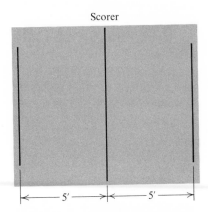

Figure 14-4.   Sidestep test floor plan.

How to Increase Agility

Agility in specific movements can be increased if the movements are practiced extensively so that the coordinations involved are improved. Strength is a contributing factor to agility. If strength is increased, the agility will increase in movements involving heavy resistance such as rapid stopping and starting, or in movements involving the force of inertia which keeps the body in motion in the same direction, such as dodging. The other factors which influence agility—speed of movement and reaction time—may be increased a limited amount by practicing fast movements.

Selected References

American Association for Health, Physical Education and Recreation, *Youth Fitness Test Manual*, 1961.

Edgren, H. D., "An Experiment in Testing Ability and Progress in Basketball," *Research Quarterly* III, 1, March 1932, p. 159.

Gates, Donald D., and Sheffield, R. P., "Tests of Change of Direction as Measurement of Different Kinds of Motor Ability in Boys of the 7th, 8th, and 9th Grades." *Research Quarterly*, 1940, *11*, 3, 136–47.

Johnson, Barry L., and Nelson, Jack K., *Practical Measurements for Evaluation in Physical Education*. Minneapolis: Burgess Publishing Company, 1969, pp. 100–14.

McCloy, Charles H., and Young, Norma D., *Tests and Measurements in Physical Education*, 3rd ed., New York: Appleton-Century-Crofts, 1954, p. 80.

Seils, L. G., "Agility-Performance and Physical Growth." *Research Quarterly*, 1951, *22*, 244.

15

Measures
of Flexibility

Adequate flexibility allows for a full range of motion in the joints and is often limited by the amount of extensibility of the muscles, tendons, and ligaments. A frequent cause of improper movement is poor flexibility.

Relationship of Flexibility to Performance

Flexibility is important to several types of performance, such as modern dance, ballet, gymnastics, diving, swimming, hurdling, and high jumping. In these activities the body must be extremely flexible to assume certain positions which determine good form. However, such activities as basketball, football, and soccer require only normal flexibility.

In addition to those persons who need unusual amounts of flexibility for certain performances, all individuals should develop sufficient flexibility to follow the normal living activities of working, playing, and resting without undue muscular strain.

Flexibility Tests

The tests presented in this section specifically measure flexibility in the regions of the body that rely on great flexibility for good performance. Although validity and reliability coefficients for these tests have not been computed, the tests are valid and reliable measures of flexibility. In addition to the tests described, the Wells sit and reach test (Wells and Dillon 1952) and the Leighton flexometer test (Leighton 1955) are also useful measurements of flexibility.

Forward Bend of Trunk

This test measures flexion of the trunk and hips, since most movement occurs in the lower spine and hip joints. A small measuring tape is the only equipment needed. About 40 students can be tested in a 40-minute period.

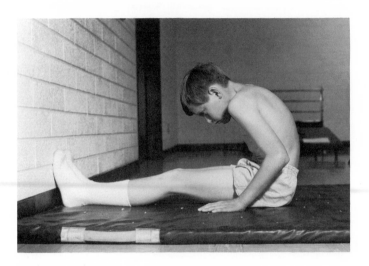

Figure 15-1.   Forward bend of trunk test.

Procedure: The student sits on a table or on the floor with his feet flat against the wall, hip width apart, and his legs straight and rigid. He bends the trunk forward and downward as far as possible, reaching his hands toward the heels of his feet (see Figure 15-1). As the student holds this position, the examiner measures the vertical distance from the table to the top of the student's sternum (suprasternal notch).

Scoring: The score is the distance measured, to the nearest quarter inch. As flexibility increases the measured distance will become shorter. Because achievement scales are not available, the measurement is meaningful only when compared to measurements of other students or to measurements of the same student on different occasions. If the examiner needs another indication of flexibility, he may determine how near the student can come to touching his heels with his fingers.

Upward–Backward Movement of Arms

This test measures flexibility of the shoulders and shoulder girdles. The equipment and time required are the same as that for the forward bend of trunk test, with the addition of a stick two feet long.

Procedure: The student lies in a prone position on a table with his chin touching the table and his arms reaching forward directly in front of his shoulders. He holds the stick horizontally with both hands. Keeping his elbows and wrists straight and his chin on the table, he raises his arms upward as far as possible (see Figure 15-2).

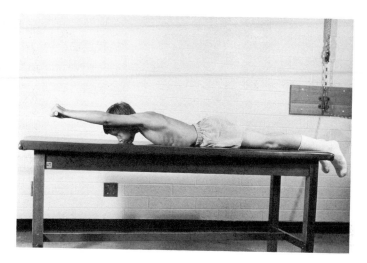

Figure 15-2.   Upward–backward arm movement test.

Scoring: The examiner measures the vertical distance from the bottom of the stick to the table. For interpretation he compares the student's score with the scores of other students or with the scores of the same student on different occasions.

Sideward–Backward Movement of Arms

This test (Cureton 1941) measures flexibility of the same body region as the upward-backward movement of arm test, except that the movement is in a different direction.

Procedure: To perform the test the student stands with his back against a wall, places his palms forward, and raises his arms until they are horizontal. Keeping his arms horizontal and the fifth finger of each hand in contact with the wall, he moves his back forward, away from the wall, as far as possible (see Figure 15-3).

Scoring: The examiner measures the horizontal distance, to the nearest quarter inch, from the wall to the spine at arm level. The examiner should interpret scores as described for the forward bend of trunk test.

Plantar-Dorsal Flexion of Foot

This test (Cureton 1941) measures flexibility in the ankle and foot regions. A paper pad, a pencil, and a protractor are necessary.

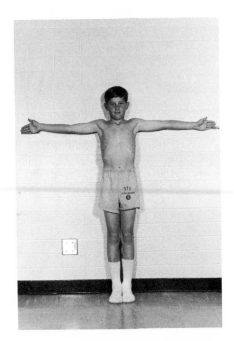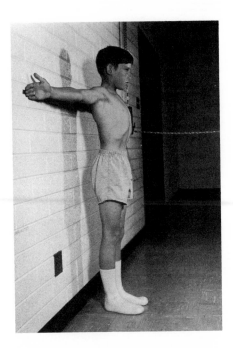

Figure 15-3.   Sideward–backward arm movement test.

Procedure: The student sits on a table with his legs straight and together. Keeping his heels and backs of his knees on the table, he plantar flexes the foot as far as possible. With a pad of paper placed in a vertical position at the inside of the foot, the examiner places a dot on the paper at the end of the toenail of the great toe. The student then dorsi flexes his foot as far as possible, and the examiner places a second dot on the paper in a similar manner. Finally the student relaxes his ankle, and the examiner places a third dot on the paper where the ankle bends at the top of the instep (see Figure 15-4).

Scoring: The examiner removes the pad and draws lines from the third dot to each of the other two dots. Using a protractor or goniometer, he measures the angle of each of the lines from the horizontal and interprets the scores as described for the forward bend of trunk test.

Trunk Extension

This (Cureton 1941) test measures trunk extension. A small measuring tape is the only equipment necessary to test 40 students in 40 minutes.

Procedure: The student takes a prone position on a table or the floor with his hands clasped together near the small of his back. With a partner pressing

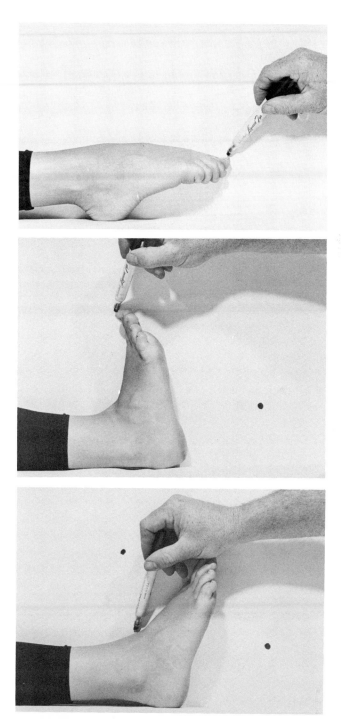

Figure 15-4.   Plantar-dorsal flexion test.

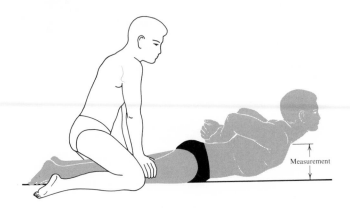

Figure 15-5.   Trunk extension test.

downward on the back of his legs, the student lifts his chest from the floor as high as possible (see Figure 15-5).

Scoring: For the raw score the examiner measures the distance, to the nearest quarter inch, from the suprasternal notch to the floor. For the final score, which is more meaningful, the examiner multiplies the raw score by 100 and divides the product by trunk length measured in inches.

Bridge Up

This test measures the student's ability to extend his back and hips and to reach backward with his arms, under force. Only a tape measure is needed to test about 40 students in a 40-minute period.

Procedure: From a supine position on the floor or mat the student extends his hips upward by arching his back and walks on his hands and feet, keeping them as close together as possible (see Figure 15-6).

Scoring: The examiner measures the distance between the fingertips and the heels to the nearest quarter inch. The lesser the distance, the better the score.

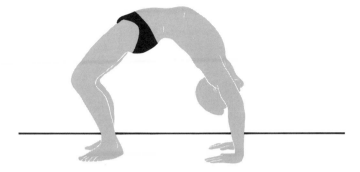

Figure 15-6.   Bridge up test.

Leighton Flexometer

Jack Leighton devised a reliable and objective instrument (see Figure 15-7) for measuring flexibility in 30 joint movements. The Leighton flexometer consists of a weighted 360-degree dial and a weighted pointer mounted in a case about four and a half inches in diameter. The case is secured to the body segment by a strap. In the operating position the dial and pointer coincide and point upward. With separate locking devices the dial is locked in place when the segment is positioned to begin a test action. The pointer may be locked in the point of finished movement. The direct dial reading represents the arc or range of motion. Leighton also devised various flexibility tests (Leighton 1955).

Figures 15-8 through 15-12 illustrate observation measures of flexibility.

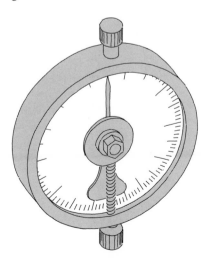

Figure 15-7.   Leighton flexometer.

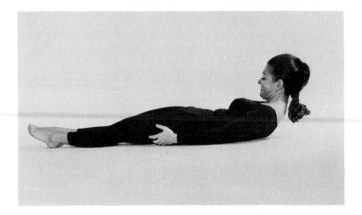

Figure 15-8.   Normal flexibility of the neck allows the chin to move close to the upper chest.

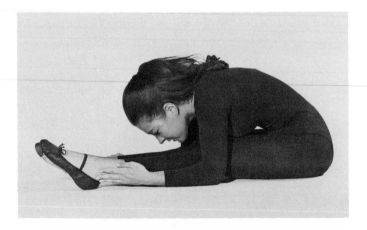

Figure 15-9.   Normal flexibility in the hips and lower back allows flexion to about 135 degrees in the young adult. Children should be even more flexible.

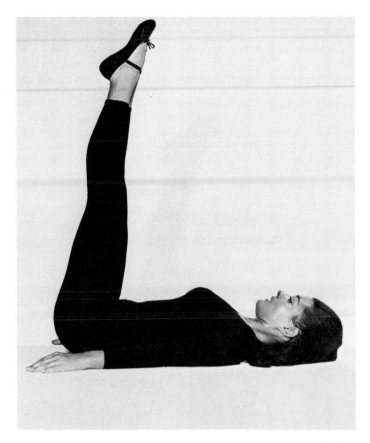

Figure 15-10.   Normal flexibility of the hamstring muscles allows straight leg raising from a back-lying position to 90 degrees.

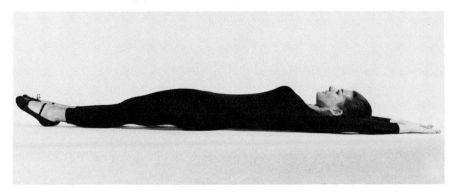

Figure 15-11.   Normal flexibility of the chest muscles allows the arms to be flexed at the shoulders to 180 degrees.

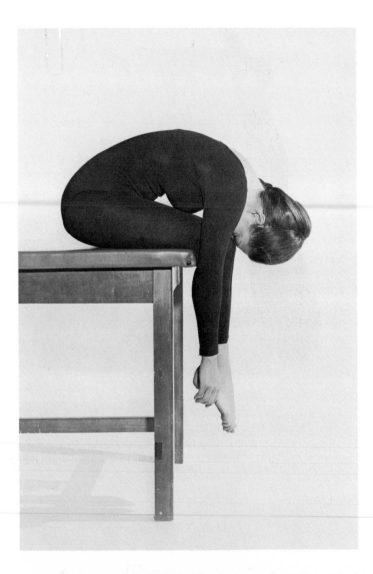

Figure 15-12.   Normal flexibility in the back with the knees bent allows the face to meet the knees.

How to Increase Flexibility

Flexibility may be increased by regular stretching of the muscles and other connective tissues. Traditionally rapid tension movements, such as bobbing, were used to increase flexibility, but now slow tension is known to be a more effective means. Slow tension movements give the muscles under stretch a chance to relax and extend to their maximum, without activating the stretch reflex.

It is generally recommended that the student move slowly through the particular movement until he feels the stretch pain in his muscles. As he holds the position for five to ten seconds, he should consciously cause the muscles to relax and stretch. Best results occur when the student repeats the exercise five to six times daily.

Selected References

Barney, Vermon S., Hirst, Cynthia C., and Jensen, Clayne R., *Conditioning Exercises*. St. Louis: C. V. Mosby Company, 1969.

Broer, Marion, and Galles, Naomi, "Importance of Relationship Between Various Body Measurements in Performance of the Toe-Touch Test." *Research Quarterly*, 1958, *29*, 262.

Burley, Lloyd R., and others, "Relation of Power, Speed, Flexibility, and Certain Anthropometric Measures of Junior High School Girls." *Research Quarterly*, 1961, *32*, 443.

Cureton, Thomas K., Jr., "Flexibility as an Aspect of Physical Fitness." *Research Quarterly Supplement*, 1941, *12*, 388–89.

DeVries, Herbert, "Evaluation of Static Stretching Procedures for Improvement of Flexibility." *Research Quarterly*, *33*, 1962, pp. 222–29.

Forbes, Joseph, "Characteristics of Flexibility in Boys." Microcarded doctoral dissertation, University of Oregon, 1950.

Hupprich, Florence L., and Sigerseth, Peter, "The Specificity of Flexibility in Girls." *Research Quarterly*, 1950, *21*, 32.

Hutchins, Gloria Lee, "The Relationship of Selected Strength and Flexibility Variables to the Anteroposterior Posture of College Women." *Research Quarterly*, 1965, *36*.

Johnson, Barry L., and Nelson, Jack K., *Practical Measurements for Evaluation in Physical Education*. Minneapolis: Burgess Publishing Company, 1969.

Leighton, Jack, "An Instrument and Technique for the Measurement of Range of Joint Motion." *Archives of Physical Medicine*, 36, 9, p. 571.

McCue, Betty F., "Flexibility Measurements of College Women." *Research Quarterly*, 1953, *24*, 323–24.

Olsen, Barbara H., An Investigation of the Relationship of Ankle, Knee, Trunk, and Shoulder Flexibility to General Motor Ability. Microcarded master's thesis, University of Oregon, 1956.

Sigerseth, Peter O., and Haliski, Chester, "The Flexibility of Football Players." *Research Quarterly*, 1950, *21*, 398.

Tyrance, Herman J., "Relationship of Extreme Body Types to Ranges of Flexibility." *Research Quarterly*, 1958, *29*, 248.

Wells, Katherine F., and Dillon, Evelyn K., "The Sit and Reach—A Test of Back and Leg Flexibility," *Research Quarterly*, 1952, *23*, 118.

16

Measures of
Reaction Time and Speed

Reaction time, response time, and running speed are three factors to consider in determining speed in performance.

Relationship of Reaction Time and Speed to Performance

Reaction time is the time lapse between the external stimulus and the initial response to that stimulus. It is extremely important in all performances requiring quick responses. It has special significance in events in which individuals must defend against each other and thereby respond to each other's movements. A performer who reacts slowly is left behind at the start of a running event. A person with slow reactions is hapless in his defensive efforts against a person with faster reactions. Slow reactions also hinder offensive play because the performer is not able to demonstrate the necessary quickness.

Response time is determined by reaction time and movement time (rate of muscle contraction). The relative speed of contraction of different muscles varies greatly among individuals. For example, person A may have faster leg actions while person B has faster arm actions. Moreover person A's arm extensor muscles may contract relatively fast while his arm flexors contract slowly. In other words speed varies with individual body movements. Although a person is a slow runner, he may have fast arm and finger movements or vice versa. Speed of response of the body as a whole or in part is important in a variety of performances; it determines how quickly a performer can respond completely and correctly to a given situation.

Running speed is not only an athletic event itself, but it is also an important factor in numerous other sports. Running speed and maneuverability are important in almost all court and field games. It can make the difference in whether a performer is able to gain an advantage over his opponent.

Tests of Reaction Time

Nelson Finger and Foot Reaction Tests

These tests (Nelson 1967) are designed to measure how quickly a person reacts to a visual stimulus. They are equally useful for boys and girls of any age group.

The tests have not been validated, probably because there is no suitable criterion measure against which to compare them. Their validity is accepted at face value. Reliability coefficients of .89 for the hand test and .85 for the foot test have been produced for the test-retest method. A Nelson reaction timer, a desk chair or a table and chair are needed; however a yardstick made of hard wood may be substituted for the Nelson reaction timer. About 15 students can be tested on each test in a 40-minute period.

Procedure for the finger reaction test: The student sits on the chair with his forearm and hand resting comfortably on the edge of the desk. He holds his index finger and thumb about two inches apart and beyond the edge of the desk (see Figure 16-1).

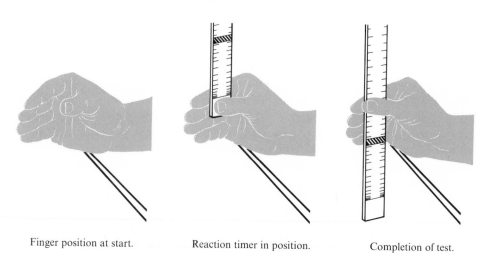

Finger position at start.   Reaction timer in position.   Completion of test.

Figure 16-1.   Nelson finger reaction test.

The thumb and index finger should be in a horizontal position, and the base line of the reaction timer should be even with the upper surface of the thumb. Ready to grip the reaction timer when it is released, the student looks directly at the concentration zone, a black shaded area. On the command "ready" the test administrator releases the reaction timer and the student grasps it, as quickly as possible, with his thumb and index finger. He has 20 trials.

Scoring: The score for each trial is the number at the upper edge of the thumb. The score is recorded in hundredths of a second. The five slowest and five fastest trials are discarded, and an average of the middle ten trials is recorded as the score.

Procedure for the foot reaction test: The student sits on a table or bench about one inch from a wall. With his shoe removed, the student positions his foot so that the ball of the foot is about one inch from the wall with the heel resting on the edge of the table about three inches from the wall. The test administrator holds the reaction timer next to the wall so that it hangs between the wall and the student's foot, with the base line at the end of the big toe (see Figure 16-2). The student looks directly at the concentration zone, and when the administrator drops the timer, the student presses the stick against the wall as quickly as possible with the ball of his foot.

Scoring: The student is scored the same as for the finger reaction test.

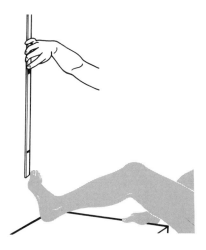

Figure 16-2.   Nelson foot reaction test.

Hand and Arm Reaction Test

This test (Nelson 1967) is designed to measure the hand and arm reaction time. It is suitable for both boys and girls of any age group. A Nelson reaction timer (or a yardstick), a table and a chair are needed. About 15 students can be tested in 40 minutes.

Procedure: The student sits at the table, as illustrated in Figure 16-3, with his hands one foot apart and the ends of his little fingers on the table. He looks directly at the concentration zone on the reaction timer, and when the administrator drops the timer, he slaps his hands together on the timer as quickly as possible.

Scoring: The student is scored the same as for the finger reaction test.

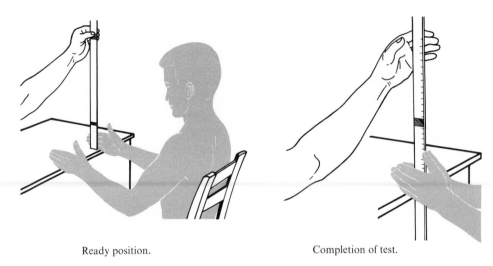

Ready position.   Completion of test.

Figure 16-3.   Hand and arm reaction test.

Tests of Response Time

Four-Way Alternate Response Test

This test (Jensen 1969) is designed to measure how quickly a person can complete a response to a signal to move in a given direction. Its validity and reliability have not been established; however, because of the nature of the test they can be accepted at face value. The test is suitable for both boys and girls of any age group. A floor area should be marked according to Figure 16-4. Only a stopwatch is needed to test about 20 students in 40 minutes.

Procedure: The student stands at point X on the floor and concentrates on the right hand of the test administrator standing at point Y on the floor. After giving the preparatory command "ready," the test administrator makes an obvious movement with his hand in one of four directions. On the signal the student moves in the designated direction as rapidly as possible and crosses over the line five yards from point X. Hence if the tester were to move his hand up, the student would move forward across the line. If he were to move his hand down, the student would move backward. If he were to move his hand to either side, the student would move in the direction of his motion. The student is given 20 trials, five in each direction. The trials in the different directions may come in any order the tester chooses.

Scoring: The tester holds a stopwatch which he starts at the beginning of each hand movement. He stops the watch when the student crosses the correct line, and

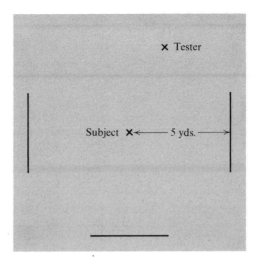

Figure 16-4.   Floor area for four-way alternate response test.

records the time to the nearest tenth of a second. The score is the total of the times on all 20 trials. Achievement scales are not available.

Two-Way Alternate Response Test

This test (Smith 1964) is the same as the four-way alternate response test except the student is required to respond to either the right or the left. Ten trials are given, five to each side. The score is the total time for the 10 trials.

Hand and Arm Response Test

This test (Jensen 1969) is designed to measure how quickly the student can respond with his arm and hands. Its validity and reliability are accepted at face value. The test may be used with men and women of any age group. Equipment needed is the same as that for the hand and arm reaction test. About 15 students can be tested in 40 minutes.

Procedure: The procedure is the same as that for the hand and arm reaction test except the student's hands are placed on the table three feet apart instead of one foot apart. This additional distance places emphasis on both reaction time and speed of movement time and therefore indicates response time.

Scoring: The student is scored the same as for the hand and arm reaction test.

Tests of Speed

Sprint for Speed Test

This test is to measure a person's ability to run a prescribed distance in the shortest time possible. Necessary equipment includes a starting pistol or a whistle and as many stopwatches as there are contestants in each heat. Four to six students can be tested at one time if enough watches and timers are available. Timers should be trained to time correctly. Students should receive thorough instruction on correct starting techniques and should be allowed adequate practice. Starting blocks should be used if they are available.

Procedure: On the starter's command the student takes the "on-the-mark" position. On the second command he moves to the "set" position. On the starting signal (pistol shot or whistle) he sprints as fast as possible to the finish line.

Scoring: A student's score is the time, measured to the nearest tenth of a second, that lapses between the starting signal and the time the student crosses the finish line. Achievement scales for the 50-yard run for girls and women appear in Appendix B. Scales for the 100-, and 440-yard runs for boys appear in Appendix C. In Appendix D are scales for the 100- and 440-yard runs for college men.

Running Maneuverability Test

Chapter 14 describes tests that measure a person's ability to maneuver while running. Among the better tests of running maneuverability are the dodging run, the shuttle run, and the right-boomerang run.

How to Improve
Reaction Time and Speed

Even a small improvement in reaction time may produce significant results in certain performances for which quick reactions are essential. There is evidence that reaction time in specific movements will improve a limited amount as a result of extensive practice of those movements. For example, practice of starting to a pistol shot will result in faster reactions to that stimulus. Even though reaction time for specific acts can be improved by practice, the improvement by training of reaction time in general has not been established.

Running speed is determined by the length of stride and frequency (speed) of stride. To increase his running speed, the student must increase one or both of these factors. Length of stride is dependent primarily upon leg length and the power of the stride. Leg speed (frequency) is dependent mostly upon speed of muscle contractions and neuromuscular coordination (skill) in running. A student's speed can be measured accurately by recording the time it takes him to run an appropriate distance. For high school boys and college men the 50- and 100-yard sprints are considered to be the best measure of pure speed. Shorter distances are influenced too much by the start, and distances longer than 100 yards are influenced by a student's endurance. These longer distances are too strenuous for students who are not well-conditioned athletes. The 50- or 60-yard sprint is considered the most desirable distance for girls and women and elementary school boys.

Selected References

Endres, John P., The Effect of Weight Training Exercise Upon the Speed of Muscular Movements. Microcarded master's thesis, University of Wisconsin, 1953.

Fairclough, Richard H., "Transfer of Motivated Improvement in Speed of Reaction and Movement." *Research Quarterly*, 1952, *23*.

Gibson, Dennis A., Effect of a Special Training Program for Sprint Starting on Reflex Time, Reaction Time and Sargent Jump. Microcarded master's thesis, Springfield College, 1961.

Gottshall, Donald R., The Effects of Two Training Programs on Reflex Time, Reaction Time and the Level of Physical Fitness. Microcarded master's thesis, Springfield College, 1962.

Henry, Franklin M., "Increase in Speed of Movement by Motivation and by Transfer of Motivated Improvement." *Research Quarterly*, 1951, *22*.

Henry, Franklin M., "Independence of Reaction and Movement Ties and Equivalency of Sensory Motivators of Faster Response." *Research Quarterly*, 1952, *23*.

Henry, Franklin M., "Reaction Time-Movement Time Correlations." *Perceptual and Motor Skills*, 1961, *12*.

Howell, Maxwell L., "Influence of Emotional Tension on Speed of Reaction and Movement." *Research Quarterly*, 1953, *24*.

Jensen, Clayne R., Practical Measurements of Reaction Time, Response Time and Speed. Unpublished study, Brigham Young University, 1969.

Johnson, Barry L., *Practical Measurements for Evaluation in Physical Education*. Minneapolis: Burgess Publishing Company, 1969.

Keller, Louis F., "The Relation of Quickness of Bodily Movement to Success in Athletics." *Research Quarterly*, 1942, *13*.

Masley, John W., Hairabedian, Ara, and Donaldson, Donald N., "Weight Training in Relation to Strength, Speed, and Coordination." *Research Quarterly*, 1953, *24*.

Michael, Charles E., The Effects of Isometric Contraction Exercise on Reaction and Speed of Movement Times. Unpublished doctoral dissertation, Louisiana State University, 1963.

Nelson, Fred B., "The Nelson Reaction Timer." Instructional leaflet, 1965. P.O. Box 51987, Lafayette, Louisiana.

Nelson, Jack K., Development of a Practical Performance Test Combining Reaction Time, Speed of Movement and Choice of Response. Unpublished study, Louisiana State University, 1967.

Smith, Leon E., "Effect of Muscular Stretch, Tension, and Relaxation Upon the Reaction Time and Speed of Movement of a Supported Limb." *Research Quarterly*, 1964, *35*.

Thompson, Clem W., Nagle, Francis J., and Dobias, Robert, "Football Starting Signals and Movement Times of High School and College Football Players." *Research Quarterly*, 1958, *29*.

17

Tests of Balance
and Kinesthetic Perception

Balance and kinesthetic perception are quite different from each other. However perception is an important contributor to balance. Tests of balance and tests of perception are combined into one chapter more for convenience than for any other reason.

Relationship of Balance
and Perception to Performance

Certain performances depend directly upon balance: Among them are gymnastic events such as balance beam performances, floor exercise routines and dismounting from various gymnastic apparatus; Diving, rebound tumbling, and some forms of dancing also require unusual amounts of balance. Stability (firmness of balance) is of special importance in all body contact sports such as wrestling, football, rugby, and soccer and in some supposedly noncontact sports such as basketball and hockey. In an off-balance position a performer is in a poor position to respond to the act of an opponent, to execute an act requiring accuracy, and to resist force or apply force in any direction except the direction in which he is off-balance. In many cases increased balance will result in improved performances.

Kinesthetic perception is important to both balance and accuracy. In certain activities an individual is at a disadvantage if he is unable to judge accurately the position of his body parts or the amount of force applied by his muscles. A high degree of kinesthetic sense results in better coordination and a more accurate "touch."

Static Balance Tests

Balance is defined as the ability to remain in equilibrium. When the body is in equilibrium, an even adjustment exists among all opposing forces, and the body remains balanced. The state of equilibrium may be stable or precarious. A balance center located in the inner ear, the kinesthetic sense, and the eyes all play important roles in maintaining balance.

For an individual to maintain his balance in any stationary position his center of gravity must remain over the base of support. Whenever the center of gravity moves outside the supporting base, the body is off-balance in that direction. This fact applies to all body positions, including upright, inverted (hands forming the base of support), and three-, four-, or six-point positions. If the center of gravity moves outside the base of support, the individual must make a quick adjustment to regain his balance. He may move or enlarge the base, or he may shift a body part to return the center of gravity to a position over the base. After he has made the adjustment

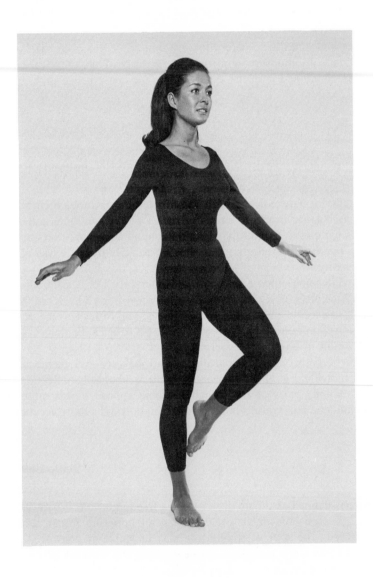

Figure 17-1. Stork stand balance test.

the performer is more stable and less susceptible to another loss of balance if he lowers the center of gravity.

Balance tests are either static or dynamic. Static tests measure ability to remain in balance in a stationary position (see Figure 17-1), while dynamic tests measure ability to remain in balance while in motion. The two types of balance tests are arranged according to their difficulty. These tests can be given to a large number of students in a 40-minute period if the students are arranged in pairs so they can score each other.

The following tests of static balance are useful in educational programs.

The objective of these tests is to measure the individual's ability to balance in a stationary, upright position while standing on a small base.

1. *Stork Stand (Foot)*. This test (Jensen 1970a) has produced a reliability coefficient of .85 when the test-retest method was employed. Its validity is accepted at face value. To perform the test the student stands on the flat foot of the dominant leg and places the other foot on the inside of the supporting knee. He then puts his hands on his hips and holds this position as long as possible. The student is scored on the length of time, in seconds, that he is able to maintain his balance. The best of three trials is recorded.

2. *Stork Stand (Toes)*. The student performs this test as the previous test except he balances on the ball of his foot instead of on the whole foot. This test has produced a reliability coefficient of .87 with the test-retest method. Its validity is accepted at face value.

3. *Bass Stick Test (Lengthwise)*. This test (Bass 1939) has produced a reliability coefficient of .90. Its validity is accepted at face value. Necessary equipment is a stick one inch wide and twelve inches long, a stopwatch, and adhesive tape to fasten the stick to the floor. To perform the test the student places the ball of the dominant foot lengthwise on the stick and lifts the opposite foot from the floor maintaining his balance in that position as long as possible (see Figure 17-2). He performs the test three times on the right leg and three times on the left leg. His score is the total time, in seconds, for all six trials.

4. *Bass Stick Test (Crosswise)*. The student performs this test (Bass 1939) the same as the previous test except he places his foot crosswise to the stick and balances on the ball of his foot (see Figure 17-3).

The objective of these tests is to measure the performer's ability to remain in balance while in the inverted position.

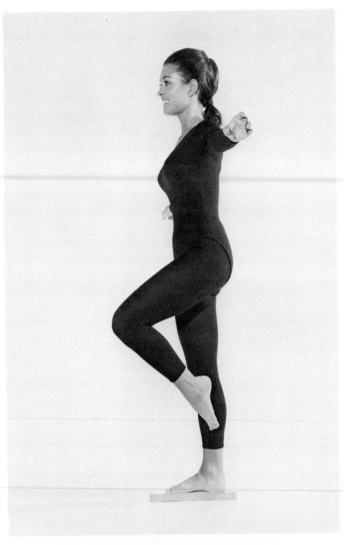

Figure 17-2. Bass stick test (lengthwise).

1. *Tripod Test.* From a squat position the student places his hands shoulder width apart with his fingers pointing straight ahead. He then leans forward bending at the elbows and places the backs of his knees against and slightly above the outside of the elbows. He continues to lean forward until his feet come off the floor with his forehead resting on the mat (see Figure 17-4). Balancing in this position as long as possible, he is scored on the length of time he maintains his balance measured to the nearest second. He is permitted three trials.

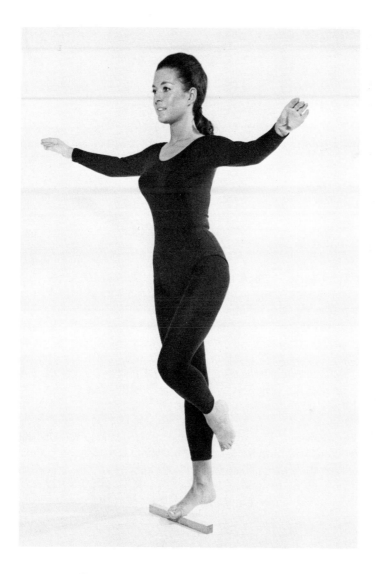

Figure 17-3. Bass stick test (crosswise).

2. *Tip-Up Test.* This test is the same as the tripod test except the student does not rest his head on the mat, but instead balances on both hands with his face several inches above the floor (see Figure 17-5).

3. *Head and Hand Balance.* The student puts his forehead on the mat several inches in front of his hands. He kicks upward, one foot at a time and maintains his balance, keeping his back slightly arched, his legs straight and together, and his toes pointed. With his body weight primarily on his hands and some weight on his

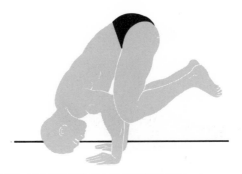

forehead, the student balances in this position for as long as possible (see Figure 17-6). His score is the best time of three trials recorded to the nearest second. To get out of this position the student pushes with his hands, ducks his head, and rolls forward, or he steps down one foot at a time.

4. *Head and Forearm Balance.*   The student places his forearms on the mat and brings his hands close enough together for the thumbs and forefingers to form a cup for his head. He then puts his head in the cup and kicks upward one foot at a time, balancing in this position for as many seconds as possible (see Figure 17-7). His score is the best time of three trials.

5. *Two-Hand Balance.*   The student bends forward and places his hands on the mat about shoulder width apart. He leans his shoulders over his hands and places one foot ahead of the other. Then swinging his rear foot upward as the front foot pushes from the mat, he maintains a balanced position with his feet overhead for as many seconds as possible (see Figure 17-8). His score is the best time of three trials.

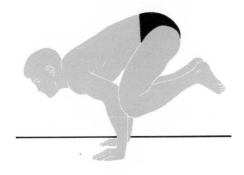

Figure 17-5.   Tip-up test.

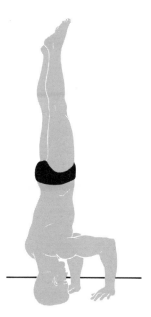

Figure 17-6.   Head and hand balance.

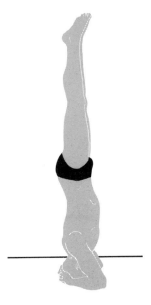

Figure 17-7.   Head and forearm balance.

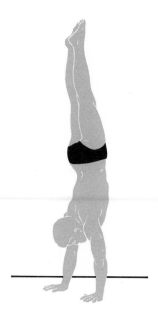

Figure 17-8.   Two-hand balance.

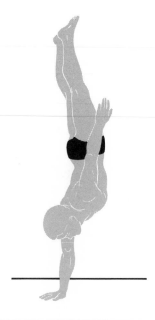

Figure 17-9.   One-hand balance.

6. One-Hand Balance. The student performs the same as for the two-hand balance test except he balances on one hand instead of on two. He moves into the one-hand balance from the two-hand balance position (see Figure 17-9). He is scored the same as for the two-hand balance test.

Dynamic Balance Tests

The following dynamic balance tests have proved useful in school programs.

Upright Dynamic Tests

The objective of these tests is to measure how well the performer can balance while in motion in an upright position.

1. Balance Beam Walk. A regulation balance beam is the only equipment needed for this test. Starting from the standing position on one end of the beam, the student walks slowly the full length of the beam, pauses for five seconds, turns around, and walks back to the starting position (see Figure 17-10). He is allowed three trials and is scored either "pass" or "fail." (For a more difficult test a balance beam two inches wide and 12 feet long may be used.)

2. Johnson Modification of the Bass Test of Dynamic Balance. Validity of this test (Johnson and Leach 1968) is accepted at face value. With the test-retest method it produced a reliability coefficient of .75. A stopwatch, masking tape, and a yardstick are needed. The floor plan is according to Figure 17-11.

To perform the test the student stands with his right foot on the starting mark. He then leaps to the first tape mark and lands on the left foot, balancing on the ball of his foot as long as possible up to five seconds. Then he leaps to the next tape mark, landing on the right foot and balancing again for five seconds. He continues this procedure, balancing on each tape mark as long as possible up to five seconds.

The student scores five points each time he lands successfully on the tape mark, plus one point for each second he balances on the mark up to five seconds. Thus he could score ten points for each mark with a total of one hundred points possible for the test. However, he could lose five points for an improper landing from the leap if he commits any of the following errors:

1. Failure to stop upon landing.

2. Failure to keep his heel or any part of his body other than the ball of the supporting foot from touching the floor.

3. Failure to cover the mark completely with the ball of the foot.

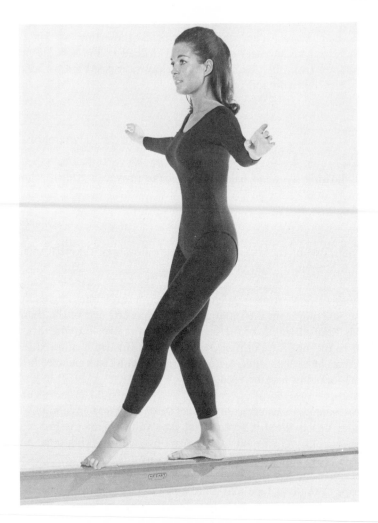

Figure 17-10.   Balance beam walk.

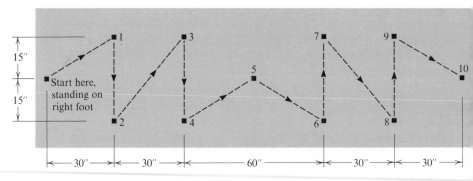

Figure 17-11.   Floor plan for the modified Bass test.

(He is allowed to reposition himself for the five-second balance on the ball of his foot after making a landing error.)

In addition the student sacrifices the remaining points at the rate of one point per second if he commits any of the following errors prior to the completion of the five seconds:

1.   Failure to keep any part of his body other than the ball of the supporting foot from touching the floor.

2.   Failure to hold his foot steady while in the balance position.

(When he loses his balance, the student must step back on the proper mark and then leap to the next mark.)

3. *Modified Sideward Leap Test.*   The validity of this test (Scott and French 1959) is accepted at face value. The original (unmodified) test has produced reliability coefficients ranging from .66 to .88 at different age levels. The floor plan is according to Figure 17-12.

The student starts the test by standing on one foot on spot X. He leaps to spot A, landing on the same foot, and balances in that position for five seconds. Then he leaps to either spot B or spot C and balances for five seconds. He repeats the test four times, twice to each side.

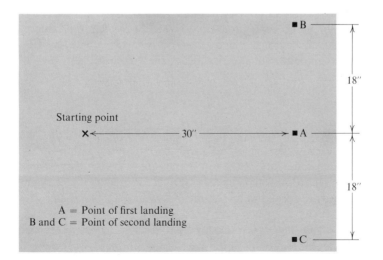

A = Point of first landing
B and C = Point of second landing

The student can earn up to 20 points on each trial for a total score of 80 points. He is awarded five points for landing correctly on spot *A*, five points for balancing five seconds on spot *A*, five points for landing correctly on either spot *B* or spot *C*, and five points for balancing five seconds on spot *B* or spot *C*.

Inverted Dynamic Tests

The objective of these tests is to measure how well the performer can balance while in motion in an inverted position.

1. *Tip-Up Walk Test.*   This test is the same as the tip-up test previously described in this chapter, except the student walks on his hands while in the tip-up position. His score is the number of feet he walks before losing his balance.

2. *Hand Walk Test.*   This test is the same as the two-hand balance test, except the student walks on his hands as far as possible. His score is the number of feet he walks before losing his balance.

Tests of Kinesthetic Perception

Kinesthetic perception is the sense that gives us an awareness of the body and its parts in space so that we can cause desired movements without using our five basic senses of smell, taste, touch, sight, and hearing; hence it is sometimes referred to as the sixth sense or the muscle sense. With this sixth sense we are aware of muscle contractions—the degree of contraction and the force of the contraction.

Tests of kinesthetic perception are designed to measure our ability to judge the positions and movements of our body parts without the use of the five basic senses. Hence these tests measure the effectiveness of the "sixth sense."

Distance Perception Jump

This test (Scott 1955) was designed to measure the ability of the performer to perceive distances without the use of his eyes, by concentrating on the feel of the jump. Validity and reliability of the test are accepted at face value. The test is useful for both sexes, age 10 through college age. A measuring tape, blindfolds, chalk, and marking tape are needed to test about 30 students in 40 minutes at each station.

Procedure: Two lines are placed on the floor 24 inches apart as illustrated in Figure 17-13. The student stands at the starting line and visually reviews the situation. Then he closes his eyes, pauses for five seconds, and jumps from the starting position trying to judge the distance of the jump so that his heels land on the target line (see Figure 17-13).

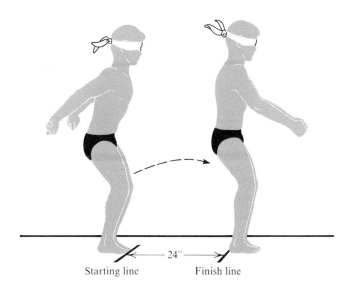

Starting line   Finish line

Figure 17-13.   Distance perception jump.

Scoring: The number of inches the student jumps between the target line and the heel farthest from the line is measured to the nearest quarter inch. The student has two trials, and his score is the total inches measured for the two trials.

Pedestrial Tests
of Size and Vertical Space

The purpose in these tests (Weibe 1951) is to measure the ability of the performer to position his feet without the use of his eyes. Validity and reliability of the test are accepted at face value. The test is useful for both sexes from age 10 through college age. With the same equipment as for the distance perception test and a 12-inch ruler about 30 students can be tested in 40 minutes at each station.

Procedure for the test of size: With his eyes closed or with a blindfold placed over his eyes, the student tries to spread his heels so the inside of the heels are 12 inches apart; at the same time he concentrates on the length of a 12-inch ruler and attempts to place his heels the correct distance from each other (see Figure 17-14).

Scoring: The student has three trials, and his score for each trial is the distance that the heels deviate from the preferred distance of 12 inches, measured to the nearest quarter inch. His final score is the total of the scores on the three trials.

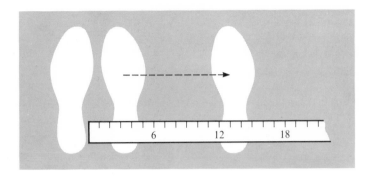

Figure 17-14.   Pedestrial test of size.

Procedure for the vertical space test: While blindfolded the student attempts to place the bottom edge of the shoe sole of one foot on top and parallel with a line drawn on a wall 14 inches above the floor (see Figure 17-15).

Scoring: The student has three trials, and his score for each trial is the farthest distance that the sole of the foot deviates from the line, measured to the nearest quarter inch. His final score is the total scores of the three trials.

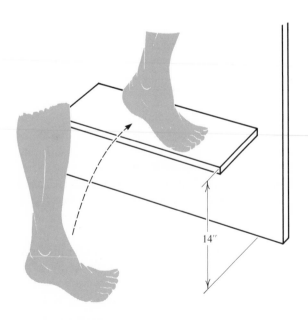

14''

Figure 17-15.   Pedestrial test of vertical space.

Tests of Horizontal
and Vertical Distances

The purpose in these tests (Wiebe 1951) is to measure the kinesthetic ability to determine specific positions along horizontal and vertical lines. The tests are suitable for both sexes age 10 through college age. With a measuring tape, yardstick, blindfolds, and marking tape about 25 students can be tested in 40 minutes at each station.

Procedure for horizontal space test: Figure 17-16 illustrates the physical arrangement for this test. The yardstick is placed on the wall so that it is at approximately

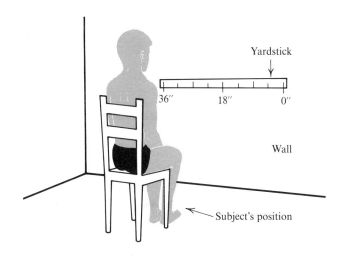

Figure 17-16. Horizontal space test.

eye level while the student is in the sitting position. The student sits on the chair facing the yardstick and attempts to establish in his mind a sense of its position. Then while blindfolded and without a practice trial he attempts to point the index finger of the right hand to the mark on the yardstick indicated by the instructor.

Scoring: The score is the deviation from the desired mark, measured to the nearest quarter inch. The final score is the total of the deviations on three trials.

Procedure for the vertical space test: Figure 17-17 illustrates the arrangement for this test. The yardstick is placed so that the 16-inch mark is about eye level for the student while he is sitting. The student sits on the chair facing the yardstick and attempts to establish in his mind a sense of its position. Then while blindfolded and

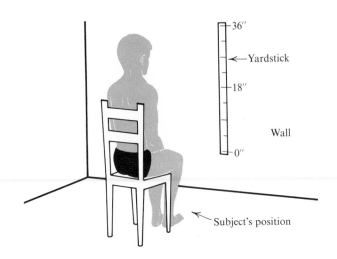

Figure 17-17.   Vertical space test.

without a practice trial he points the index finger of his right hand to the point indicated by the instructor.

Scoring: The score procedure is the same as for the horizontal space test.

Basketball Foul Shot Test

The purpose of this test (Jensen 1970b) is to measure the performer's ability to shoot foul shots accurately without using his eyes. In other words, the test measures kinesthetic perception in connection with foul shooting. Twenty-five students can be tested in 40 minutes at each station. The equipment includes a basketball standard, basketball, and blindfold at each testing station.

Procedure: The student stands at the foul line and shoots three trial shots. Then without moving from the line he blindfolds himself and shoots five additional shots.

Scoring: The student is scored for each shot as follows: 3 points if the ball goes through the hoop; 2 points if it strikes the hoop but fails to go through; 1 point if it strikes the backboard but misses the hoop; 0 points if it misses the backboard and the hoop. The final score is the total for the five trials.

Ball Throw Test

The purpose of this test (Jensen 1970b) is to measure the performer's ability to throw a ball a specified distance without using his eyes. In other words, the test

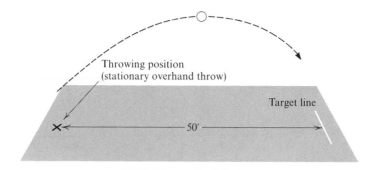

Figure 17-18.   Ball throw test of kinesthetic perception.

measures kinesthetic perception as it relates to throwing. Figure 17-18 illustrates the physical arrangement. Equipment needed is a softball and blindfold at each testing station. Thirty students can be tested in 40 minutes at each station.

   Procedure: The student stands on the starting line in a throwing position and reviews the situation carefully, trying to develop a sense of the distance to the target line. Then while blindfolded he attempts to throw a softball in such a way that it lands on the target line.

   Scoring: The student is allowed three trials, and his score for each trial is the distance the ball misses the target line, measured to the nearest foot. The final score is the total of the scores for three trials.

Bass Kinesthetic Stick Tests (Lengthwise and Crosswise)

   These tests (Young 1945) measure kinesthetic perception as it relates to balance. The tests are performed the same as the Bass stick tests (lengthwise and crosswise), except in this case the performer is blindfolded. The student is allowed three trials; the score for each trial is the number of seconds he maintains his balance, measured to the nearest second. The final score is the sum of the scores for the three trials.

How to Improve Balance and Perception

   Balance in certain positions is strongly dependent upon strength because the supporting muscles must be able to hold the weight and the body parts firmly in position. Therefore, in some cases balance will improve a limited amount as a result of increased strength. Agility, reaction time, and specific neuromuscular coordinations also contribute to balance. Agility, reaction, and coordination can all be increased limited amounts as discussed in Chapters 14, 16, and 18 respectively.

Once a person understands the basic principles that influence balance, the best way he can improve is through extensive practice of balancing in the particular position. In balance, as in many other aspects of performance, correct practice makes perfect.

In addition to agility, reaction, coordination, and strength, kinesthetic perception contributes to balance. Perception will increase with extensive and varied use of the neuromuscular system; however, the amount that perception can be increased and the best approach to increasing it are yet undetermined.

Selected References

Bass, Ruth I., "An Analysis of the Components of Tests of Semi-Circular Canal Function and of Static and Dynamic Balance." *Research Quarterly*, 1939, *10*.

Espenschade, Ann, et al., "Dynamic Balance in Adolescent Boys." *Research Quarterly*, 1953, *24*.

Estep, Dorothy O., "Relationship of Static Equilibrium to Ability in Motor Activities," *Research Quarterly*, 1957, *28*.

Jensen, Clayne R., Unpublished Studies of Tests of Balance, Brigham Young University, 1970a.

Jensen, Clayne R., Unpublished Studies of Tests of Kinesthetic Perception, Brigham Young University, 1970b.

Johnson, Barry L., and Leach, John, A Modification of the Bass Test of Dynamic Balance. Unpublished study, East Texas State University, 1968.

Russell, Ruth I., A Factor Analysis of the Components of Kinesthesis. Unpublished doctoral dissertation, State University of Iowa, 1954.

Scott, M. Gladys, "Measurement of Kinesthesis." *Research Quarterly*, 1955, *26*.

Scott, M. Gladys, and French, Esther, *Measurement and Evaluation in Physical Education*. Dubuque, Iowa: W. C. Brown Company, 1959.

Wiebe, Vernon R., A Study of Tests of Kinesthesis. Unpublished master's thesis, State University of Iowa, 1951.

Witte, Faye, A Factorial Analysis of Measures of Kinesthesis. Unpublished doctoral dissertation, Indiana University, 1953.

Young, Olive G., "A Study of Kinesthesis in Relation to Selected Movements," *Research Quarterly*, 1945, *16*.

18
Skill Tests

An individual's skill is his ability to perform a series of movements smoothly and efficiently, using all his muscles—agonists, antagonists, neutralizers, and stabilizers—in coordination. In other terms skill is the ability to use the correct muscles with the exact force necessary to perform the desired movements in the correct sequence and timing.

Relationship of Skills to Performance

Performance in any activity includes several specific skills. For example, good performance in basketball requires skill in jumping, shooting, running, throwing, catching, and dribbling. In soccer a player must be able to dribble, pass, screen, dodge, and kick effectively. Regardless of his other traits a person must learn the skills specific to a particular sport in order to become an effective performer. The development of specific skills is a paramount concern of physical education.

A skill test is used to measure specific skills which are essential to a particular activity. Once estimates of skill have been obtained this information can serve as a basis for determining the rate of student progress toward skill development for classifying students into groups for instruction and competition, and for selecting content of instruction. A highly useful skill test is relatively short, valid, and reliable. The following tests are useful to measure skill in particular activities.

Archery

Hyde Archery Test

Edith Hyde (1936) constructed standards of archery performance for college women in the Columbia Round. The Columbia Round, a standard event in archery, consists of 24 arrows shot at 50 yards, 24 arrows shot at 40 yards, and 24 arrows shot at 30 yards. The achievement scales which Hyde developed consist of three parts:

1. A scale for evaluating achievement in the first Columbia Round. This scale is used to evaluate the student's total score made in the first round after a minimum of practice, which might include 120 arrows shot at each distance—30, 40, and 50 yards.

2.   A scale for evaluating the student's score made in the final Columbia Round after an undetermined amount of practice in the event. It is best used toward the end of the archery season or at the end of an archery course.

3.   A scale consisting of three separate sections for evaluating the student's achievement at each of the distances (50, 40, and 30 yards) included in the round.

Procedure: The progress of beginning as well as advanced female students may be evaluated using the Columbia Round directions:

The student shoots the arrows in ends of six arrows each. She is allowed only one practice end for each distance and must shoot 24 arrows at each distance. She does not have to complete the entire test or round in one day but should finish at least one distance (24 arrows) each session.

Scoring: A standard 48-inch target face, shown in Figure 18-1, is used. The

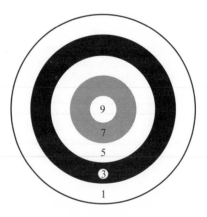

Figure 18-1. Archery target.

target has a gold center worth 9 points, an adjacent red circle worth 7 points, a blue circle worth 5 points, a black circle worth 3 points, and an outside white circle worth 1 point. The center of the gold circle is four feet from the ground. The student is given the higher value in scoring an arrow which cuts two colors. If an arrow goes completely through the target or if it bounces off the target, she receives an arbitrary score of 5 points for that arrow. Achievement scales for college women appear in Appendix B.

Badminton

Lockhart–McPherson
Badminton Volleying Test

This test (Lockhart and McPherson 1949) measures the badminton playing ability of college women. It may also be used effectively to classify college men and high school girls and boys for instruction and measurement of progress in skill development. As a test of badminton skill it has produced validity coefficients on two different occasions of .72 and .60. It has a reliability coefficient of .90.

A stopwatch, badminton racket, indoor shuttlecock (bird), and unobstructed wall space at least 10 feet by 10 feet are necessary. (If sufficient wall space is available, several students can be tested simultaneously.) One scorer is needed for each student being tested. Two to three minutes are required to administer the test to one person.

Procedure: A net line is marked on the wall at a height of five feet. A starting line is marked on the floor six feet six inches from the wall, and a restraining line is marked parallel to the starting line and three feet from the wall. The student stands behind the starting line. On the signal "go" she puts the shuttlecock into play against the wall with an underhand stroke, volleying the bird against the wall as many times as possible in 30 seconds. For a volley to count, the shuttlecock must strike the wall on or above the net line. The student may move up to the restraining line after serving the shuttlecock, but if she crosses the restraining line, the hit will not count. If she loses control of the shuttlecock, she should pick it up as quickly as possible and put it into play again with an underhand stroke from behind the starting line.

Scoring: The student has three trials, with each trial 30 seconds in length. The combined number of good hits during the three trials is the final score. A score may be interpreted in comparison with scores made by other students or with scores made by the same student on different occasions. The following scale rates college women:

Rating	Test Score
Superior	126 and up
Good	90–125
Average	62–89
Poor	40–61
Inferior	39 and below

French Short Serve Test

This test (Scott and French 1959) measures a student's ability to serve accurately and low in badminton. The test was originally designed for college women, but it may be used effectively for college men and high school boys and girls. A validity coefficient of .66 was reported with tournament rankings as the criterion measure. Reliability coefficients ranging from .51 to .89 have been obtained on different occasions.

A clothesline rope long enough to stretch between two net standards, a badminton racquet, and at least five shuttlecocks are needed at each testing station. Marks are placed on the badminton court as illustrated in Figure 18-2. About 10 students can be tested in 40 minutes at each station.

Procedure: The student stands in the service court diagonally opposite the target (see Figure 18-2). She takes 20 serves either consecutively or in groups of ten, trying on each serve to send the shuttlecock between the net and the rope, which is two feet above the net, into zone 5, near the intersection of the center line and the short service line.

Scoring: The zones are given point values of 5, 4, 3, 2, and 1, as indicated in Figure 18-2. The value of the area in which the serve hits is recorded as the score for that serve. A serve that does not pass between the net and the rope counts zero;

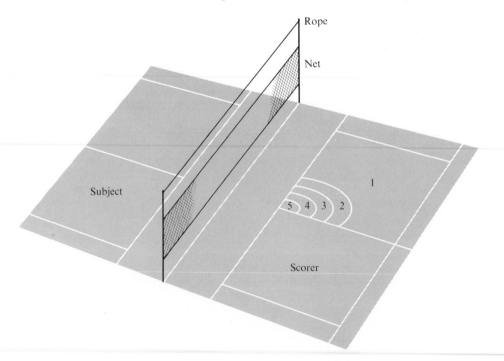

Figure 18-2.   French short serve test floor plan.

a serve that does not land in one of the five designated zones counts zero; and a serve that lands on one of the division lines counts the higher value. If the shuttlecock hits the rope, the trial does not count, and the serve is taken again. The final score is the total of the values made on the 20 serves.

Scott–Fox Long Serve Test

This test (Scott and French 1959) measures the student's ability to serve high and deep into the court in badminton. It is useful for college men and women and high school boys and girls. The test has a validity coefficient of .54 when compared to the subjective judgments of badminton experts. Reliability coefficients of .68 and .77 have been obtained.

Each testing area needs a racquet, at least five shuttlecocks, a rope, and two extra standards from which the rope can be stretched across the court at a height of eight feet and a distance of 14 feet from the net. Floor markings are placed on the court as illustrated in Figure 18-3. Ten students can be tested in 40 minutes at each station.

Procedure: The student stands in the service court diagonally opposite the target and serves the shuttlecock over the rope and into the corner of the court containing the target. He is allowed a total of 20 trials.

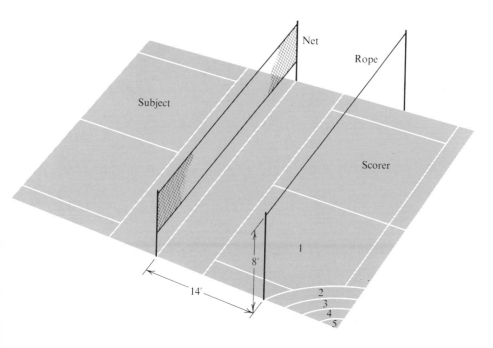

Figure 18-3. Scott–Fox long serve test floor plan.

Scoring: A score corresponding to the number of the zone in which the shuttle-cock lands is given for each serve. The final score is the sum of the scores for the 20 different serves. A serve that does not pass over the rope or one that falls outside the five zones is scored zero. Only legal serves count as trials.

French Clear Test

This test (French and Stalter 1949) measures a student's ability to perform the clear shot in badminton. It was originally designed for college women but can be used for college men and high school boys and girls. The test has produced a validity coefficient of .60 when correlated with tournament rankings. Its reliability rating is .96.

Each testing station needs a racquet, five shuttlecocks, a rope, and an extra set of standards from which the rope can be stretched across the court at a height of eight feet and a distance of 14 feet from the net. The court is marked as illustrated in Figure 18-4. About 10 students can be tested in 40 minutes at each station.

Procedure: The student stands behind the short service line on the court opposite the target. An experienced player serves the shuttlecock to the student who stands between two marks on the court. The student attempts to return the shuttle-cock using a clear shot that goes over the rope and lands near the end line. This procedure is repeated for 20 trials. The serve to the student should fall between the

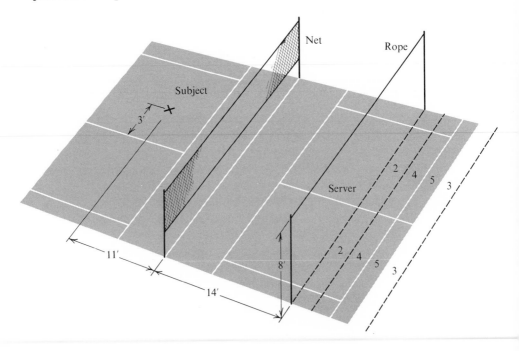

Figure 18-4.   French clear test floor plan.

two marks; if it is too short, too long, or falls outside the two marks, she should not return it. Only those serves that are played count as trials.

Scoring: The score for each trial is determined by the number of the zones in which the shuttle lands. The total score is the sum of the scores for the 20 trials. If the shuttlecock fails to pass over the rope, or if it lands outside the scoring areas, it counts zero.

Genevie Dexter (1949) checklist to rate performance in badminton

---

Student's Name_____Date_____Rated by_____
    Directions: Check appropriate items as you watch the student play badminton.

Desirable Performance	*Undesirable Performance*

_____Grips racket correctly	_____Fails to look at shuttlecock
_____Keeps eyes on shuttlecock	_____Strokes with stiff wrist or elbow
_____Uses wrist snap	_____Fails to return to good court position
_____Sends short serves low over net	after stroking
_____Sends high clear within three feet of	_____Runs around shuttlecock to avoid
back line	backhand shots
_____Places shots strategically	_____Uses drive strokes excessively
_____Starts strokes with same preliminary	_____Returns most shots to center of
movements	opponent's court
_____Uses variety of shots and a change of	_____Fails to use a variety of strokes
pace	_____Gives away direction and type of
_____Displays good footwork	shot to be made
_____Uses effectively a doubles system of	_____Starts late and moves slowly
teamwork	_____Gives no indication of definite
	partnership play in doubles

Other Useful Badminton Tests

There are other tests of skill in badminton in addition to those described here: the French–Stalter badminton test for college women (French and Stalter 1949) and the Miller wall volley test (Miller 1951).

Basketball

Stroup Basketball Test

This test (Stroup 1955) measures basketball playing ability of college men and high school boys. According to Stroup a high correlation exists between scores on this test and basketball playing ability in the game situation.

A regulation basketball standard, three basketballs, seven Indian clubs (or substitute markers), a running area 100 feet long, a solid wall against which a basketball may be bounced, and three stopwatches are necessary for each testing area. If one testing station is used for each test item, about 20 students can be tested in a 40-minute period.

Procedure: The test consists of three items to be performed as follows:

1. Standing at any position on the court, the student shoots as many baskets as possible in one minute. He must retrieve the ball himself after each shot. He is scored 1 point for each basket; his final score is the total number of points

2. Standing behind a line six feet from the wall, the student passes the ball against the wall as many times as possible in one minute. A pass is not counted if the student bats the ball instead of catching it or if he steps over the restraining line as he makes the pass. His score is the number of legal passes he makes in one minute.

3. The student dribbles the ball as he zigzags alternately to the left and right of seven Indian clubs placed in a line 15 feet apart for a 90 foot distance. He circles the end club each time and continues dribbling for one minute. A miss is counted if he knocks over a club, or if the club is not passed on the proper side. His score is the number of clubs he passes properly within the time limit. The starting line is 15 feet from the first Indian club.

Scoring: The raw scores for the three phases are converted to standard scores which may be averaged to obtain a final standard score. Achievement scales for boys and men are found in Appendix D.

Lehsten Basketball Test

The purpose of this test (Lehsten 1948) is to measure general basketball playing ability. It was developed for high school boys but is also useful for college men and women and high school girls. The original test consisted of eight items which were correlated with basketball playing ability as rated by five expert judges. The test has produced a validity coefficient of .80. When five of the eight items were correlated with all eight items, a coefficient of .986 resulted; therefore the final test consists of the five test items. Each item is administered at a separate station. About 25 students can be tested in 40 minutes at each station.

Procedure: The five specific test items are performed as follows:

1.   *Dodging Run.* See description on page 181.

2.   *Forty-Foot Run.* The student takes a position behind the out-of-bounds line at the end of the basketball floor. He starts from an upright position and runs 40 feet as rapidly as possible. His score is the time it takes him to run the distance, recorded to the nearest tenth of a second.

3.   *Wall Bounce.* A rectangular target two feet wide and four feet high is placed on a smooth wall with the lower limit of the rectangle three feet above the floor. The student stands six feet from the wall in front of the target. On the starting signal he bounces the basketball against the wall inside the target and then catches the ball on the rebound. (The ball should not bounce on the floor after the rebound.) The student repeats this bouncing and catching as many times as possible in 10 seconds. His score is the number of times he catches the ball as it rebounds from the wall within the 10-second period.

4.   *Vertical Jump.* See description on page 172.

Scoring: Each of the five tests are scored separately. Achievement scales for high school boys appear in Appendix C.

Leilich Basketball Test

This battery of tests (Leilich 1952) was designed for college women but is also appropriate for high school girls. Its purpose is to measure general basketball playing ability. The battery resulted from a factor analysis study covering all basketball tests available at the time. The factors included in the analysis were basketball motor ability, speed, accuracy in ball handling, speed in passing, and accuracy in goal shooting. Validity and reliability of the test have not been determined. When all stations operate simultaneously, about 25 students can be tested in 40 minutes.

Procedure: The three individual test items are conducted as follows:

1.   *Bounce and Shoot.* This test measures agility, ball handling ability, and speed and accuracy of shooting. Two marks are placed on the floor 18 feet from a basket as illustrated in Figure 18-5. Two basketballs are placed on two chairs adjacent to the two marks. On the starting signal the student picks up the ball from chair *A*, bounces the ball once as

he moves toward the basket, and then shoots. He catches the ball on the rebound and passes it to the person standing behind chair *A*. Then he runs to chair *B* and repeats the procedure until he has completed ten shots. He is allowed three trials and is scored on the best of these for accuracy and speed. His accuracy score is the total number of points he accumulates from his shots: two points for each basket, one point for hitting the rim but missing the basket, and no points for missing the rim and basket. His speed score is the total number of seconds he takes to complete the test.

2.   *Half-Minute Shooting.* This test measures accuracy and speed of shooting. The student stands near the basket, holding a basketball. On the signal he begins shooting and continues shooting for 30 seconds from any position on the floor. His score is the number of baskets he makes in 30 seconds. He is allowed two trials, and the better trial is the final score.

3.   *Push Pass.* This test measures speed and accuracy of passing. Figure 18-5, illustrates the arrangement for the test. The student stands behind the restraining line and passes the ball to the target using a two-hand push pass. He repeats this passing as many times as possible in a 30-second period. He must keep both feet behind the restraining line

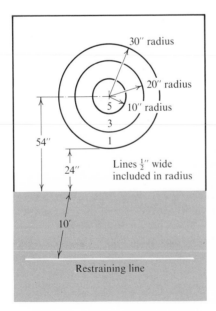 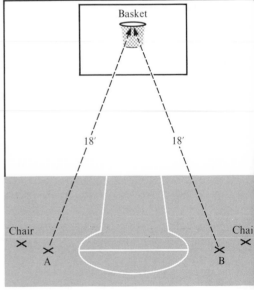

Figure 18-5.   Leilich basketball test floor plan.

when he passes the ball but may move forward of the restraining line to retrieve the ball. A ball that hits inside a given circle is scored by the value of that circle. A ball that strikes a line scores the higher value. The student is allowed two trials, and the better trial is recorded as the final score.

Scoring: Each of the three tests is scored separately. Achievement scales for college women appear in Appendix B.

In addition to the aforementioned tests the following tests are also useful measures of basketball skill: Achievement levels for women (Miller 1954), Albion basketball rating scale for college men (Voltmer 1940), Edgren basketball test for college men (Edgren 1932), Friermood basketball progress test for boys and men (Friermood 1934), Johnson basketball ability test for high school boys (Johnson 1934), Knox basketball test for high school boys (Knox 1947), LSU basketball passing test (Nelson 1967), and LSU long and short test (Nelson 1967).

Bowling

There have been no actual bowling skill tests reported. Performance in the game itself is the best measure of bowling skill. However, some interesting and useful norms have been developed and may be found in the Phillips–Summers bowling achievement scales for college women (Phillips and Summers 1950) and the Martin bowling norms for college men and women (Martin 1960).

Field Hockey

Friedel Field Hockey Test

This test (Friedel 1956) measures ball control and maneuverability of high school girls. The test is also useful for college women. It has a validity coefficient of .87 when correlated with the Schmithals–French hockey achievement test (Schmithals and French 1940). A reliability coefficient of .90 has been produced.

A field at least 30 yards long and 15 yards wide is needed as a testing area. (Several testing areas are recommended.) With a trained assistant who knows how to roll the ball into play the teacher can test five students at each station in a 40-minute period.

Procedure: The field arrangement should be according to Figure 18-6. An

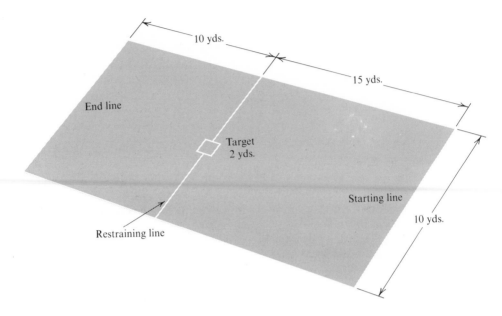

Figure 18-6. Friedel hockey test floor plan.

assistant to the teacher throws a ball either from the right or left corner, aiming toward the target area. (If it is not accurately aimed, the ball should be rolled again.) The student stands behind the starting line holding her hockey stick. On the signal she runs toward the target area to receive the ball which the assistant has rolled from one of the corners. Controlling the ball, the student passes the restraining line on the way to the end line. At the end line she turns around and drives the ball back to the starting line, keeping it within the 10-yard lane. She may follow the ball to drive it a second time if necessary. The student has 20 trials, 10 from each side.

Scoring: Each trial is timed from the beginning signal until the ball crosses the starting line on the return trip. The final score is the student's total times for the 20 trials.

Strait's Field Hockey Rating Scale

This scale, based on a five-point plan, is to be scored as follows:
Excellent (5 points)

1.   Is superior in stickwork

2.   Controls footwork consistently

3.   Controls ball excellently

4.   Passes are well timed and accurate

5.   Fouls very rarely

6.   Positions herself well

7.   Cuts to receive passes

8.   Takes advantage of nearly all opportunities

Good (4 points)

1.   Shows ability to make proper use of the stick

2.   Uses feet to good advantage most of the time

3.   Has ball under control most of the time

4.   Passes are well timed and accurate

5.   Fouls rarely

6.   Positions herself well most of the time

7.   Is able to see opportunities and take advantage of them

8.   Cuts to receive passes

Average (3 points)

1.   Shows skill in driving and fielding but lacks fine control of the ball for consistent dodges and tackles

2.   Does not make full use of the feet

3.   When in possession of the ball, occasionally loses it because of poor control

4.   Passes well on some occasions but is not well timed or accurate on others

5.   Fouls moderately often

6.   Is not sure as to where her position should be many times

7.   Misses some available opportunities

8.   Does not consistently cut for passes

Low (2 points)

1.   Drives weakly

2.   When fielding, often misses the ball

3.   Rarely tries dodges

4.   Tackles unsuccessfully

5.   Has feet sometimes in the way

6.   Has small degree of ball control

7.   Frequently passes with poor timing and accuracy

8.   Fouls fairly often

9.   Lacks good positioning

10.   Usually fails to take advantage of opportunities

11.   Is slow in getting to the ball.

Poor (1 point)

1.   Lacks general control of the stick

2.   Has feet in the way

3.   Rarely controls the ball

4.   Passes with poor timing and direction

5.   Fouls often

6.   Appears not to realize the benefits of good positioning

7.   Rarely takes advantage of opportunities

8.   Usually does not move to meet the ball

9.   Generally lacks body control

In addition to the aforementioned tests, the Schmithals–French Field Hockey Test for College Women (Schmithals 1940) is a useful test of skill in field hockey.

Football

There has been little done toward the development of objective skill tests in football. The only current work in this area is the AAHPER football skill test (see page 262). In addition the Borleske touch football test for college men (Borleske 1937) and the Brace football achievement test for college men (Brace 1943) may prove useful.

Golf

Clevett Golf Putting Test

This test (Clevett 1931) measures golf putting accuracy. It is useful for either men or women of practically any age.

A smooth carpet 20 feet long and 27 inches wide is marked as illustrated in Figure 18-7. Each zone is nine inches square; square 10 represents the hole. A putter and at least 10 golf balls are required. Validity and reliability of the test have not been determined. About 25 students can be tested at each station in 40 minutes.

Procedure: The student stands at the starting mark, which is approximately 15 feet from the hole and attempts to putt the ball into square 10. He is allowed 10 trials.

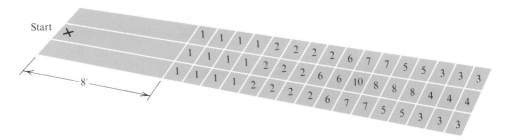

Figure 18-7.   Clevett golf putting test floor plan.

Scoring: The square in which the ball stops is the score for that putting trial. The total of the ten trials is the final score. Balls resting on a line are given the higher point value.

Nelson Golf Pitching Test

This test (Nelson 1967) measures the ability of the golfer to use the short irons in pitching close to the pin and it is suitable for men and women of practically any age. It has produced a validity coefficient of .86 when compared to judges' ratings and .79 when compared to golf scores. A reliability coefficient of .83 has been obtained with the test-retest method.

A target should be marked on the field as shown in Figure 18-8. The inner

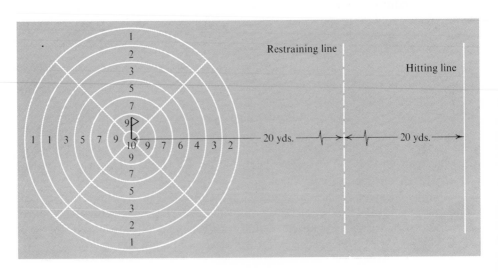

Figure 18-8.   Nelson golf pitching test floor plan.

circle of the target is six feet in diameter, and from the center of the target the radius of each circle is five feet wider than the radius of the previous circle. Hence diameters are 6, 16, 26, 36, 46, 56 and 66 feet. The target is divided into equal quadrants. A restraining line is marked 20 yards from the flag, and the hitting line is marked 40 yards from the flag. (As many as four stations can be set up around one flag.) The numbers for the particular sectors of the circle are shown in Figure 18-8. About 15 students can be tested at each station in a 40-minute period.

Procedure: The student stands behind the hitting line with the appropriate club (usually an 8 iron, a 9 iron or a wedge) and at least 13 balls. He is allowed three practice balls and then has ten official trials, trying to knock each ball as close to the flag as possible. A legal ball must be airborn until it passes the restraining line. Each swing is counted regardless of how far the ball goes or how poorly the ball was hit.

Scoring: The scorer stands close to the flag and records the value of each hit. The point value of the area in which the ball comes to rest is the recorded score. A ball resting on a line is given the higher point value. The score is the total point value for the 10 trials.

In addition to the Clevett golf putting test and the Nelson golf pitching test, the following tests are also useful measures of golf skills:

Cochrane indoor golf skills test (Cochrane 1960), McKee golf test (McKee 1950), Vanderhoof golf test (Vanderhoof 1956), and Vanderhoof rating scale for girls (Vanderhoof 1956).

Handball

Cornish Handball Test

Clayton Cornish (1949) developed this test to measure specific skills in handball. He selected five test items (30-second volley, front wall placement, back wall placement, service placement, and the power test) which correlated .694 with actual playing ability. Alone the power test correlated .58 with the criterion, and in combination with the 30-second volley test the power test correlated .67 with the criterion measure. Therefore, Cornish recommends that the power test be used with the 30-second test. About 15 students can be tested at each station in 40 minutes.

Procedure: The two recommended tests are performed as follows:

1.   *Power Test.* The floor of a court is divided into five playing areas as illustrated in Figure 18-9. The student stands in the service zone and

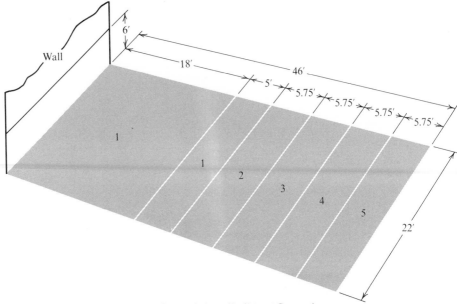

Figure 18-9. Cornish handball test floor plan.

throws the ball against the front wall, letting it hit the floor on the rebound before striking it. He then hits the ball as hard as possible, making sure it strikes the front wall below the six-foot line. He repeats this procedure until he has made five strokes with each hand. He has another trial if he steps into the front court or if the ball fails to hit the wall below the six-foot line. The score for each trial is the value of the scoring zone on the floor where the ball lands. The final score is the total points for the 10 trials.

2.   *Thirty-second Volley.* The student stands behind the service line, drops the ball to the floor, and volleys it against the front wall as many times as possible in 30 seconds. He should make all strokes from behind the service line, but if the ball fails to return to the service line, he may step forward of the line to play that particular stroke and then return behind the service line for the succeeding stroke. If he misses the ball, the instructor hands him another ball and he continues volleying. His score is the total number of times the ball hits the wall in 30 seconds.

Scoring: Each test is scored separately. Achievement scales are not available.

Rhythm Tests

Heaton Dance Rating Scale

This rating scale (Heaton 1965) applies to all dancers—beginners through advanced. One couple at a time dances across the floor. A maximum of nine points is possible for each fundamental. The points can be converted letter grades if one point is considered an F (failing), three points a D, five points a C, seven points a B, and nine points an A (excellent).

	1	2	3	4	5	6	7	8	9	Points	Grade
Posture											
Walking											
Rhythm											
Etiquette											
Position											
Leading											
Following											
Styling											
Relaxation											
Steps											

Total =

Square Dance Performance Test

In this test (Jensen 1968) the student performs each movement in the order listed. A check is placed on his score card opposite each movement performed correctly. (94–100 = excellent, 86–93 = good, 78–85 = fair, below 78 = poor).

A.   With a partner perform the following (4 points each):

_____1.   Do-si-do   _____5.   Balance

_____2.   All around left-hand lady   _____6.   Courtesy turn

_____3.   Seesaw   _____7.   Sashay

_____4.   Half-promenade   _____8.   Box the gnat

_____ 9. Swat the flea   _____11. Star thru

_____10. Frontier whirl   _____12. California twirl

B. With a partner and another couple do the following (4 points each):

_____1. Two ladies chain   _____ 8. Ocean wave

_____2. Pass thru   _____ 9. Swing thru

_____3. Cross trail   _____10. Bend the line

_____4. Right and left thru   _____11. Dixie chain

_____5. Right-hand star   _____12. Do-si-do

_____6. End turn in   _____13. Ends turn out

_____7. Substitute

Soccer

McDonald Soccer Test

This test (McDonald 1951) measures general soccer playing ability of college men, but it is also useful for high school boys. When results of the test were correlated with coaches' ratings of playing ability, validity coefficients ranging from .63 to .94 were obtained on different occasions. Reliability has not been established.

A wall or backboard 30 feet wide and at least $11\frac{1}{2}$ feet high is needed. A restraining line is drawn nine feet from the wall. With a stopwatch and three soccer balls about 15 students can be tested at each station in 40 minutes.

Procedure: At the signal, the student begins kicking the ball against the wall from behind the restraining line and continues to do so as many times as possible in 30 seconds. He may kick the ball on the fly or on the bounce, and may use his hands to retrieve it. However, to score a point he must make the kick from behind the restraining line. If the ball goes out of control, he has the option of playing one of the spare balls instead of retrieving the loose ball. The two spare balls are placed nine feet behind the restraining line. The student is given four trials.

Scoring: The score is the highest number of legal kicks in any one of the four trials.

This test (Johnson 1963) measures general soccer playing ability of college men. It is also useful for high school boys. The test has produced validity coefficients ranging from .58 to .98 on various occasions. It has a reliability coefficient of .92.

A backboard 24 feet wide and at least eight feet high is required. (This dimension is the same as that for a regulation soccer goal.) The restraining line is placed 15 feet from the wall. A ball container for spare balls is placed 15 feet behind the restraining line. About 18 students can be tested at each station in 40 minutes.

Procedure: The student holds a soccer ball while standing behind the restraining line. On the starting signal, he kicks the ball against the backboard, either on the fly or after a bounce. When the ball rebounds, he kicks it again and continues kicking the ball against the backboard as many times as possible in 30 seconds. He must kick the ball from behind the restraining line with a legal soccer kick. If the ball goes out of control the student may use a spare ball rather than chase the loose ball. The student has three 30-second trials.

Scoring: The score is the total number of legal kicks during the three trials.

In addition to the aforementioned tests the following are useful measures of soccer ability: Bontz soccer test for boys and girls (Bontz 1942), Shaufele soccer test for girls (Shaufele 1940), and Warner test of soccer skills (Warner 1950).

Softball

O'Donnell Softball Test

Doris O'Donnell (1950) designed this test to measure basic softball playing skills of high school girls. The test is also useful for college women and there is no reason why it could not be used for college men and high school boys. The total test consists of six items. O'Donnell suggests that two simplified versions should be considered, consisting of test items three, four, and six or test items three and four. With all six items included, the test has produced a validity coefficient of .91. Its reliability has not been established. When all six stations are operated simultaneously, about 30 students can be tested in 40 minutes.

Procedure: The six specific tests are performed as follows:

1.   *Speed Throw.* The student stands behind a restraining line 65 feet from the wall. On the starting signal she throws a ball as fast as possible at the wall. The score is the time that elapses from the starting signal

until the ball hits the wall. The student is allowed three trials, and the best is recorded to the nearest tenth of a second.

2. *Fielding Fly Balls.* Holding a softball, the student stands behind a restraining line six feet from the wall. On the signal she throws the ball against the wall and catches the rebound on the fly. She repeats this procedure as many times as possible in 30 seconds. The ball must strike the wall above a line 12 feet from the floor. The student must throw the ball from behind the restraining line but may catch it in front of the line if she desires. She is allowed one practice trial. Her score is the number of legal catches she makes in one official trial.

3. *Throw and Catch.* A rope is stretched eight feet directly above a starting line which is drawn on the floor. The student stands behind the starting line, throws a softball over the rope, and then runs and catches the ball. The objective is to cover the maximum distance and still catch the ball. The score is the distance from the rope to the position of the heel of the student's front foot at the time she catches the ball. The student is allowed one practice throw and three official throws. The score of the best official throw is recorded.

4. *Repeated Throws.* The student stands behind the restraining line which is 15 feet from the wall. On the signal she throws the ball against the wall, attempting to hit the wall above a line placed seven and one-half feet from the floor. She catches the ball on the rebound and repeats throwing the ball above the seven-and-one-half foot line as many times as possible in 30 seconds. She must make each throw from behind the restraining line. The score is the number of legal throws in 30 seconds.

5. *Fungo Batting.* Standing in the batter's box, the student tosses a softball into the air and bats it. A ball that lands in the outfield counts five points; one that lands in the infield, three points; and a foul ball, one point. The score is the sum of the points on 10 trials. Only tosses that are swung at count as trials.

6. *Overhand Accuracy Throw.* A target is drawn on a wall consisting of four circles with the center of the target two feet from the floor. The inner circle has a radius of three inches. The radii of the other circles are 11 inches, 21 inches, and 33 inches. The value of each circle from the center is four, three, two and one respectively. From a restraining line 45 feet from the target, the student throws 10 softballs at the target. The score is the number of points in the 10 trials.

Scoring: Each of the six tests is scored separately. Achievement scales are not available.

Fox–Young Batting Test

This test (Fox and Young 1954) measures batting distance and accuracy. Validity and reliability coefficients of .64 and .87 respectively have been recorded. Supplies needed at each testing station include a bat, a batting tee and eight softballs. About 20 students can be tested at each station in a 40-minute period.

Procedure: The student stands in the batter's box, places a ball on the tee, and knocks the ball as far as possible. He is allowed three practice trials and five official trials.

Scoring: Each trial is measured from the batter's box to the point where the ball first strikes the ground. The total score is the sum of the distances of the five official trials. (Experience and practice with a batting tee should be prerequisite for this test.)

Dexter Batting Test

The following scale (Dexter 1949) rates softball batting skill.

Dexter Batting Test

Student's Name_____Date_____
Rated by_____Score_____
Directions: First check the student's performance as good, fair, or poor on each item and then check deviations noted. Determine the student's score by assigning one point for poor, two for fair, and three for good; then total the points.

	Rating	*Deviations from Standard Performance*
1. Grip	_____Good _____Fair _____Poor	_____Hands too far apart _____Wrong hand on top _____Hands too far from end of bat
2. Preliminary	_____Good _____Fair _____Poor	_____Stands too near the plate _____Stands too far from plate _____Stands too far forward toward pitcher _____Stands too far backward toward catcher _____Feet not parallel to line from pitcher to catcher _____Rests bat on shoulder _____Shoulders not horizontal
3. Stride or footwork	_____Good _____Fair _____Poor	_____Fails to step forward _____Fails to transfer weight _____Lifts back foot from ground before swing

Dexter Batting Test *continued*

	Rating	Deviations from Standard Performance
4. Pivot or body twist	_____Good _____Fair _____Poor	_____Fails to "wind up" _____Fails to follow-through with body _____Has less than 90 degree pivot
5. Arm movement or swing	_____Good _____Fair _____Poor	_____Arms held too close to body _____Bat not held approximately parallel to ground _____Not enough wrist motion used _____Wrists not uncocked forcefully enough
6. General (Eyes on ball, judgment of pitches, and the like)	_____Good _____Fair _____Poor	_____Body movements jerky _____Tries too hard; "presses" _____Fails to look at center of ball _____Judges pitches poorly _____Appears to lack confidence _____Does not use suitable bat

Speedball

Buchanan Speedball Test

This test (Buchanan 1942), designed for high school girls, measures fundamental skills required in speedball. Validity and reliability ratings for the test are not available. When four stations are operated simultaneously, about 20 students can be tested in 40 minutes.

Procedure: The test consists of the following four specific tests:

1. *Lift to Others.* A volleyball, badminton, or tennis net is stretched between two standards so that the top of the net is two and one-half feet above the ground. The student stands behind a restraining line six feet from the net and attempts to lift the speedball with either foot, passing it over the net so that it lands within a three-foot square diagonally opposite from where he is standing (see Figure 18-10). He is allowed 10 trials and scores one point for each pass that lands within the proper square.

2. *Throwing and Catching.* A restraining line is marked six feet from and parallel to an unobstructed wall. On the starting signal the student throws the ball against the wall and catches it on the rebound as many times as possible in 30 seconds. The score is the average number of catches made in five trials.

3.   *Dribbling and Passing.* The field is marked according to Figure 18-10 with a starting line 60 yards from the end line of the field. Five Indian clubs or similar objects are placed in a line 10 yards apart, beginning at the starting line. At the end line two goals are marked, one to the right and one to the left of the dribbling course. The goal areas are six yards long, and their inner borders are four feet to the left and four feet to the right of the dribbling line. The student stands behind the starting line and on the signal starts dribbling the ball down the field. He dribbles to the right of the first Indian club, to the left of the second, and so on. Immediately after dribbling to the right of the last club, he attempts to kick the ball to the left into the goal area. He follows this procedure for 10 trials, five to the right and five to the left. Three scores are obtained: The dribbling score is the sum of the 10 trials in seconds; the passing score is the number of accurate passes (goals) made in the 10 trials; and the combined score is the sum of the times for the 10 trials recorded in seconds, minus 10 times the number of accurate passes (goals) on the 10 trials.

4.   *Kick-Ups.* For this test each testing station consists of a two-foot square with the inner side three feet from the sideline of the field. A

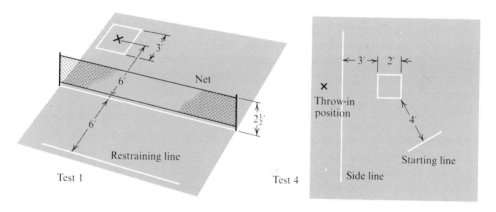

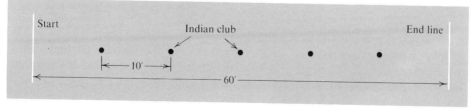

Figure 18-10.   Field plan for Buchanan speedball test (modified).

starting line is placed four feet from the outside corner of the square, following an imaginary extension of the diagonal of the square (see Figure 18-10). Two students work as partners with one student throwing the ball from behind the sideline directly opposite the square. The thrower tosses the ball from overhead so that it lands in the two-foot square. The performer (his partner) stands behind the starting line until the thrower releases the ball. At that instant, the performer runs forward and does a kick-up to himself. The score is the number of successful kick-ups in 10 trials.

Scoring: Each of the four items is scored separately. There are no achievement scales for the test.

In addition to the Buchanan speedball test the Smith speedball test (Smith 1947) is also a useful measure.

Swimming

Fox Swimming Power Test

This test (Fox 1957) measures the power of swimmers in the sidestroke and front crawl stroke. It was constructed especially for college women but is useful for high school girls and boys and for college men. Validity coefficients of .83 and .69 were reported for the sidestroke and crawl stroke respectively when the scores were compared with experts' ratings on swimming form. Reliability coefficients of .97 for the sidestroke and .95 for the crawl stroke have been reported.

A rope measuring about 20 feet longer than the width of the pool should be stretched across the pool at a distance of two feet from the end. One end of the rope should be attached to the bank while the other end remains free so that when the free end is released the rope will drop to the bottom of the pool. Adhesive tape, masking tape, or other such material is used for markers along the bank of the pool. The markers are placed at five-foot intervals beginning at the rope. About 30 students can be tested at each station in 40 minutes.

Procedure: With the starting point at the middle of the pool the rope is pulled tight so that it is about one foot under the water at the starting point. The student is in a floating position (on his side for the sidestroke, on his front for the crawl stroke) with his ankles resting on the rope. On the starting signal the rope is dropped, at which time the student begins swimming from a motionless float, taking six powerful strokes.

Scoring: The score for the sidestroke is the distance, measured to the nearest foot, from the starting line to the position of the ankles at the beginning of the recovery of the sixth stroke. The score for the front crawl stroke is the distance, measured to the nearest foot, from the starting line to the point where the ankles are when the fingers enter the water at the beginning of the sixth stroke.

Jack Hewitt (1949) constructed achievement scales for high school boys and girls, based on tests given to 1,093 high school students. To estimate the validity of the various items, Hewitt correlated the scores of the individual items with the total scores in all events. By this method the different items produced validity coefficients ranging from .60 to .94. By the test-retest method reliability coefficients of the different items ranged from .89 to .96. Hewitt recommends the sidestroke test as the best measure of high school swimming ability, in view of this test's .94 correlation with the total test scores. The number of swimming lanes available determines the number of students that can be tested in a 40-minute period.

Procedure: The test consists of three items:

1.   *Fifty-Yard Crawl Stroke for Time.* Using a racing dive the student swims the 50-yard crawl stroke as fast as possible. The time is recorded to the nearest tenth of a second.

2.   *Twenty-five Yard Flutter Kick for Time with Polo Ball.* The student holds onto the bank with one hand and the ball with the other. On the signal he pushes off from the bank, grasps the ball with both hands and swims 25 yards as fast as possible using the flutter kick only. The time is recorded to the nearest tenth of a second.

3.   *Twenty-Five Yard Glide Relaxation Swim.* Starting from in the water, the student pushes off from the bank and swims 25 yards in as few strokes as possible using the elementary backstroke. He repeats the same procedure using the sidestroke and the breaststroke. The score is the number of strokes used plus one for the push-off.

Scoring: Each test is scored separately. Achievement scales are available in Hewitt (1948).

This test (Hewitt 1948) consists of four items. Hewitt computed the validity of the individual test items by correlating each one with the total of the four items. By this method the validity coefficients for the individual tests ranged from .54 to .93. By the test-retest method the reliability coefficients ranged from .89 to .95. The number of swimming lanes available determines the number of students that can be tested in 40 minutes.

Procedure: The four test items are performed as follows:

1.   *Twenty or Twenty-five Yard Underwater Swim.* Using a regulation diving start from the bank, the student swims the full distance under water. The time is recorded to the nearest tenth of a second.

2.   *Fifteen Minute Endurance Swim.* Starting from in the water, the student swims continuously for 15 minutes, covering as much distance as possible. The score is the number of yards covered in the allotted time. The student does not receive a score if he fails to swim continuously for the time period.

3.   *Twenty-five or Fifty Yard Sprint Swims with the Crawl Stroke, Breast-stroke, and Backstroke.* Either the 25- or 50-yard distance is selected. Using a regulation diving start, the student swims the distance as fast as possible. The score for each swimming style is the time to the nearest tenth of a second.

4.   *Fifty-yard Glide Relaxation with the Elementary Backstroke, Sidestroke, and Breaststroke.* Starting from in the water, the student pushes off and swims the distance with as few strokes and kicks as possible. The score for each swimming style is the number of strokes taken plus one for each push-off. The objective is to get the lowest score possible.

Scoring: Each test is scored separately. Achievement scales are in Hewitt (1949).
In addition to the aforementioned tests the following are useful measures of swimming skill: Bennett diving test (Bennett 1942), Cureton test of endurance in speed swimming (Cureton 1935), and Wilson achievement test for intermediate swimming (Wilson 1962).

Tennis

Broer–Miller Forehand–Backhand Test

This test (Broer and Miller 1950) measures the tennis playing ability of college women. However, it can be used for college men and high school boys and girls. Validity and reliability of the test have not been determined.

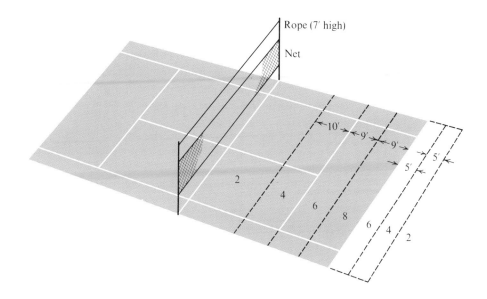

Figure 18-11.   Broer–Miller forehand–backhand test floor plan.

The court is marked with chalk lines and numbers indicating the point value of each zone, as shown in Figure 18-11. A rope is stretched across the court directly above the net at a height of seven feet. About 20 students can be tested at each station in 40 minutes.

Procedure: The student stands behind the baseline on the unmarked side of the court. He bounces the ball and hits it between the net and the rope, aiming for the nine-foot zone nearest the baseline on the opposite side of the court. He has 28 trials, 14 with the forehand and 14 with the backhand.

Scoring: Each trial counts the number of the zone in which the ball first lands. A ball that is obstructed does not constitute a trial and is taken over, but a ball that is missed on the first bounce constitutes a trial. Balls that go over the top of the rope are scored half the value of the zone in which they land.

Dyer Tennis Test

This test (Dyer 1935) measures the tennis playing ability of college women. It has also proved useful for college men and high school boys and girls. When results of the test were compared with experts' ratings, the test produced validity coefficients of .85 and .90; it has a reliability coefficient of .90.

A backboard or unobstructed wall space approximately 10 feet high and 15 feet wide is needed at each testing station as well as the following equipment: a stopwatch, a tennis racket, several tennis balls and a box for extra balls. About 15 students can be tested at each station in a 40-minute period.

Procedure: A line three inches wide is painted on the backboard to represent the height of a tennis net (36 inches from the floor to the top of the line). A restraining line 15 feet long, running parallel to the wall, is marked on the floor five feet from the wall. The box holding extra balls is placed at the left end of the restraining line (at the right end for left-handed players).

The students are divided into groups of four, and the students in each group are numbered one through four. They have the following responsibilities: student 1 takes the test; student 2 counts the points; student 3 watches for fouls at the restraining line; and student 4 collects the balls. The players rotate duties until all have performed the test three times.

Student 1 stands anywhere behind the restraining line holding a racket and two balls. At the starting signal he puts a ball into play by bouncing it on the floor and then hitting it against the wall so that it strikes above the net line. When it rebounds he hits the ball again. The objective is to volley the ball legally against the wall as many times as possible in 30 seconds. If he loses control of the ball, he quickly takes another ball from the box and puts it into play. After the ball rebounds, he may strike it again before it bounces, or he may let it bounce one or more times before striking it.

Student 2 counts the number of times the ball strikes the wall on or above the net line and enters the score of student 1 on the score card. If student 3 reports any infringements, student 2 deducts them before recording the score. A ball striking coincident with the word "stop" does not count.

Student 3 watches the player in relation to the restraining line and reports to the scorer (student 2) at the end of the trial the number of hits made while the player (student 1) was across the restraining line.

Student 4 collects the balls that have gone out of control and returns them to the box.

Scoring: The final score is the sum of the legal hits during the three trials. Ratings for college women appear below.

Ratings for Dyer Tennis Test

Rating	College Women	Women Majors Physical Education*
Superior	46 and up	79 and up
Good	38–45	58–78
Average	29–37	35–57
Poor	21–28	13–34
Inferior	20 and below	12 and below

* Based on scores made by 672 women physical education majors, Miller, Wilma, "*Achievement Levels in Tennis Knowledge and Skill for Women Physical Education Students.*" Unpublished doctoral thesis, Indiana University, 1952.

This test (Hewitt 1965) measures the general tennis playing ability of students and classifies them for instruction. It is useful for both males and females at college and high school levels. When scores on the test were compared to the results of a round-robin tournament, validity coefficients ranging from .68 to .73 were produced for beginning players and .84 to .89 for advanced players. With the test-retest method, reliability coefficients of .82 and .93 were produced for beginning and advanced players respectively.

A smooth wall 20 feet high and 20 feet wide is needed as well as the following equipment: a stopwatch, a tennis racket, and a basket with at least a dozen new tennis balls. A line one inch wide and 20 feet long is marked on the wall at a height of three feet from the floor to simulate the net. A restraining line about 20 feet long is placed 20 feet away from the wall. About 15 students can be tested at each station in 40 minutes.

Procedure: The student stands behind the restraining line with two balls in his hand. On the signal he hits one of the balls against the wall above the net line, using a stroke. When the ball strikes the wall, the timer starts the stopwatch. The student rallies the ball against the wall as many times as possible in 30 seconds, using any kind of stroke he desires. If the ball goes out of control, he serves the other ball. If the second ball goes out of control, he may take additional balls from the basket which should be close by. Each time he takes a new ball, he must put it into play with a service stroke. The student has three trials.

Scoring: One point is counted for each time the ball hits above the three-foot net line. No points are given for balls that strike the wall below the line or for balls that hit in front of the restraining line. A ball that hits on the net line counts. The average of the three trials is the final score.

This test (Hewitt 1966) measures a student's ability in the service, forehand, and backhand strokes. It can be used effectively for both males and females at college and high school levels. Based on the results with beginners, advanced, and varsity tennis players validity coefficients ranged from .52 to .93. The service placement test had the highest validity for varsity players, the revised Dyer wall test had the highest validity for advanced players, and the speed of service test had the highest validity for beginners. Reliability coefficients ranging from .75 to .94 have been obtained. About 20 students can be tested at each station in 40 minutes.

Procedure: Hewitt's achievement test consists of the following three test items:

1.   *Service Placement Test.* The court is marked as illustrated in Figure 18-12. A small rope is stretched above the net at a height of seven feet.

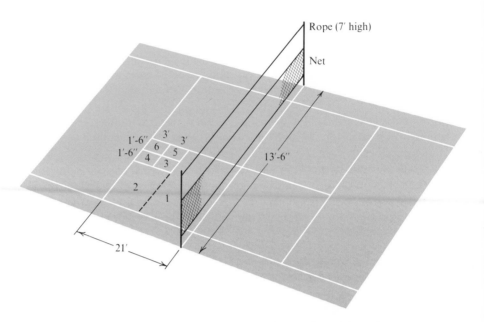

Figure 18-12.   Hewitt tennis service placement test layout.

Prior to administering the test the examiner should clearly describe it and demonstrate its procedure. A 10-minute warm-up should precede the performance of the test. From behind the baseline, the student serves 10 balls into the marked service court. The ball must pass between the net and the seven-foot rope. The score for each trial is the point value of the zone in which the ball hits. A ball that goes over the rope receives a score of zero. The student's final score is the sum of the points for the 10 trials.

2.   *Speed of Service Test.* Four zones are designated on the court as illustrated in Figure 18-13. The objective is to cause the ball to bounce a long distance after it strikes inside the service court. The student serves 10 balls. For each good serve the scorer notes the zone in which the ball hits after the first bounce. The number of that zone represents the score for that ball. The total score is the sum of the 10 serves.

3.   *Forehand and Backhand Drive Tests.* The court is marked as illustrated in Figure 18-14. A small rope is stretched above the net at a height of seven feet. The student taking the test stands at the center mark of the baseline, while the instructor, with a basket full of balls, takes a position across the net at the intersection of the center line and the service line (see Figure 18-14). The instructor (or a ball-throwing machine) hits five practice balls to the student just beyond the service court. Then the

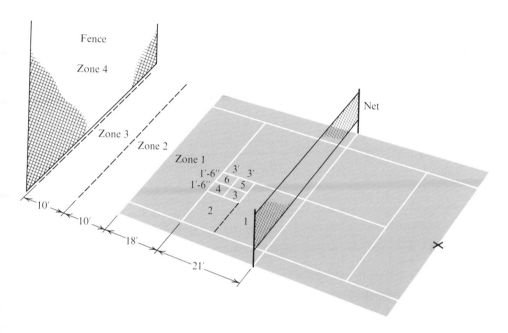

Figure 18-13.   Hewitt tennis speed service test layout

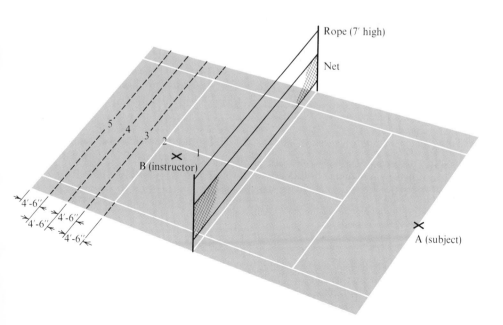

Figure 18-14.   Hewitt tennis forehand and backhand drive test layout.

student takes 20 official trials, 10 for the forehand and 10 for the back-hand. The student may choose which balls to hit forehand and which to hit backhand. He tries to hit the ball between the net and the rope so that the ball goes deep into the court. The same instructor should hit to all students in order to standardize the procedure as much as possible. The score for each trial is the number of the zone in which the ball lands.

Scoring: Each test item is scored separately. Achievement scales are not available.

Volleyball

Chamberlain
Forearm Bounce Pass Test

This test (Chamberlain 1968) measures the ability of college women to perform the volleyball bounce pass. A validity rating of 12.4 was determined with the use of Fisher's test of significance to determine the differences in performance by highly skilled and poorly skilled players. The test was found to be highly discriminative, with skilled players scoring high and poorly skilled players scoring low. The reliability coefficient was .78 with the use of the odd-even method. Both figures were significant at the .01 level of confidence.

Three ropes, standards to which the ropes can be attached, and three volleyballs are needed for each testing station. The floor markings are illustrated in Figure 18-15. About 15 students can be tested at each station in 40 minutes.

Procedure: A set-up person tosses the ball underhand between two ropes (5 feet and 7 feet high) to the student taking the test (see Figure 18-16). The performer makes a bounce pass which should go over the 10-foot rope and land on a target placed on the floor. She may move forward beyond the toss line to bounce pass the ball. The performer has 14 consecutive trials. She takes over a trial in which the ball hits any of the three ropes.

Scoring: The student scores two points if the ball travels over the 10-foot rope, and she receives additional points if the ball lands on one of the concentric circles of the target, which have point values of four, three, and two. The inner circle has the highest point value. For balls that land on a line between concentric circles the student scores the higher value. She does not score a target point if the ball fails to go over the 10-foot rope. A total of six points is possible for each trial when the height score is added to the target score.

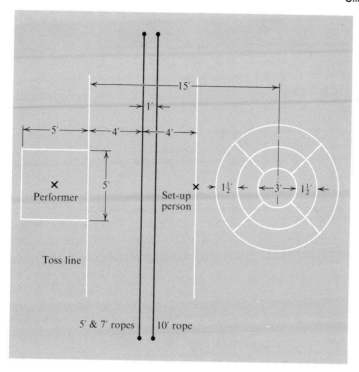

Figure 18-15. Floor plan for Chamberlain test (top view).

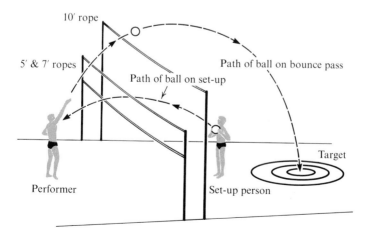

Figure 18-16. Floor plan for Chamberlain test (side view).

Brady Volleyball Test

This test (Brady 1945) is a relatively simple and practical test of general volley-ball playing ability. It is highly useful for classifying students for instruction or for measuring their progress in volleyball skill. Validity and reliability coefficients of .86 and .93 respectively have been established for the test. Each testing station should have a stopwatch, a volleyball, and a smooth wall at least 15 feet high, marked according to Figure 18-17. About two minutes is required for each person taking the test. Several testing stations may be used.

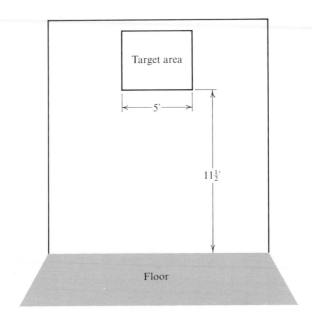

Figure 18-17.   Brady volleyball test floor plan.

Procedure: The student stands at the desired position in front of the wall. At the starting signal he throws the ball against the wall. As it rebounds he volleys the ball against the wall within the boundaries of the lines and continues the volley as many times as possible for one minute. If he catches or loses control of the ball, he starts as he did at the beginning of the test by throwing the ball against the wall. Only legal volleys that hit the wall within the rectangle on or above the 11-foot 6-inch line are counted. A legal volley is determined by the definition in the official volleyball rule book.

Scoring: The number of legal volleys in one minute constitutes the score. When the test is used for classifying students, the scores may be arranged according to size and then divided into as many subgroups as desired. As a basis for determining skill improvement, the difference in scores made by students before and after a program of instruction may be compared. When it seems desirable to take into account differences in the starting levels of the students along with the skill development, progress may be measured by computing the difference between the scores on the first test and the last test, then adding the score on the last test. For example, if a student scored 16 at the beginning of a unit of instruction and 24 at the end of the unit, his score would be $24 - 16 = 8$, plus 24. The total score would be 32. Achievement scales are not available for this test.

Clifton Single Hit Volley Test

This test (Clifton 1949) measures volleying ability of college women. It may also be used for college men and high school boys and girls. With experts' ratings of volleying as the criterion measure the test produced a validity coefficient of .70. With the test-retest method it produced a reliability coefficient of .83.

The test requires a stopwatch, an official volleyball, and a smooth wall. A line 10 feet long is placed on the wall seven and one-half feet above the floor. A restraining line ten feet long is placed on the floor seven feet from the wall. The ceiling should be high enough to permit ample space for volleying above the seven and one-half foot line. If the students are alternated so that the testing station is in continuous use, about 20 students can be tested at each station in 40 minutes.

Procedure: The student stands behind the restraining line and on the signal tosses the ball underhand against the wall. Then she volleys the ball as many times as possible above the seven and one-half foot line on the wall. All volleys must be legal hits, according to the official volleyball rules, and should be made from behind the restraining line. If she loses control of the ball, the student must recover it and put the ball back into play with an underhand toss from behind the restraining line. At the end of the first 30-second trial the student takes a two-minute rest after which she begins another 30-second trial.

Scoring: The score is the number of legal volleys touching on or above the seven and one-half foot line on the wall. No score is allowed for illegal hits or for hits made from on or in front of the restraining line. The total score is the sum of the scores for both trials.

Brumbach Volleyball Service Test

This test (Brumbach 1967) measures the student's ability to serve the volleyball low and deep into the opponent's court. A rope is stretched four feet above the volleyball net. (In most cases extensions will need to be attached to the standards.) The floor is marked as illustrated in Figure 18-18. About 20 students can be tested at each station in 40 minutes.

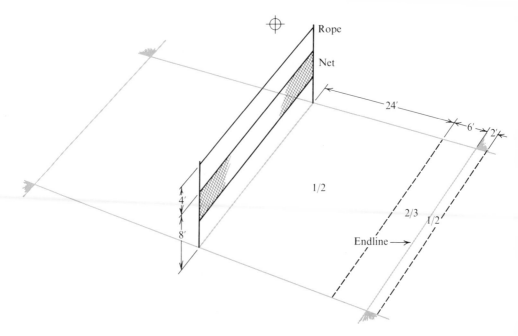

Figure 18-18.   Brumbach service test floor plan.

Procedure: The student stands behind the baseline. Without a practice trial he attempts to serve a volleyball so that the ball crosses the net without touching, goes underneath the rope, and lands in the opposite court. He tries to have the ball land as near the baseline of the court as possible.

Scoring: A ball that passes between the rope and net is given the higher of the two values for the particular zone in which the ball lands. A ball that goes over the rope receives the smaller value. A foot fault, a ball that hits the net, and a ball that lands outside the scoring zones count zero. The student is given 12 trials in two sets of six. The final score is the sum of the point values for the 10 best trials. A perfect score would be 30.

In addition to the aforementioned tests the following are also useful measures of volleyball skill: French–Cooper test for girls (French and Cooper 1937), Lamp volleyball test for boys and girls (Lamp 1954), Liba–Stauff test of volleyball pass (Liba and Stauff 1963), Russell–Lange volleyball test for girls (Russell and Lange 1954), and Wisconsin volleyball test for women (Basset, Glassow, and Locke 1937).

AAHPER Skill Tests

Under the guidance of a skill test committee appointed by the Board of Directors, the American Association of Health, Physical Education and Recreation has developed several specific skill tests and has published a manual for each test. Each test manual includes introductory information, instructions for administering the test, descriptions of the test items, and achievement scales based on a nationwide sample.[1] Manuals on the following activities are available.

Archery for Boys and Girls

10-yard shooting test
20-yard shooting test
30-yard shooting test

Basketball for Boys

Front shot
Side shot
Foul shot
Under basket shot
Speed pass
Jump and reach
Overarm pass for accuracy
Push pass for accuracy
Dribble

Basketball for Girls

Front shot
Side shot
Foul shot
Under basket shot
Speed pass
Jump and reach
Overarm pass for accuracy
Push pass for accuracy
Dribble

[1] Each manual, approximately 40 pages in length, may be obtained from **AAHPER** at a cost of $.75.

Football

Forward pass for distance
Fifty-yard run with football
Blocking
Forward pass for accuracy
Football punt for distance
Ball changing zigzag run
Catching the forward pass
Pull-out
Kick-off
Dodging run

Softball for Boys

Throw for distance
Overhand throw for accuracy
Underhand pitching
Speed throw
Fungo hitting
Base running
Fielding ground balls
Catching fly balls

Softball for Girls

Throw for distance
Overhand throw for accuracy
Underhand pitching
Speed throw
Fungo hitting
Base running
Fielding ground balls
Catching fly balls

Volleyball for Boys and Girls

Volleying
Serving
Passing
Set-up

How to Increase Skill

An individual's skill is his ability to perform a combination of specific movements smoothly and efficiently, using his agonist, antagonist, neutralizer, and stabilizer muscles in effective coordination. In other terms skill is the ability to use the correct muscles at the correct time with the exact force necessary to perform the desired movements in the proper sequence. Athletic performance consists of several specific skills, each of which involves one or more movements of body segments. Therefore, to take a systematic and effective approach to improving performance, a person must analyze the specific skills composing the performance and then attempt to improve each skill. For example, basketball is composed of such specific skills as shooting, running, rebounding, jumping, dodging, pivoting, dribbling, passing, and catching. A person may improve his basketball performance in general by improving one or all of the specific skills involved in the activity.

Hence the problem is to identify the specific skills in a performance and then to employ effective techniques in the effort to improve the skills. Essentially an individual improves his skill by determining the correct mechanics and incorporating them into the performance. The individual must practice a specific skill correctly until his pattern of movement becomes naturally smooth and efficient. In addition to such practice the performer may increase his skill by better judgment of speed, distance, and time and by better insight into the environmental circumstances related to the performance.

Selected References

Barrow, Harold M., and McGee, Rosemary, *A Practical Approach to Measurement in Physical Education*. Philadelphia: Lea & Febiger, 1966.

Basset, Gladys, Glassow, Ruth, and Locke, Mabel, "Studies Testing Volleyball Skills. *Research Quarterly*, 1937, *8*, 61.

Bennett, LaVerne Means, "Diving Ability on the Springboard." *Research Quarterly*, 1942, *13*, 109.

Bontz, Jean, An Experiment in the Construction of a Test for Measuring Ability in Some of the Fundamental Skills Used by Fifth and Sixth Grade Children in Soccer. Unpublished master's thesis, State University of Iowa, 1942.

Borleske, S. C., "A Study of Achievement of College Men in Touch Football." *Research Quarterly*, 1937, *8*, 73.

Brace, David K., "Validity of Football Achievement Tests as Measures of Motor Learning and as a Partial Basis for the Selection of Players." *Research Quarterly*, 1943, *14*, 372.

Brady, George F., "Preliminary Investigations of Volleyball Playing Ability." *Research Quarterly*, 1945, *16*, 14–17.

Broer, Marion R., and Miller, Donna M., "Achievement Tests for Beginning and Intermediate Tennis." *Research Quarterly*, 1950, *21*, 303.

Brumbach, Wayne, *Beginning Volleyball, A Syllabus for Teachers*, rev. ed. Eugene, Ore.: Wayne Baker Brumbach (distributed by University of Oregon), 1967.

Buchanan, Ruth E., A Study of Achievement Tests in Speedball for High School Girls. Unpublished master's thesis, State University of Iowa, 1942.

Chamberlain, Diane, Determination of Validity and Reliability of a Skill Test for the Bounce Pass in Volleyball. Unpublished master's thesis, Brigham Young University, 1968.

Clarke, H. Harrison, *Application of Measurement to Health and Physical Education*, 4th ed. Englewood Cliffs, N.J.: Prentice-Hall, 1967.

Clevett, Melvin A., "An Experiment in Teaching Methods in Golf." *Research Quarterly*, 1931, *2*, 104.

Clifton, Marguerite A., "Single Hit Volley Test for Women's Volleyball." *Research Quarterly*, 1949, *33*, 208–11.

Cochrane, June Fleurette, The Construction of an Indoor Golf Skills Test as a Measure of Golfing Ability. Unpublished master's thesis, University of Minnesota, 1960.

Cornish, Clayton, "A Study of Measurement of Ability in Handball." *Research Quarterly*, 1949, *20*, 215–22.

Cureton, Thomas K., "A Test for Endurance in Speed Swimming." *Supplement to the Research Quarterly*, 1935, *6*, 106.

Dexter, Genevie, *Teachers' Guide to Physical Education for Girls in High School*. Sacramento, Calif.: State Department of Education, 1949.

Dexter, Genevie, *Teachers' Guide to Physical Education for Girls in High School*. Sacramento, Calif.: State Department of Education, 1957, p. 316.

Dyer, Joanna T., "The Backboard Test of Tennis Ability." *Supplement to the Research Quarterly*, 1935, *6*, 63.

Edgren, J. D., "An Experiment in Testing Ability and Progress in Basketball." *Research Quarterly*, 1932, *3*, 159.

French, Esther L., and Cooper, Bernice I., "Achievement Tests in Volleyball for High School Girls." *Research Quarterly*, 1937, *8*, 150.

French, Esther, and Stalter, Evelyn, "Study of Skill Tests in Badminton for College Women." *Research Quarterly*, 1949, *20*, 257.

Friedel, Jean, The Development of a Field Hockey Skill Test for High School Girls. Microcarded master's thesis, Illinois State Normal University, 1956.

Friermood, John T., "Basketball Progress Tests Adapted to Class Use." *Journal of Health and Physical Education*, 1934, *5*, 45.

Fringer, Margaret Neal, A Battery of Softball Skill Tests for Senior High School Girls. Unpublished master's thesis, University of Michigan, 1969.

Fox, Margaret G., "Swimming Power Test." *Research Quarterly*, 1957, *23*, 233, 237.

Fox, Margaret G., and Young, Olive G., "A Test of Softball Batting Ability." *Research Quarterly*, 1954, *25*, 26.

Glasgow, Ruth B., Colvin, V., and Schwarz, M. M., "Studies in Measuring Basketball Playing Ability of College Women." *Research Quarterly*, 1938, *9*, 60.

Heaton, Alma, *Techniques of Teaching Ballroom Dance.* Provo, Utah: Brigham Young University Press, 1965.

Hewitt, Jack E., "An Achievement Scale in Archery." *Research Quarterly*, 1936, *7*, 64–73.

Hewitt, Jack E., "Achievement Scale Scores for High School Swimming." *Research Quarterly*, 1949, *20*, 170–79.

Hewitt, Jack E., "Hewitt's Tennis Achievement Test." *Research Quarterly*, 1966, *37*, 321–27.

Hewitt, Jack E., "Swimming Achievement Scale Scores for College Men." *Research Quarterly*, 1948, *19*, 282–89.

Hewitt, Jack E., "Revision of the Dyer Backboard Tennis Test." *Research Quarterly*, 1965, *36*, 153–57.

Hyde, Edith I., "National Research Study in Archery." *Research Quarterly*, 1936, *7*, 64–73.

Jensen, Clayne R., and Jensen, Mary Bee, *Beginning Square Dance.* Belmont, Calif.: Wadsworth Publishing Company, 1968.

Johnson, Barry L., and Nelson, Jack K., *Practical Measurements for Evaluation in Physical Education.* Minneapolis: Burgess Publishing Company, 1969.

Johnson, Joseph R., The Development of a Single-Item Test as a Measure of Soccer Skill. Microcarded master's thesis, University of British Columbia, 1963.

Johnson, L. William, Objective Tests in Basketball for High School Boys. Unpublished master's thesis, State University of Iowa, 1934.

Knox, R. O., "Basketball Ability Tests," *Scholastic Coach*, 1947, *17*, 45.

Lamp, Nancy A., "Volleyball Skills of Junior High School Students as a Function of Physical Size and Maturity." *Research Quarterly*, 1954, *25*, 189.

Lehsten, Nelson, "A Measure of Basketball Skills in High School Boys." *The Physical Educator*, 1948, *4*, 103.

Leilich, Avis, The Primary Components of Selected Basketball Tests for College Women. Unpublished doctoral dissertation, Indiana University, 1952.

Liba, Marie R., and Stauff, Marilyn R., "A Test for the Volleyball Pass." *Research Quarterly*, 1963, *34*, 56–63.

Lockhart, Aileene, and McPherson, Frances A., Development of a Test of Badminton Playing Ability. *Research Quarterly*, 1949, *20*, 402–5.

Martin, Joan L., "Bowling Norms for College Men and Women." *Research Quarterly*, 1960, *31*, 113.

Mathews, Donald K., *Measurement in Physical Education.* Philadelphia: W. B. Saunders Company, 1963.

McCloy, Charles H., and Young, Norma D., *Tests and Measurements in Health and Physical Education.* New York: Appleton-Century-Crofts, 1954.

McDonald, Lloyd G., The Construction of a Kicking Skill Test as an Index of General Soccer Ability. Unpublished master's thesis, Springfield College, 1951.

McKee, Mary E., "A Test for the Full Swinging Shot in Golf." *Research Quarterly*, 1950, *21*, 40.

Meyers, Carlton R., and Blesh, T. Erwin, *Measurement in Physical Education*. New York: The Ronald Press, 1962.

Miller, Frances A., "A Badminton Wall Volley Test." *Research Quarterly*, 1951, *22*, 208.

Miller, Wilma K., "Achievement Levels in Basketball Skills for Women Physical Education Majors." *Research Quarterly*, 1954, *25*, 450.

Nelson, Jack K., An Achievement Test for Golf. Unpublished study, Louisiana State University, 1967.

Nelson, Jack K., The Measurement of Shooting and Passing Skills in Basketball. Unpublished study, Louisiana State University, 1967.

O'Donnell, Doris J., Validation of Softball Skill Tests for High School Girls. Unpublished master's thesis, Indiana University, 1950.

Phillips, Marjorie, and Summers, Dean, "Bowling Norms and Learning Curves for College Women." *Research Quarterly*, 1950, *21*, 377.

Russell, Naomi, and Lange, Elizabeth, "Achievement Tests in Volleyball for Junior High School Girls." *Research Quarterly*, 1954, *25*, 189.

Schmithals, Margaret, and French, Esther, "Achievement Tests in Field Hockey for College Women." *Research Quarterly*, 1940, *11*, 84.

Scott, M. Gladys, and French, Esther. *Measurement and Evaluation in Physical Education*. Dubuque, Iowa: William C. Brown Company Publishers, 1959, pp. 199–202.

Shaufele, Evelyn F., The Establishment of Objective Tests for Girls of the Ninth and Tenth Grades to Determine Soccer Ability. Unpublished master's thesis, State University of Iowa, 1940.

Smith, Gwen, Speedball Skill Tests for College Women. Unpublished study, Illinois State Normal University, 1947.

Strait, C. Jane, The Construction and Evaluation of a Field Hockey Skills Test. Unpublished master's thesis, Smith College, 1960.

Stroup, Francis, "Game Results as a Criterion for Validating Basketball Skill Tests." *Research Quarterly*, 1955, *26*, 353.

Vanderhoof, Ellen R., Beginning Golf Achievement Tests. Microcarded master's thesis, University of Oregon, 1956.

Voltmer, E. F., and Watts, T., "A Rating Scale of Player Performance in Basketball." *Journal of Health and Physical Education*, 1940, *11*, 94.

Warner, Glenn F. H., "Warner Soccer Test," *Newsletter of the National Soccer Coaches Association of America*, 1950, *6*, 13–22.

Wilson, Marcia Ruth, A Relationship Between General Motor Ability and Objective Measures of Achievement in Swimming at the Intermediate Level for College Women. Unpublished master's thesis, The Women's College of the University of North Carolina, 1962.

Young, Genevieve, and Moser, Helen, "A Short Battery of Tests to Measure Playing Ability in Women's Basketball." *Research Quarterly*, 1934, *5*, 3.

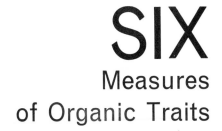

SIX
Measures
of Organic Traits

Organic measures are concerned with the efficiency of the organic systems. The more useful measures deal with the efficiency of the circulatory and the respiratory systems, which function in direct support of muscular functions.

19

Tests of
Circulorespiratory Endurance

The trait that enables a person to continue a vigorous activity over a period of time is referred to as endurance. It is the ability of an individual to resist fatigue and to recover quickly after fatigue. Circulorespiratory endurance is the ability of the individual's circulatory and respiratory systems to resist fatigue while they effectively support vigorous muscular activity.

Relationship of Endurance to Performance

Physiologists generally agree that the main limitation in short duration endurance performances is the supply of oxygen to the working muscles. The circulorespiratory system is directly responsible for supplying oxygen to the tissues and to keep the tissues free of carbon dioxide and other waste products. Therefore circulorespiratory endurance is essential to prolonged vigorous exercise. When endurance gives way to fatigue as a result of exercise, several elements important to good performance diminish: strength, coordination, timing, speed of movement, reaction time, and alertness. Increased endurance prolongs the onset of fatigue; therefore endurance contributes to improved performance in activities where fatigue is a limiting factor.

Circulorespiratory Tests

The measurement of circulorespiratory endurance has proved difficult because endurance can be measured accurately only if the organism is worked to complete fatigue—neither a feasible nor a prudent practice. As a substitute, tests estimating endurance have been devised, but they do not always furnish highly accurate results. At best they are only indicators of endurance. This word of caution is not to imply that the tests are not useful; they are valuable as screening devices to identify extreme weakness in endurance, and they serve as an endurance indicator for the performer. With wise use and interpretation these tests serve a worthwhile purpose in school programs.

Circulorespiratory tests measure the durability and efficiency of the circulatory and respiratory systems. In other words they measure the ability of these systems to carry on their functions under strenuous demands. Circulorespiratory tests are usually based on the variables of pulse rate and blood pressure. Supposedly the amount of change in these variables, as a result of a given amount of work, indicates the condition of the total circulorespiratory system. The condition of the circulorespiratory system is generally a good indicator of endurance of the total body.

Measuring Pulse
Rate and Blood Pressure

Certain circulorespiratory tests should be administered and interpreted cautiously because rest, food intake, body position, activity, time of day, and emotional changes may alter pulse rate and blood pressure.

Pulse Rate.   The average pulse rate of adults in general is 72 beats per minute, with a range of about 35 to 110 beats per minute. Children have faster than average pulse rates, as do elderly people. On the average, men have slower pulse rates than women, and well-conditioned people have slower pulse rates than poorly conditioned people. Pulse rate can best be measured by lightly pressing the middle finger against the axillary artery in the wrist (see Figure 19-1) or against the carotid artery in the

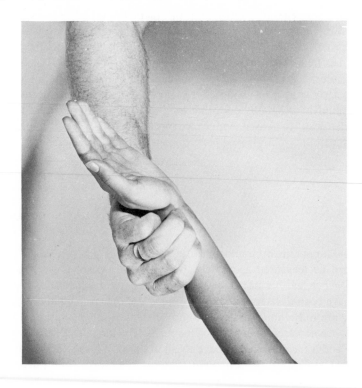

Figure 19-1.   Pulse rate being taken at the wrist.

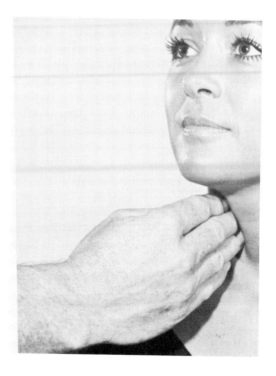

Figure 19-2. Pulse rate being taken at the neck.

neck (see Figure 19-2). The beat should be counted for 30 seconds; then the number of beats multiplied by two to give the pulse rate per minute.

Blood Pressure. The measurement of systolic and diastolic blood pressure is relatively simple with the use of a sphygmomanometer and a stethoscope; however, like most testing, such measurement requires considerable practice for proficiency.

The tester wraps the cuff of the sphygmomanometer around the bare arm above the elbow of the person being tested. With the earphones of the stethoscope in his ears tester places the bell of the stethoscope on the brachial artery just above the hollow of the elbow of the person being tested and pumps up the cuff until the artery collapses and he hears no pulse beat (see Figure 19-3). Then the tester slowly releases pressure as he watches the gauge or mercury column. When he hears the first sound of the pulse, he notes the reading in millimeters of mercury at that instant. This reading is the systolic pressure. The tester continues slowly to release pressure until he notes a dull, weak beat. At that instant he notes the pressure in millimeters of mercury. This reading represents the diastolic pressure. He records the measures, with the systolic pressure first and then the diastolic pressure. A typical reading might be 120/80.

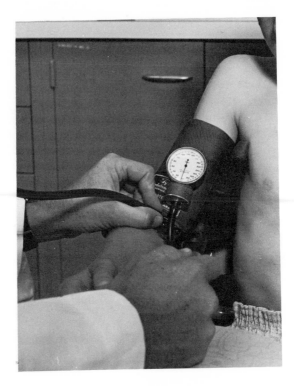

Figure 19-3.   Measurement of blood pressure.

Cooper Twelve Minute Run–Walk Test

Kenneth Cooper (1968) did extensive research on which to base a rating scale for evaluating activities in terms of circulorespiratory conditioning. His research showed the importance of such vigorous activities as running, swimming, cycling, walking, handball, basketball, and squash in the development of circulorespiratory endurance. Cooper developed the 12-minute run–walk test and scale as a simple method of self-evaluation of circulorespiratory fitness. A validity coefficient of .90 has been reported when maximum oxygen uptake was used as the criterion. Using the test-retest method a reliability coefficient of .94 has been reported.

Procedure: The test consists of running, or running and walking, as great a distance as possible in 12 minutes. The route can be measured by running around a standard length track, by using an automobile odometer, or by carrying a pedometer.

Scoring: The score is the total distance covered in 12 minutes. The score may be interpreted by applying it to the following scale:

12-Minute Run–Walk—Scoring Scale*

Distance covered	Fitness level
Less than 1 mile	Very poor
1–1.25 miles	Poor
1.25–1.50 miles	Fair
1.50–1.75 miles	Good
More than 1.75 miles	Excellent

* For men over 35, 1.4 miles is good; for women, 1.3.

600-Yard Run–Walk

This test (*Youth Fitness Test Manual* 1961) measures a combination of running speed and endurance. It requires a track or large field, a starting pistol or whistle, and a stopwatch for each contestant. Several students can perform the test at once. Often one watch is used to time more than one student by reading the times as each student crosses the finish line. Validity and reliability of the test have not been established.

Procedure: On the starting signal the student begins to run at his desired pace. He may interchange running and walking as he desires. His objective is to cover the distance in the shortest possible time.

Scoring: The score is the time required to cover the distance, measured in minutes and seconds. Percentile scales for girls and women appear in Appendix B; for boys in Appendix C; and for college men in Appendix D.

440-Yard Run

This test measures a combination of running speed and endurance, with considerable emphasis on speed. It requires the same equipment and same organization as the 600-yard run–walk test.

Procedure: On the starting signal the student begins to run at a pace he considers best for over a 440-yard distance. He runs the distance in the shortest possible time.

Scoring: The score is the time required for the student to run the distance, measured to the nearest tenth of a second. Achievement scales for high school boys and men appear in Appendix C and D respectively.

Squat Thrust for One Minute

Squat thrusts for 10 seconds is considered a test of agility. When they are performed for one minute, squat thrusts measure endurance. Validity and reliability of the test have not been established. A large number of students can be tested at one time if they are arranged in pairs so they can score each other.

Procedure: A description of how to organize the students for the test and how to execute the squat thrust may be found on page 178.

Scoring: The score is the number of squat thrusts the student performs in one minute. Achievement scales are not available.

Harvard Step Test

The Harvard step test (Brouha 1943) measures the ability of adult males to perform hard muscular work. The test consists of the student's stepping up and down on a bench in the prescribed manner for a period of five minutes. There must be one examiner for each student being tested. The examiner stands close to the student to make sure the student performs the test correctly. Scoring is based on the student's pulse rate taken at prescribed times after exercise, combined with the length of time that the student performs. A stopwatch and bench or platform 20 inches high are necessary. If a group of students is to be tested, a wall clock with a sweep second hand may be preferred. With the necessary number of benches and leaders several students can be tested every 10 minutes. The test may be administered in slightly less than 10 minutes if the rapid form of scoring is used. Testing more than 20 students at one time is not recommended. Ratings of validity and reliability have not been established.

Procedure: The student stands facing the bench and at the starting signal begins the exercise (see Figure 19-4). He places one foot on the bench, then steps up and places the other foot beside the first one. He straightens his back and legs to an erect standing position, then immediately steps down again, one foot at a time, leading with the foot that stepped up first. The student continues to step up and down in this manner, keeping time with the cadence of 30 steps per minute, which is counted aloud as, Up, 2, 3, 4, Up, 2, 3, 4, and so on. He may change his lead foot if one leg tires. The student continues this procedure until he is halted at the end of five minutes or until he can continue no longer; he then turns around and sits quietly on the bench.

Forty-five seconds after the end of the exercise, the examiner locates the pulse

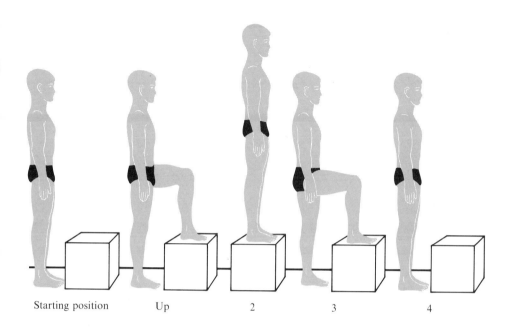

Figure 19-4.   Harvard step test procedure.

and prepares to count. The count starts at exactly one minute after exercise and continues for one-half minute. (If the student did not last five minutes, the count starts one minute from the time he terminated his exercise.) Locating the pulse in advance, the examiner again counts for 30 seconds, beginning at two minutes after exercise, and again at three minutes after exercise. He records each count.

After hard exercise, it is easier to count the pulse at the subclavian artery or the carotid artery than at the wrist. The subclavian artery can be located by holding the fingers vertically and placing them alongside the neck just in back of the clavical bone. The carotid artery can be located by placing the fingers horizontally and pressing on the front of the neck alongside the trachea.

Scoring: The formula for computing the final score is:

$$\text{Score} = \frac{\text{duration of exercise in seconds} \times 100}{2 \text{ times the sum of the 3 pulse counts}}$$

The score is then interpreted according to the following scale:

Excellent Condition	90 and above
Good	80–89
High Average	65–79
Low Average	55–64
Poor Condition	54 and below

To illustrate, if a person finished five minutes (maximum length) of exercise and if his three pulse counts were 90, 80, 70, then his score would be:

$$\frac{300 \text{ seconds} \times 100}{2 \times (90 + 80 + 70)} = 62.5$$

A score of 62.5 is rated low average.

To simplify calculations, a scoring scale has been computed which gives the scores for those students who continue for five minutes. Achievement scores may be found in Appendix D. To use the scale, the examiner simply totals the number of heart beats counted during the three 30-second periods and reads the score opposite that number. For example, for the man whose three pulse counts were 90, 80, 70, the examiner would find the sum of the counts (240) and, using the scoring scale in Appendix D, look for the score opposite the sum (62).

A rapid form for scoring the Harvard step test has been developed based on the duration of exercise and a single pulse count taken from one to one and one-half minutes after exercise. The formula:

$$\text{Score} = \frac{\text{duration of exercise in seconds} \times 100}{5.5 \times \text{pulse count}}$$

The scores for the rapid form may be interpreted as follows:

Poor condition	49 and below
Average condition	50–80
Good condition	81 and above

Modification of the Harvard Step Test

J. Roswell Gallagher and Lucien Brouha (1943a, 1943b) modified the Harvard step test for use by high school students, ages 12 to 18. The test measures the same factors as the Harvard step test and, except for a few exceptions, is administered the same way. Validity and reliability ratings have not been established.

Procedure: For high school boys the duration of exercise is shortened to four minutes and the height of the bench is reduced to 18 inches. Boys with body surface areas of more than 1.85 square meters use the standard 20-inch bench.

Using standard body surface charts the examiner can easily determine surface area from the student's height and weight. For high school girls the height of the bench is reduced to 16 inches and the duration of exercise is four minutes.

Scoring: The procedure for pulse counts and the formula for scoring the tests are the same as for the Harvard step test. The following example determines the score of a 16-year-old-boy who finished four minutes of exercise and whose pulse rates were 80, 70, and 60.

$$\text{Score} = \frac{240 \text{ seconds} \times 100}{2(80 + 70 + 60)} = \frac{24,000}{420} = 57.1$$

According to the classification plan for boys a score of 57 indicates poor condition. A classification of scores for girls is not available.

Superior condition	91 or more
Excellent condition	81–90
Good condition	71–80
Fair condition	61–70
Poor condition	51–60
Very poor condition	50 or less

This test (Sloan 1959) is a modification of the Harvard step test, designed for women. It deviates only slightly in procedure from the Harvard step test.

Procedure: The student steps up and down on an 18-inch bench at the rate of 30 steps per minute for a total exercise period of five minutes or until she is unable to continue the exercise.

Scoring: The pulse rate is counted for 30 seconds at three different times, beginning at one minute, two minutes, and three minutes after completion of the exercise. The fitness index (*FI*) is computed as follows:

$$FI = \frac{\text{duration of exercise in seconds} \times 100}{2 \times \text{sum of pulse counts after exercise}}$$

The standards for interpreting fitness index scores are as follows:

Excellent condition	90 and above
Good condition	80–89
Average condition	56–79
Poor condition	55 and below

Carlson Fatigue Test

This test (Carlson 1945) is based on the fatigue curve. The test consists of ten 10-second bouts of inplace running combined with pulse rates taken at five different times. The only equipment needed is a stopwatch, pencils, and score cards. One examiner can administer the test to 25 students at one time. About 15 minutes are required to explain and conduct the test. Ratings of validity and reliability have not been established.

Procedure: The examiner keeps accurate time with the stopwatch and gives commands to the students at exactly the right time. Each student performs ten 10-second bouts of inplace running with a 10-second rest between bouts. On the starting command the student begins to run in place, moving his feet as rapidly as possible while clearing the floor with each step. He counts the number of times the right foot strikes the floor during each 10 seconds of running, and at the end of each bout quickly records on his score card the number of right foot contacts. Then he gets ready for the next bout and repeats this procedure for 10 bouts.

The student, while in a sitting position, takes his pulse before exercise, ten seconds after completion of exercise, two minutes after exercise, four minutes after exercise, and six minutes after exercise. Each pulse count is taken for 10 seconds and multiplied by six to give the pulse rate per minute.

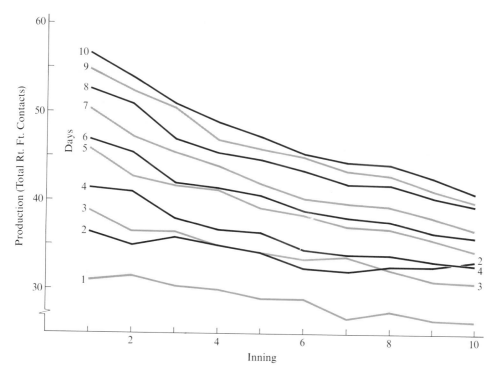

Figure 19-5.   Composite fatigue curves improving for ten consecutive days. Carlson, H. C., "Fatigue Curves." *Research Quarterly,* 1945, *16*, 173.

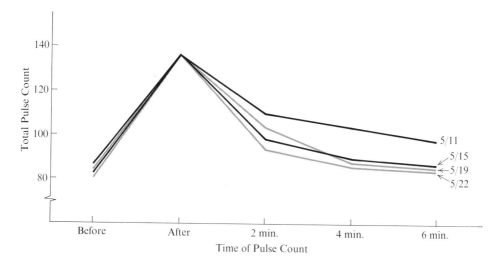

Figure 19-6.   Composite curves of condition corresponding to four of the days shown in Figure 19-5. Carlson, H. C., "Fatigue Curves." *Research Quarterly,* 1945, *16*, 173.

Scoring: The number of right foot contacts during the 10 bouts is summed to indicate the total work accomplished. The rate at which the student's pulse returns to normal indicates his condition. If a student is able to maintain high consistency in his rate of inplace running throughout the 10 bouts and if his pulse rate returns to normal relatively soon, then he is considered to be in good condition. The extent to which these two conditions do not occur indicates poor condition. A comparison of the student's scores made on different occasions indicates changes in his condition (see Figures 19-5 and 19-6). Achievement scales are not available. We recommend that the test be administered to the same group of students 10 days in succession and that records be kept of the students' progress on the test.

Moyle's Test of Swimming Endurance (Speed–Endurance Ratio)

In this test (Moyle 1936) the final score results in a quotient that is easy to interpret. The test is useful for boys and girls of all ages. A stopwatch for each performer and a whistle or starting pistol are necessary equipment. Twenty to 25 performers can be tested in a 40-minute period.

Procedure: Two marks are made on the side of the pool at five and 15 yards from the starting mark. On the starting signal the student begins in the water with a push-off as used following a swimming turn and swims at full speed until he passes the 15-yard mark. His time from the five- to the 15-yard mark is recorded. The watch is started as his head reaches the five-yard mark and is stopped as his head reaches the 15-yard mark. Three trials are given and the best time is recorded. After a 20-minute rest the student uses the same starting procedure as for the 15-yard test and swims 100 yards for time, pacing himself according to his judgment of endurance.

Scoring: The best time of the three trials on the short swim is recorded to the nearest tenth of a second. The time for the 100-yard swim is recorded in the same manner. A quotient is obtained by dividing the 100-yard time by the 10-yard time. A relatively low quotient indicates a large amount of swimming endurance. A quotient is meaningful when compared to quotients obtained by other students, or when compared to quotients by the same student on different occasions. Achievement scales are not available.

In addition to the aforementioned tests the following tests are also useful measure of circulorespiratory endurance: Balke treadmill test (Balke 1954); Barach energy index test (Barach 1914); Crampton blood ptosis (heart rate and blood pressure) test (Crampton 1905), Foster's heart rate test (Foster 1923), Schneider pulse rate and blood pressure test (Schneider 1920), and Tuttle pulse ratio test (Tuttle 1931).

How to Increase
Circulorespiratory Endurance

Physiologists agree that in short-duration endurance performances the main limitation is the oxygen supply to the working tissues—in other words circulorespiratory endurance. Endurance of the circulorespiratory system is increased by applying overload. In this case overload means exercising until the heart rate and the rate and depth of breathing increase a significant amount. The most effective method for increasing endurance is interval training, which consists of a number of short bouts of vigorous exercise with a brief recovery period following each bout.

Interval training for endurance makes good sense from the physiological point of view because the prime objective of an endurance training program is to expose the person to the greatest work load before the onset of fatigue. Research results show that when work is done continuously, a work level which can be tolerated for an hour with the interval training technique will bring about exhaustion in nine minutes. Thus the total work accomplished before fatigue is more than three times greater if the interval training technique is used instead of the continuous training method. This greater output of work during a particular training session results in a stronger endurance stimulus.

The interval training technique is used extensively for swimmers and distance runners and can be used successfully for total body conditioning of performers in activities such as wrestling, baseball, basketball, and various field sports. Interval training has been found to produce the best results when each exercise bout consists of approximately 30 seconds of vigorous work (running, swimming, or other forms of exercise), followed by light exercise or rest for two to three minutes or less. According to Herbert deVries (deVries 1966) the rest interval is adequate when the resting heart rate returns to 120 beats per minute. (This figure undoubtedly varies for different individuals.) He also points out that training can be hampered if the organism is worked to total fatigue. The person should be able to recover from a workout within a few hours.

Endurance overload may result from interval training when the program is adjusted in any of the following ways:

1.   increase in the intensity of the work in each bout

2.   increase in the duration of each work bout

3.   a shortening of the interval between work bouts

4.   an increase in the number of work bouts in a particular training session

Suppose a workout consists of fifteen 220 yard runs at three-fourths full speed with a two to three minute rest between runs. In this case, overloading could be caused by increasing the speed of each run, by increasing the distance of each run, by shortening the rest period between runs, or by increasing the total number of runs in a single workout.

Selected References

Balke, Bruno, "Work Capacity After Blood Donation." *Journal of Applied Physiology*, 1954, *7*.

Barach, J. H., "The Energy Index." *Journal of American Medical Association*, 1914, *512*.

Brouha, Lucien, "The Step Test: A Simple Method of Measuring Physical Fitness for Muscular Work in Young Men." *Research Quarterly*, 1943, *14*.

Carlson, H. C., "Fatigue Curve Test." *Research Quarterly*, 1945, *16*.

Cooper, Kenneth H., *Aerobics*. New York: Bantam Books, 1968.

Crampton, C. Ward, "A Test of Condition: Preliminary Report." *Medical News*, 1905, *537*.

DeVries, Herbert A., *Physiology of Exercise* (Dubuque, Iowa: William C. Brown Company, 1966).

Doolittle, T. L., and Bigbee, Rollin, "The Twelve-Minute Run-Walk: a Test of Cardio-respiratory Fitness of Adolescent Boys." *Research Quarterly*, 1969, *30*.

Foster, W. L., "A Test of Physical Efficiency." *American Physical Education Review*, 1914, *19*. (See also J. F. Williams, *The Organization and Administration of Physical Education*. New York, The Macmillan Company, 1923, p. 294.)

Gallagher, J., and Brouha, Lucien, "A Functional Fitness Test for High School Girls." *Journal of Health and Physical Education*, 1943a.

Gallagher, J. Roswell, and Brouha, Lucien, "A Simple Method of Testing the Physical Fitness of Boys." *Research Quarterly*, 1943b, *14* (1).

Moyle, William J., A Study of Speed and Heart Size as Related to Endurance in Swimming. Unpublished master's thesis, State University of Iowa, 1936.

Schneider, Edward C., "A Cardiovascular Rating as a Measure of Physical Fitness and Efficiency." *Journal of the American Medical Association*, 1920, *524*.

Sloan, A. W., "A Modified Harvard Step Test for Women." *Journal of Applied Physiology*, 1959, *14*.

Taylor, Craig, "A Maximal Pack Test of Exercise Tolerances." *Research Quarterly*, 1944, *15* (4).

Tuttle, W. W., "The Use of the Pulse-Ratio Test for Rating Physical Efficiency." *Research Quarterly*, 1931, *2*.

Youth Fitness Test Manual. American Association for Health, Physical Education and Recreation, 1961.

SEVEN
Measurements
of Multiple Traits

A test of multiple traits consists of a battery of several test items, each of which measures a specific trait. These tests are used to measure general characteristics that cannot be measured by a single test item, such as general athletic (motor) ability, motor educability, and motor fitness. This section describes the more useful tests of multiple traits.

20

General Athletic
(Motor) Ability Tests

General athletic ability is used synonymously with general motor ability. It includes several items such as strength, endurance, power, ability, speed, reaction time, and flexibility. An abundance of these traits enables a person to perform well in such basic activities as running, jumping, climbing, throwing, and dodging. If a performer has a large amount of general athletic ability, he is said to be a natural athlete.

Relationship of General
Athletic Ability to Performance

A person with a high level of general athletic ability possesses the basic physical components necessary to achieve excellence in a number of activities. But in spite of this general ability he will still be unable to perform well in a particular sport until, through long hours of practice, he develops the skills specific to that sport. Endurance, agility, reaction time, power, and speed are general components of performance in basketball, soccer, football, baseball, track and field, and various other sports. But because a person possesses these basic physical components does not make him an expert in basketball. He must also be able to dribble, rebound, shoot, pass, and catch.

A decathlon champion possesses considerable general athletic ability along with the specific skills required in the 10 decathlon events. But he will not do well in tennis until he develops the specific skills required in tennis. He will not bowl a high score until he develops accuracy in bowling, and he will do poorly in soccer until he learns to handle the ball, play correct field positions, and execute specific defensive and offensive techniques effectively. His general athletic ability will assist him in learning the specific skills and will serve as a solid base from which he can develop excellence in various athletic performances.

Tests of General Athletic Ability

General athletic ability tests consist of a battery of items especially selected to measure motor traits that are common to several performances.

Barrow Motor Ability Test

Harold Barrow (1954) designed this test in 1953 to measure general motor ability of college men and junior and senior high school boys. There are two separate test batteries. The outdoor battery has produced a validity coefficient of .95. It includes six items: the standing long jump, the softball throw, the zigzag run, the wall pass, the medicine ball put, and the 60-yard run. The indoor battery has a validity rating of .92. It includes three items: the standing long jump, the medicine ball put, and the zigzag run. If all stations are operating simultaneously, about 25 students can be tested in 40 minutes.

Procedure: The test items should be taken in the order they are listed.

1.   *Standing Long Jump.* See description on page 173. The student is given three trials and the best distance is recorded.

2.   *Softball Throw.* See description on page 174. The student is given three throws and the longest distance is recorded.

3.   *Zigzag Run.* A stopwatch and five obstacles, such as jump standards or chairs, are needed. The course is laid out according to Figure 20-1. On the command to start the student runs the course as directed in Figure 20-1 without touching the obstacles. He continues running until he has gone through the course three complete times. The score is the

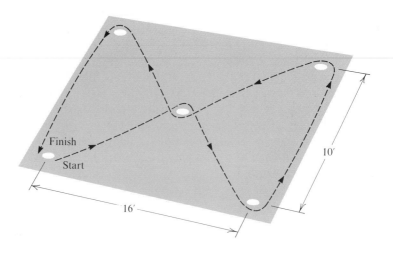

Figure 20-1.   Zigzag run course for the Barrow motor ability test.

time it takes to run three complete circuits, recorded to the nearest tenth of a second. If he makes an error, the student may take a second trial after a sufficient rest.

4.   *Wall Pass.* A stopwatch, one or more regulation basketballs, and sufficient wall space are necessary. A restraining line is marked on the floor nine feet from a smooth wall. The student stands behind the restraining line and on the signal to start he passes the basketball against the wall in any manner desired. Catching the ball on the rebound, he returns it to the wall as rapidly as possible, keeping both feet behind the restraining line. If he misses the ball, he retrieves it and returns to the line before continuing the test. He repeats this procedure for 15 seconds. The score is the number of times the ball hits the wall in the 15-second period.

5.   *Medicine Ball Put.* A six-pound medicine ball and a measuring tape are needed. The student stands no more than 15 feet behind the restraining line, approaches the restraining line in any manner he desires and puts the six-pound medicine ball as far as possible. He should execute the skill in a manner similar to putting the shot. The student is allowed three trials, and the longest distance is recorded to the nearest half foot.

6.   *Sixty-Yard Run.* A stopwatch and whistle are necessary equipment. The student is allowed only one trial for this dash, and his time is recorded to the nearest tenth of a second.

Scoring: The total general motor ability score (GMAS) is computed by means of the following equation:

$$\text{GMAS} = 2.2 \ (\text{standing broad jump}) + 1.6 \ (\text{softball throw}) + 1.6 \ (\text{zigzag run}) + 1.3 \ (\text{wall pass}) + 1.2 \ (\text{medicine ball put}) + 60\text{-yard run.}$$

In the original source Barrow presented the following rating scale based on a sample of college men. He recommends that the users of the test establish their own norms.

| Physical Education Majors | | | Nonmajors | |
Six Items	Three Items	Rating	Six Items	Three Items
586 and above	197 and above	Excellent	550 and above	185 and above
534–585	180–196	Good	481–549	163–184
480–533	161–179	Average	410–480	138–162
428–479	143–160	Poor	341–409	116–137
427 and below	142 and below	Inferior	340 and below	115 and below

Cozens General Athletic Ability Test

This test (Cozens 1936) was designed to serve as a basis for classifying college male students for instruction and to identify strengths and weaknesses in relation to athletic achievement. The test consists of seven items: baseball throw, football punt, bar snap, standing long jump, dips, dodging run, and quarter-mile run. One person can be tested in about 20 minutes. If all stations are operating simultaneously, about 25 students can be tested in 40 minutes.

Procedure: The two throwing events should be performed just inside the two sidelines of a football field so the yardage lines may be used for measuring distances. The other events may be performed on a grass area in the end zone or along the side of the field. The student is allowed a one minute warm-up for each test item.

1.   *Baseball Throw for Distance.* The equipment consists of several regulation baseballs and a measuring tape. See the description of the procedure for the softball throw on page 261.

2.   *Football Punt for Distance.* See description on page 175.

3.   *Bar Snap.* See description on page 175.

4.   *Standing Long Jump.* See description on page 173.

5.   *Dips.* See description on page 153.

6.   *Dodging Run.* See description on page 181.

7.   *Quarter-Mile Run.* If possible the run should be done on a quarter-mile track. The time is recorded to the nearest tenth of a second.

Scoring: Raw scores are transposed into standard scores by use of standard scales (Cozens 1936). For the final score of each test item the seven standard scores are multiplied by the weights (multipliers) in Table 20-1. The seven final scores are summed, and the total is compared to the five category classification in Table 20-1.
    Table 20-1 is an example of how to compute and interpret scores for a short, slender boy if his obtained raw scores are those listed in the raw score column. His final score rates above average.

Table 20-1
Sample Scores on the Cozens General Athletic Ability Test

	Raw Score	Standard Score	Multi-plier	Final Score	Classification	
Baseball throw	190 feet	75	1.5	113	Superior	496 and above
Football punt	40 yards	75	1.0	75	Above average	399–495
Bar snap	6 feet	62	.5	31	Average	302–398
Standing long jump	8 feet	69	.9	62	Below average	205–301
Dips	10	55	.8	44	Inferior	204 and below
Dodging run	25	42	1.0	42		
Quarter-mile run	60	87	1.3	113		
				Total $\overline{480}$ = above average		

Larson Motor Ability Test

After performing a study involving 25 test items Leonard Larson (1941) constructed a test of motor ability for college men and high school boys. The test includes an indoor and an outdoor version as follows:

Indoor Test	Outdoor Test
Chins (pull-ups)	Chins (pull-ups)
Vertical jump	Vertical jump
Dips	Bar snap
Dodging run	Baseball throw
Bar snap	

Based on the 25 items included in Larson's study the indoor and outdoor tests produced validity ratings of .97 and .98 respectively. Reliability ratings have not been established. If all testing stations are operating simultaneously, about 30 students can be tested in 40 minutes.

Procedure: The following items are included in both the indoor and outdoor tests.

1.   *Chins.* See description of pull-ups on page 155.

2.   *Vertical Jump.* See description on page 172.

3.   *Dips.* See description on page 153.

4.   *Dodging Run.* See description on page 181.

5.   *Bar Snap.* See description on page 175.

6.   *Baseball Throw.* See description of softball throw on page 174.

Scoring: Each raw score is converted into a weighted score by use of the scoring tables. The standard scores can be averaged to produce a score for the total test. Achievement scales appear in Appendix D.

Newton Motor Ability Test

Based on extensive experimentation the Newton (named after Newton High School in Massachusetts) test (Powell and Howe 1939) measures motor ability of high school girls. The test is also useful for college women. From a list of 18 test items the following three items were finally selected; standing long jump, hurdle run, and scramble. Validity and reliability of the test have not been determined. If all three testing stations are operating simultaneously, about 25 students can be tested in 40 minutes.

Procedure: The test items should be taken in the following order:

1.   *Standing Long Jump.* See description on page 173.

2.   *Hurdle Run.* To administer this test item ten gymnasium benches, five bamboo sticks for the hurdles, an Indian club, and a stopwatch are needed. The first hurdle is placed five yards from the starting line, the others at three-yard intervals beyond the first, with the Indian club three yards beyond the last hurdle. The hurdles should be 15 inches in height.

       On the signal to start the student runs at top speed over the hurdles, around the Indian club, and back over the hurdles to the starting line.

There is no penalty for a displaced hurdle. The score is recorded to the nearest fifth of a second.

3. *Scramble.* To administer this test item a jumping standard with the peg set at four feet above the floor, a small bell or substitute, and a stopwatch are needed. The bell is fastened securely to the peg on the jumping standard which is placed 10 feet from the wall.

    The student takes a supine position on the floor with both feet against the wall and arms stretched sideways at shoulder level, palms down. On the signal to start he scrambles to his feet, runs and taps the bell twice, and then returns to the starting position. He slaps his hands on the floor twice, runs back to the bell and rings it twice, and repeats the performance as rapidly as possible until he has completed the fourth double tap of the bell. The time is recorded to the nearest fifth of second.

The tests should be administered twice on successive days to increase the reliability of the second-day scores and to allow students an opportunity to improve their initial scores.

Scoring: Each raw score is converted into a standard score by use of the scoring tables in Appendix B. The three standard scores may be averaged to produce a final score.

Scott Motor Ability Test

Based on a rather thorough study Gladys Scott (1939, 1943) selected five items to measure the general motor ability of college women and high school girls. With the five items she constructed two tests. Test 1 consists of four items: basketball throw, four-second dash, wall pass, and standing long jump. Test 2 consists of three items: basketball throw, standing long jump, and obstacle run. Validity coefficients of .91 and .87 have been established for Test 1 and Test 2 respectively. Reliability of the tests has not been reported, but the validity coefficients indicate high reliability. If all stations are operating simultaneously, about 25 students can be tested in 40 minutes.

Procedure: The following items are used in both Test 1 and Test 2.

1. *Basket Throw.* One or more regulation basketballs and a long measuring tape are necessary equipment. While standing behind a restraining line the student throws the ball as far as possible using any technique she desires. The best of three trials is recorded, measured to the nearest foot from the restraining line to the point where the ball first strikes the surface.

2.   *Four-Second Dash.* To administer this test a stopwatch and whistle are necessary equipment. A running lane (85 to 90 feet long and 4 feet wide) is marked with lines placed every yard. The student takes any starting position she desires. On the command she begins to run, dashing as far as possible by the end of four seconds. The starter blows a whistle to start and again at four seconds. An assistant records the distance in yards from the starting line to the place the student reached at the sound of the second whistle. The distance is recorded to the nearest foot.

3.   *Wall Pass.* See description under Barrow's test on page 287.

4.   *Standing Long Jump.* See description on page 173.

5.   *Obstacle Run.* A stopwatch, a jumping standard, and a six-foot crossbar with supports are required for this test to measure speed, agility, and total body coordination. The student starts in a supine position on the floor with her heels at the starting line. On the command to start she scrambles to her feet and runs to the first square that is marked on the floor (see Figure 20-2). She steps on this square and on each of the next two squares, with both feet, and then runs twice around the jump standard and proceeds to the crossbar. She crawls under the bar, gets up and runs to the end line, touches it with her hand, runs back to line F, touches it, runs and touches the end line, runs back to line F, then sprints across the end line. The student is allowed only one trial.

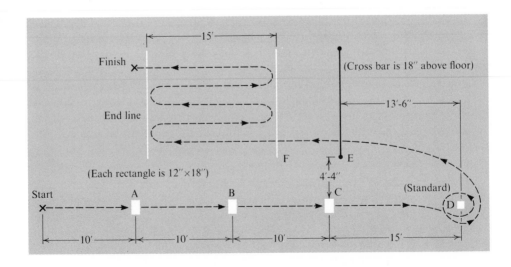

Figure 20-2.   Obstacle run course for the Scott motor ability test.

Scoring: Achievement scales have been developed for high school girls and college women. They appear in Appendix B. A final achievement score is arrived at by averaging the *T* scores for the individual items (see the sample score card shown in Table 20-2).

Table 20-2
Score Card for a High School Girl on the Scott Motor Ability Test

Name		Age	Grade
	Test	Raw Score	*T* Score
	Basketball throw	50.0	66
	Four-second dash	22.0	55
	Wall pass	14.0	73
	Standing long jump	72.0	52
		Total	246

Final score $= \dfrac{246}{4} = 61.5$

Sigma Delta Psi Test

This test (Bovard 1949) represents the entrance requirements for membership in a national athletic fraternity organized in 1912 at Indiana University.[1] To become a member a person must pass the following tests:

1. 100-yard dash   11.6 seconds

2. 120-yard low hurdles   16 seconds

3. Running high jump   Height–weight classification (chart may be obtained from Sigma Delta Psi)

4. Running long jump   17 feet

5. 16-pound shot put   30 feet

[1] Membership application forms may be obtained by writing to Sigma Delta Psi, Indiana University, Bloomington, Indiana.

6.	20-foot rope climb or golf test	12 seconds 4 out of 5 shots must land on the fly in a circle (10-foot radius) from a distance of 75 feet.
7.	Baseball throw or javelin throw	250 feet on fly 130 feet on fly
8.	Football punt	120 feet on fly
9.	100-yard swim	1 minute, 45 seconds
10.	1-mile run	6 minutes
11.	Front handspring, landing on feet	
12.	Handstand or bowling test	10 seconds 160 average (3 games)
13.	Fence vault	Chin high
14.	Good posture	Erect and attractive
15.	Scholarship	Eligible for varsity competition

A candidate who has won a varsity letter or an intramural championship in any sport may substitute this award for any test except swimming. A substitution may be made only once for a sport; for example, the candidate may substitute only one football award even though he may have earned three letters. The privilege of substitution is limited to two varsity sports and one intramural championship.

Tests of Motor Educability

Tests of motor educability serve as estimates of how well people can learn motor skills. However, whether educability can be measured with acceptable accuracy is questionable. Many authorities view motor educability tests simply as general motor ability tests, using the test results that indicate present status to estimate a person's ability to learn motor skills. In physical education a person's educability is his capacity to learn movement skills. Capacity, which depends upon heredity plus other factors, changes with time. Through activity the person develops ability within his capacity limits. Performance records indicate ability, but the examiner never knows where the scores fall on an individual or a universal capacity scale. David K. Brace's term *native ability* implies innate skill and is therefore inaccurate. Frederick Cozens also used this term in his doctoral study. Two tests called tests of motor educability are discussed in this section. They are useful tests for purposes of development.

Iowa–Brace Test

This test (McCloy 1937) consists of 21 individual stunts which were selected from an original list of 40 stunts. Validity and reliability of the test have not been clearly established, perhaps because of the difficulty in the definition and measurement of motor educability. The test can be administered to a large group of students in about 30 minutes.

Each test battery consists of 10 of the 21 stunts. Different batteries have been selected for each age group. The following stunts are used for the various grade levels.

	Boys				
Elementary Grades 4–6		Junior High School Grades 7–9		Senior High School Grades 10–12	
1st half	2nd half	1st half	2nd half	1st half	2nd half
10	2	1	2	1	3
4	3	14	3	11	14
13	7	13	12	16	15
11	16	19	16	5	17
8	17	6	17	20	21
	Girls				
10	1	2	1	3	2
18	3	12	13	11	18
8	16	15	11	7	16
19	15	19	16	17	9
11	6	17	20	19	20

Procedure: The students stand in two lines facing each other. They are arranged so that each student has a partner. The examiner reads the description of each stunt exactly as it is written here; then he demonstrates the stunt correctly and points out common mistakes. After the examiner has demonstrated the stunts, the students in the first group perform while their partners score them. There are 10 stunts in the battery. The first group performs the first five stunts, the second group performs all ten stunts and then the first group performs their remaining five stunts. In this manner both groups have the advantage of witnessing five of the stunts before performing.

Test 1: One Foot–Touch Head. Stand on your left foot. Bend forward and place both hands on the floor. Raise the right leg and stretch it back. Touch the head to the floor and regain the standing position without losing your balance. It is a failure: (a) not to touch your head to the floor, (b) to lose your balance, (c) to have to touch your right foot down or step about.

Test 2: Side Leaning Rest. Sit down on the floor, legs straight out and feet together. Put your right hand on the floor behind you. Turn to the right and take a side leaning rest position, resting on your right hand and right foot. Raise your left arm and keep this position for five counts. It is a failure: (a) not to take the proper position, (b) not to hold the position for five counts.

Test 3: Grapevine. Stand with both heels tight together. Without losing your balance bend down, extend both arms down between your knees, around behind your ankles, and clasp your fingers together in front of your ankles. Hold this position for five seconds. It is a failure: (a) to fall over, (b) not to touch and hold the fingers of both hands together, (c) not to hold the position for five seconds.

Test 4: One-Knee Balance. Face to the right. Kneel down on one knee with your other leg raised from the floor and your arms stretched out at the side. Hold your balance for five counts. It is a failure: (a) to touch the floor with any part of the body other than your one leg and knee, (b) to fall over.

Test 5: Stork Stand. Stand on your left foot. Hold the bottom of your right foot against the inside of your left knee. Place your hands on your hips. Shut both eyes and hold the position for ten seconds without shifting your left foot about on the floor. It is a failure: (a) to lose your balance, (b) to step down on your right foot, (c) to open your eyes or remove your hands from your hips.

Test 6: Double Heel Click. Jump vertically, click your feet together twice, and land with your feet apart (any distance). It is failure: (a) not to click your feet together twice, (b) to land with your feet touching each other.

Test 7: Cross-Leg Squat. Fold your arms across your chest. Cross your feet and sit down cross-legged. Get up without unfolding your arms and without having to move your feet about to regain balance. It is a failure: (a) to unfold your arms, (b) to lose your balance, (c) to be unable to get up.

Test 8: Full Left Turn. Stand with your feet together. Jump vertically, make a full turn to the left, and land on the same spot without losing your balance or moving your feet after they strike the floor. It is a failure: (a) not to turn all the way around, (b) to move your feet after they strike the floor.

Test 9: One Knee–Head to Floor. Kneel on one knee with your other leg stretched out behind and raised from the floor, your arms out at your side parallel to the floor. Bend forward and touch your head to the floor. Raise your head from the floor without losing balance. It is a failure: (a) to touch the floor with your raised leg or with any part of the body other than your knee before completing the stunt, (b) not to touch your head to the floor, (c) to drop your hands.

Test 10: Hop Backward. Stand on either foot. Close your eyes and take five hops backward. It is a failure: (a) to open your eyes, (b) to drop your other foot.

Test 11: Forward Hand Kick. Jump upward, swinging your legs forward; bend forward and touch your toes with both hands before landing. Keep your knees as straight as possible. It is a failure: (a) not to touch both feet while in the air, (b) to bend the knees more than 45 degrees.

Test 12: Full Squat–Arm Circles. Take a full squat position with your arms out sideways. Wave your arms so that your hands make a circle about 12 inches across, and jiggle up and down at the same time for 10 counts. It is a failure: (a) to move your feet about on the floor, (b) to lose your balance and fall.

Test 13: Half-Turn Jump—Left Foot. Stand on your left foot and jump a half turn to the left, keeping your balance. It is a failure: (a) to lose your balance, (b) not to complete the half turn, (c) to touch the floor with the other foot.

Test 14: Three Dips. Take a front leaning rest position; that is, place your hands on the floor, with arms straight, and extend your feet back along the floor until your body is straight (in an inclined position to the floor). Bend your arms, touch your chest to the floor, and push up again until your arms are straight. Do this dip three times in succession. Do not touch the floor with your legs or waist. It is a failure: (a) not to push up three times, (b) not to touch your chest to the floor each time, (c) to rest your knees, thighs, or waist on the floor at any time.

Test 15: Side Kick. Throw your left foot sideways to the left, jumping upward from your right foot; strike your feet together in the air and land with them apart. Your feet should strike outside the left shoulder line. It is a failure: (a) not to swing your feet enough to the side, (b) not to strike your feet together in the air, (c) not to land with your feet apart.

Test 16: Kneel, Jump to Feet. Kneel on both knees. Extend the toes of both feet out flat behind; swing your arms and jump to your feet without rocking back on your toes and without losing balance. It is a failure: (a) to have your toes curled under and rock back on them, (b) not to execute the jump, (c) not to stand still on both feet.

Test 17: Russian Dance. Squat as far down as possible and stretch one leg forward. Do a Russian dance step by hopping to this position with first one leg extended and then the other. Do this dance twice with each leg. The heel of your forward foot may touch the floor. It is a failure: (a) to lose your balance, (b) not to do the stunt twice with each leg.

Test 18: Full Right Turn. Stand with both feet together. Swing your arms and jump in the air, making a full turn to the right. Land on the same spot without losing your balance, that is, without moving your feet after they first strike the floor. It is a failure: (a) not to make a full turn and to land facing in the same direction as at the start, (b) to lose your balance and have to step about to keep from falling.

Test 19: The Top. Sit down; put your arms between your legs and under and behind your knees; grasp your ankles. Roll rapidly around to the right with your weight first over your right knee, then over your right shoulder, then on your back, then over your left shoulder, then over your left knee. Then sit up facing in the opposite direction from that which you started. Repeat the roll from this position and finish facing in the same direction from which you started your first roll. It is a failure: (a) to let go of your ankles, (b) not to complete the circle.

Test 20: Single Squat Balance. Squat as far down as possible on either foot. Stretch your other leg forward off the floor and put your hands on your hips. Hold this position for five counts. It is a failure: (a) to remove your hands from your hips, (b) to touch the floor with your extended foot, (c) to lose your balance.

Test 21: Jump Foot. Hold the toes of either foot in the opposite hand. Jump up putting your free foot over the foot that is held, without letting go. It is a failure: (a) to let go of the foot that is held, (b) not to jump through the loop made by holding the foot.

Scoring: The student gets two points for correct performance of each stunt on the first trial (maximum = 20 points), one point for correct performance on the second trial, and no points after the second trial. The student should not practice stunts prior to the test. Achievement scales for girls appear in Appendix B and for boys in Appendix C.

Johnson–Metheny Test

This test is Eleanor Metheny's revision (1948) of the original Johnson test of motor educability. It is considerably shorter and more practical than the Johnson test (which included ten items), and it produced a high correlation with the Johnson test (.87). Metheny's revised test consists of four items for boys and three items for girls. A canvas marked according to Figure 20-3 should be placed on top of the tumbling mats. About 25 students can be tested in 40 minutes.

Procedure: The first three items are used for girls; all four items are used for boys. Prior to administering each item the examiner should read the description of the item as written here and demonstrate the stunt correctly.

1.   *Front Roll.* Start from a standing position at one end of the canvas. Perform one front roll within the limits of the first half of the lane; then do another front roll within the second half of the lane. Each roll is worth five points maximum. Two points are deducted each time you stray beyond the boundary of either side of the lane. One point is deducted each time you do not complete the roll within the designated half of the lane. Five points are deducted if you fail to perform a true roll. If you fail on the first roll, you are allowed to try a second roll in the last half of the lane.

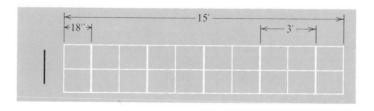

Figure 20-3. Floor markings for the Johnson–Metheny Test.

2. *Back Roll.* Start from the end of the canvas and perform two back rolls—one roll within the first half of the lane, the other roll within the second half of the lane. The scoring is the same as for the front roll test.

3. *Jumping Half Turn.* Stand on the first three-inch line. Jump upward and execute a half turn in either direction, landing on the second three-inch line. Now facing the starting line, jump upward making a half turn in the opposite direction from which you made the first turn. Proceed in this manner, alternating directions of the turns, until you have completed four jumps. From a possible 10 points, two points are deducted for each jump if you do not land on the line with both feet or if you turn in the wrong direction.

4. *Jumping Full Turn.* Stand at the end of the lane, jump upward with feet together, and execute a full turn in either direction and land in the second section. Then jump and make another full turn in the same direction and land in the fourth section. Continue the length of the mat in this manner for five turns. From a possible 10 points, two points are deducted if you do not land on both feet, if you fail to land in the designated section, if you turn too far or not far enough, or if you move your feet upon landing.

Scoring: Each stunt is worth a maximum of 10 points. Points are deducted for errors as explained in the description of each stunt. Achievement scales are not available.

In addition to the aforementioned tests the following tests are also useful measures of athletic ability: Carpenter motor ability test for grades 1–3 (Carpenter 1943), Latchaw motor achievement test for grades 4–6 (Latchaw 1954), McCloy general motor ability tests (McCloy and Young 1954), Humiston motor ability test for college women (Humiston 1937), Newton motor ability test for high school girls (Powell and Howe 1939), and Oberlin college test for college women (1936).

How to Improve General Athletic Ability

General athletic ability includes strength, endurance, agility, power, reaction time, and flexibility. If a performer excels in his general athletic ability, he is referred to as a natural athlete. However, the term *natural athlete* does not necessarily mean "inborn." Although capacity to perform is inherited, use of a person's motor skill greatly influences his level of general athletic ability development. A gifted person may have developed relatively low levels of this ability, while other less endowed persons may have developed considerable motor ability from experience. General motor ability is increased by concentrating on its specific components. Strength, a fundamental component of motor ability, can be increased rapidly and significantly by following the procedure described in Chapter 12, "Muscular Strength Tests." Endurance can be increased significantly as a result of training as described in Chapter 19 on circulorespiratory endurance. Power, another component fundamental to motor ability, can be increased by following the procedure described in Chapter 13 on power testing. In addition agility, running speed, reaction time, and flexibility can be increased by following the procedure described in Chapters 14, 15 and 16.

Selected References

Barrow, Harold M., "Test of Motor Ability for College Men." *Research Quarterly*, 1954, *25*, 253–60.

Bovard, John F., Cozens, Frederick W., and Hagman, Patricia, *Tests and Measurements in Physical Education*, 3rd ed. Philadelphia: W. B. Saunders Company, 1949.

Carpenter, Aileen, "The Measurements of General Motor Capacity and General Motor Ability in the First Three Grades." *Research Quarterly*, 1942, *13*, 444–65.

Cozens, Frederick W., *Achievement Scales in Physical Education Activities for College Men*. Philadelphia: Lea & Febiger, 1936.

Humiston, Dorothy A., "A Measurement of Motor Ability in College Women." *Research Quarterly*, 1937, *8*, 181–85.

Larson, Leonard A., "A Factor Analysis of Motor Ability Variables and Tests, with Tests for College Men." *Research Quarterly*, 1941, *12*, 499–517.

Latchaw, Marjorie, "Measuring Selected Motor Skills in Fourth, Fifth, and Sixth Grades." *Research Quarterly*, 1954, *25*, 439–49.

McCloy, Charles H., "An Analytical Study of the Stunt Type Test as a Measure of Motor Educability." *Research Quarterly*, 1937, *8*, 46–55.

McCloy, Charles H., and Young, Norma D., *Tests and Measurements in Health and Physical Education*, 3rd ed. New York: Appleton-Century-Crofts, 1954, ch. 17.

Metheny, Eleanor, "Studies of the Johnson Test as a Test of Motor Educability." *Research Quarterly*, 1938, *9*, 105–14.

Oberlin College Test, "Qualifying Test for Elective Program in Physical Education." *Journal of Health and Physical Education*, 1936, *7* (8).

Powell, Elizabeth, and Howe, Eugene C., "Motor Ability Tests for High School Girls." *Research Quarterly*, 1939, *10*, 81–88.

Scott, M. Gladys, "The Assessment of Motor Abilities of College Women Through Objective Tests." *Research Quarterly*, 1939, *10*, 63–83.

Scott, M. Gladys, "Motor Ability Tests for College Women." *Research Quarterly*, 1943, *14*, 402–5.

21

Measures
of Motor Fitness

A person's total fitness is his ability to function in his overt and covert activities. He demonstrates part of his total fitness in his ability to perform in vigorous motor activities. This phase of fitness, often referred to as motor fitness, consists of a number of individual traits and is similar to general athletic ability. The extent to which a person possesses such traits as strength, endurance, power, agility, flexibility, and speed determines his fitness for motor performance. In efforts to develop motor fitness emphasis is usually placed on strength and endurance.

Relationship of Motor Fitness to Performance

Motor fitness and general athletic ability contribute to performance in much the same way. When a person is fit, the various systems of the body are well conditioned so that each system can do its part toward effective performance. Fitness serves as a general base for excellence in performance, but it does not include all essentials. An excellent performer in a specific activity must possess, in addition to motor fitness, the specific skills that are part of that activity.

Motor Fitness Tests

Several tests to measure motor fitness have been developed in recent years. These tests measure a person's ability to exhibit motor traits basic to good performance. Each test consists of several items.

AAHPER Fitness Test

In 1957 the American Association for Health, Physical Education and Recreation launched a youth fitness project (*Youth Fitness Test Manual* 1965). One result was the construction of a seven-item test to measure the general fitness of youth. The seven items in the test are: pull-ups, sit-ups, 40-yard shuttle run, 50-yard run, standing long jump, softball throw for distance, and 600-yard run–walk.

The tests should be administered during two class periods: Pull-ups, sit-ups, standing long jump, and shuttle run should be tested in the first period; 50-yard run, softball throw for distance, and 600-yard run–walk should be tested in the second period. With the battery of tests spread over two class periods and test items administered simultaneously, 40 students can be tested in two 40-minute periods. Validity and reliability ratings have not been established for the test.

Procedure: The test items should be administered in the order in which they are described.

1.   *Pull-ups.* See description on page 155 (boys). Girls do the flexed arm hang (see page 156).

2.   *Sit-Ups.* See description on page 157. One point is allowed for each completed sit-up to a maximum of 50 points for girls and 100 points for boys.

3.   *Standing Long Jump.* See description on page 173.

4.   *Shuttle Run.* See description on page 182.

5.   *50-Yard Run.* This event measures sprinting speed and is therefore an indication of power. The test is conducted as a standard 50-yard run and is timed to the nearest tenth of a second.

6.   *Softball Throw for Distance.* See description on page 174.

7.   *600-Yard Run–Walk.* See description on page 273.

Scoring: Two sets of scoring scales are printed in the AAHPER *Youth Fitness Test Manual.*[1] One set of scales is based on age and the other one on the Neilson–Cozens Age–Height–Weight Classification Plan. The achievement scales appear in Appendixes B, C, and D.

Youth Fitness Test

In 1961 the President's Council on Youth Fitness designed this test for screening purposes (*Youth Physical Fitness Manual* 1961). It consists of three items primarily

---

[1] The manual is available from the AAHPER office at 1201 Sixteenth Street, N.W., Washington, D.C.

to measure strength and agility. One subject can be tested in 10 minutes. With three stations operating simultaneously, 30 students can be tested in a 40-minute period. Validity and reliability coefficients for the test have not been established.

Procedure: Each test item is scored as *pass* or *fail*.

1.   *Pull-Ups.* See description on page 155 (boys), and page 156 (girls, modified).

2.   *Sit-Ups.* See description on page 157.

3.   *Squat Thrusts.* See description on page 158.

Scoring: To pass each test item, a boy or a girl must perform the exercise the number of times indicated in the following table:

Table 16
Passing Standards for Youth Fitness Screening Test

Exercise	Girls Ages 10–17	Boys Ages 10–13	Boys Ages 14–15	Boys Ages 16–17
Pull-ups	8 modified	1	2	3
Sit-ups	10	14	14	14
Squat thrusts	3	4	4	4

Division of Girls' and
Women's Sports (DGWS) Test

The DGWS, a division of the American Association of Health, Physical Education and Recreation, selected eight test items to compose a motor fitness test for high school girls. The test is also useful for college women. The standing long jump, basketball throw and agility run were selected to measure general athletic ability. Sit-ups, push-ups, and pull-ups were selected to measure strength. The 10-second squat thrust test was included as a measure of agility, and the 30-second squat thrust test was selected to measure endurance. Validity and reliability ratings have not been established for the test. The committee that prepared the test recommends that if all eight items cannot be administered, the battery may be shortened to the standing long jump, the basketball throw, the agility run or 10-second squat thrust, the sit-up, and the push-up or pull-up.

Procedure: The items may be taken in any order provided the agility run is separated from the squat thrust test and the pull-up and push-up tests are separated. The following order is recommended:

1.   *Basketball Throw.* Marks should be placed on the floor at five-foot intervals from the restraining line. The only equipment necessary is a regulation basketball. The student stands one step behind the restraining line and throws the ball as far as possible using any throwing method she desires. If necessary she may take one approach step. The score is the distance from the restraining line to the spot where the ball first strikes the floor. The better distance of two trials is recorded to the nearest foot.

2.   *Agility run.* Same as the shuttle run in the AAHPER Fitness Test. See description on page 182.

3.   *Push-Ups (modified).* See description on page 155.

4.   *Standing Long Jump.* See description on page 173.

5.   *Squat Thrusts* (10 *seconds*). See description on page 178.

6.   *Sit-Ups.* See description on page 157.

7.   *Pull-Ups.* A pull-up bar (or one side of a parallel bar) is placed three and one-half feet above the floor. The student grasps the bar using a reverse grip (palms up) and moves under the bar until her shoulders are directly underneath. Her arms should be straight; her body should be straight from the shoulders to the knees; and her knees should be bent almost to a right angle with her feet flat on the floor (see Figure 21-1). Keeping her trunk straight, she pulls up from this position until her chest touches the bar. She does as many pull-ups in succession as possible.

8.   *Squat Thrusts* (30 *seconds*). See description of squat thrusts for 10 seconds on page 178.

Scoring: Achievement scales appear in Appendix B. The standard scores for the individual items may be averaged to obtain a standard score for the total test.

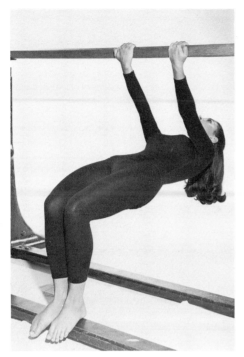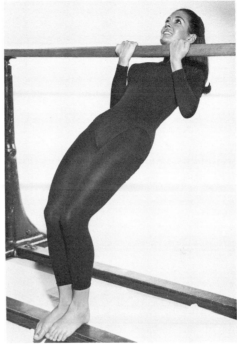

Figure 21-1.   Pull-ups for the DGWS test.

Jumping, Chinning,
Running (JCR) Test

This test (Phillips 1947) measures the student's ability to perform fundamental athletic activities such as jumping (J), chinning (C), running (R), and changing direction. It consists of three items: vertical jump, pull-ups (chins), and a 100-yard shuttle run. Validity coefficients of .90 and .81 were obtained when scores on the test were compared with scores on 19 and 25 general athletic ability test items. Reliability ratings are not available. One student can complete the test in five minutes. Using two jump boards, two chinning bars, and four running lanes, approximately 50 students can be tested in a 40-minute period.

Procedure: The test items should be administered in the following order:

1.   *Vertical Jump.* See description on page 172.

2.   *Pull-ups (Chins).* See description on page 155.

3.   *Shuttle Run.* A stopwatch for each lane and a shuttle run area as illustrated in Figure 21-2 are needed. This test measures running speed and agility (the ability to change direction rapidly). The student stands

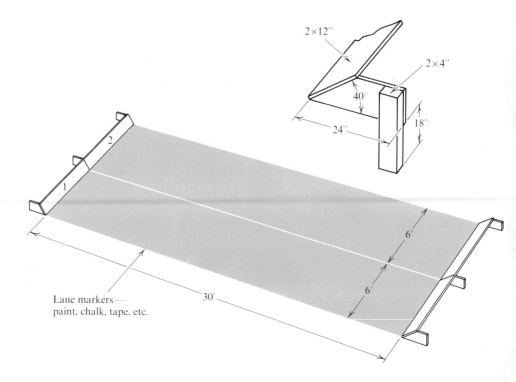

Figure 21-2. Shuttle run floor plan for JCR test. If a structure of this type is not available the run can be done back and forth between two lines 30 feet apart marked on the floor or grass.

inside the starting line with one foot on or touching the backboard. On the signal to start the student runs back and forth between the turning blocks, making five complete round trips. The examiner should keep the runner informed of the number of laps completed. The student's score is the time he takes to complete the run, measured to the nearest half second.

Scoring: The height of the vertical jump in inches, number of pull-ups, and shuttle-run time are the raw scores. With the use of scoring scales in Appendix D, the raw scores for men ages 16 to 24 may be converted to standard scores averaged to obtain a single standard score. The final score is applied to the rating scale found in Appendix D.

Rogers' Physical Fitness Index (PFI)

The *PFI* relates to Rogers' strength test (see page 161). This index has been used extensively in research and as a screening test to identify students who are low in fitness. The PFI expresses a relationship between a person's achieved strength index

(*SI*) score (see Rogers' strength test) and his strength norm. The *PFI* is computed by use of the following formula:

$$PFI = \frac{\text{achieved strength index}}{\text{normal strength index}} \times 100$$

If a person's *SI* were equal to the norm for his age and weight, his *PFI* would be equal to 100. A PFI of 100 is average; therefore a score below 100 is below average and a score above 100 is above average.

In addition to the tests already described several other fitness tests have been constructed. These tests are not used extensively throughout the nation, but they are useful in certain locales.

Motor Fitness Test for Oregon Schools

This test (1962) includes different batteries of test items for different age groups as follows:[2]

Boys Grades 4–6	*Boys Grades 7–12*	*Girls Grades 4–12*
Standing long jump	Pull-ups	Standing long jump
Floor push-ups	Vertical jump	Hang in arm-flexed position
Sit-ups	160-yard agility race	Cross-arm curl-ups

California Physical Performance Test

This test (1962) is for boys and girls ages 10 to 18.[3] The test items are the standing long jump, the knee bent sit-up, the 50-yard run, the softball throw, the pull-up (boys), and the knee push-up (girls).

Indiana Motor Fitness Test for High School and College Men

This test (Bookwalter and Bookwalter 1953) includes four indexes:[4]

Motor Fitness Index I = (chins + push-ups) × (vertical jump)
Motor Fitness Index II = (chins + push-ups) × (standing long jump)
Motor Fitness Index III = (straddle chins + push-ups) × (vertical jump)
Motor Fitness Index IV = (straddle chins + push-ups) × (standing long jump)

---

[2] A copy of the test manual, which includes achievement scales, may be obtained from the Oregon State Department of Education, Portland.

[3] A test manual, which includes achievement scales, may be obtained from the California State Department of Education, Sacramento.

[4] A copy of the complete test, including achievement scales, may be obtained from the Indiana State Department of Public Instruction in Indianapolis.

Indiana Physical Fitness
Tests for High School Boys and Girls

These tests (1944) are based on an age – height – weight classification and each test includes four test items: straddle chins, squat thrusts (20 seconds), push-ups, and vertical jump.[5]

Elementary School Motor Fitness Test

This test (Franklin and Lehsten 1948) is an adaptation, for use in the elementary schools, of the Indiana physical fitness tests. The same test items are used.[6]

New York State Physical Fitness Test

The test (1958) is for boys and girls in grades four through twelve.[7] It includes tests of posture, strength, speed, endurance, accuracy, agility, and balance.

Army Physical Efficiency Test

This test (*War Department Field Manual*) was developed during World War II for use by Army personnel. It includes five test items: pull-ups, squat jumps, 300-yard run, push-ups, and sit-ups. Achievement scales are based on performance by Army personnel.

Navy Standard Physical Fitness Test

The test includes five test items: sit-ups, squat-thrusts (1 minute), squat jumps, push-ups, and pull-ups. Achievement scales are based on performance by Navy personnel.

How to Improve Motor Fitness

An individual's motor fitness is dependent upon the fitness of his various body systems, especially his muscular and circulorespiratory systems. To improve his

---

[5] A copy of the complete test, including achievement scales, may be obtained from the Indiana State Department of Public Instruction in Indianapolis.

[6] The test, including achievement scales, may be obtained from the Indiana State Department of Public Instruction in Indianapolis.

[7] A test manual, with achievement scales, may be obtained from the New York State Education Department, Albany.

fitness an individual should engage in activities which emphasize development of these systems. He can improve his muscular strength and endurance by doing strength–endurance type conditioning (see Chapter 12). He can develop his circulorespiratory system by emphasizing circulorespiratory endurance training (see Chapter 19). In general, motor fitness results from regular participation in a variety of vigorous activities, along with good nutrition and other healthful practices.

Selected References

Bookwalter, Karl W., and Bookwalter, Carolyn W., *A Measure of Motor Fitness for College.* Bulletin of the School for Education, Indiana University, 1953, *19*, (2).

California Physical Performance Tests, Sacramento, Calif.: State Department of Education, Bureau of Health Education, Physical Education, and Recreation, 1962.

Franklin, C. C. and Lehsten, Nelsen G., "Indiana Physical Fitness Tests for the Elementary Level (Grades 4–8)." *The Physical Educator*, 1948, *5* (3).

Metheny, Eleanor, "Physical Performance Levels for High School Girls." *Journal of Health and Physical Education*, 1945, *16*, 32–35.

Motor Fitness Tests for Oregon Schools. Salem, Ore.: State Department of Education, 1962.

New York State Physical Fitness Test: A Manual for Teachers of Physical Education. Albany, N.Y.: State Department of Education, Division of Health, Physical Education and Recreation, 1958.

Phillips, B. E., "The JCR Test." *Research Quarterly*, 1947, *18*, 12–29.

Physical Fitness Manual for High School Boys. Indianapolis, Ind.: Department of Public Instruction, Bulletin No. 136, 1944.

Physical Fitness Manual for High School Girls. Indianapolis, Ind.: Department of Public Instruction, Bulletin No. 137 (revised), 1944.

Physical Fitness Manual for the U.S. Navy, Bureau of Naval Personnel, Training Division, Physical Section, 1943, ch. 4.

Rogers, Frederick R., *Physical Capacity Tests in Administration of Physical Education.* New York: Bureau of Publications, Teachers College, Columbia University, 1926.

Tunney, John J., "The Physical Fitness Program of the U.S. Navy." *Journal of Health and Physical Education*, 1942, *13* (10).

War Department Field Manual, FM 21–20, Department of the Army, Washington, D.C.

Youth Fitness Test Manual, 3rd ed. American Association for Health, Physical Education and Recreation, 1965.

Youth Physical Fitness Manual. Washington, D.C.: President's Council on Youth Fitness. Superintendent of Documents, U.S. Government Printing Office, July 1961.

EIGHT

Construction of
Tests and Application of Test Results

This section includes valuable information on how to construct written tests and motor performance tests, how to establish norms in order to make test results more useful, as well as how to apply test results effectively in the school program.

22

Construction
of Tests

Before he can measure skill or knowledge, the teacher must either select a test from the available standardized tests or construct one specifically to serve his purpose. He may need either a written test or a motor performance test, both of which are important yet serve different purposes. The construction of such tests is a difficult task requiring great concentration and effort.

Written Tests

Written tests fall into two general categories, standard tests and teacher-made tests. Standard tests are usually designed to measure general traits, such as intelligence, personality, general academic achievement, and general knowledge. A standard test, such as an IQ (intelligence quotient) test supposedly produces comparable results when it is administered to different people at different times and in different localities. Conversely a teacher-made test is highly local in nature, that is, designed for a specific group of people who have had particular experiences which prepare them for the test. For example, a teacher-made test may be constructed to evaluate the learning that occurred as a result of a unit of instruction on tennis.

Construction of
Standardized Written Tests

Construction of a standard written test is an involved project because the test must be designed to produce valid and reliable results when administered at different times and places. Thus the test items may not be localized or confined to a particular situation or group of people. Usually these tests evolve from extensive research projects which are supervised or completed by testing experts.

To develop a standard written test:

1. Determine the purpose and define its scope and delimitations.

2. Determine the type of test items to be considered: multiple choice, true–false, matching, or completion.

313

3.   Accumulate all test items that should be considered for inclusion in the test.

4.   Administer the test items to groups of people who represent the population for which the test is to be constructed. From the results determine the relative validity and reliability of the test items by correlating the results of each item with a selected criterion measure.

5.   Eliminate weak items and items that cause duplication.

6.   Select the items to be included in the semifinal draft.

7.   Administer the semifinal draft twice to a randomly selected sample of the population for which the test is designed.

8.   On the basis of the results make a final check for validity and reliability of each item. Check validity by correlating the results with the best criterion available; check reliability by correlating the results of the first administration of the test with results of the second administration of the test to the same people.

9.   Arrange the items in order from the least difficult to the most difficult items.

10.   Prepare the test in final form and include standard written instructions and score sheets.

11.   Develop norms for the test.

12.   Make a sufficient number of copies of the test and make known their availability to the potential users.

For examples of standardized written tests see Chapter 10.

Construction of Teacher-Made Written Tests

No standard written tests have been designed to measure the progress students have made during a five-week unit of instruction in tumbling, soccer, or any other activity. Such tests must be carefully prepared on the basis of what has been included in the unit. Only the teacher, perhaps with the help of the students, is in a position to design such tests because only he knows what has been covered and what should have been learned. Even though such tests are constructed to measure the students' knowledge of important facts and concepts, they may also stimulate additional interest in the subject, help the students evaluate themselves, as well as reemphasize the most important information.

To construct a teacher-made test:

1. Thoroughly review the curricular content which the test will cover and select the specific points that should receive emphasis in the test. The test should reflect approximately the same emphasis as the instruction.

2. Determine the type of questions to be used: true–false, multiple choice, matching, completion, or essay.

3. Formulate more questions than you plan to include in the test; then carefully evaluate each question and select the better ones.

4. Arrange the questions into logical sequence on the basis of type and difficulty.

5. Make a final appraisal of the test before administering it; then reappraise the test after each administration to determine if it can be improved. In appraising the test retain each test item only on the basis that it contributes to the intent and purpose of the test.

Types of Written Test Items

Written test items may be either subjective or objective. Essay questions are subjective: the answers are not clearly correct or incorrect but require critical evaluation and subjective judgment by the person correcting the test. True–false (or other alternate choice questions such as yes–no, right–wrong, preferred–not preferred, same–opposite), multiple choice, matching, and completion questions are objective; they involve the use of facts and are clearly correct or incorrect without the distortion of a person's opinion.

Examples of each type of question follow:

Sample essay questions about kinesiology. Directions: Respond to each of the following by writing concise statements using well chosen words.

1. Describe the all-or-none law of muscle contraction.

2. Describe the differences between first, second, and third class levers in the human body.

3.   Explain how increased strength of certain muscle groups may improve a person's speed in swimming.

4.   Elaborate on the meaning of the statement: "The stability of any body is dependent upon its height, mass, and size of the base of support."

Sample true–false questions about skiing.   Directions: Indicate whether each statement is true or false by writing T or F in the space opposite the statement. Any statement that is not completely true should be marked false.

_____   1.   Skiing is an activity invented and developed during the last century.

_____   2.   The American ski technique, used almost universally as the instructional technique in the United States, is dissimilar to other standard ski techniques.

_____   3.   The herringbone is a climbing technique on skis.

_____   4.   When the temperature is below freezing, soft wax is the best kind to use on skis.

_____   5.   In most turning techniques correct weight transfer is the main turning force.

_____   6.   During the traverse most of the weight should be carried on the uphill ski, and that ski should be slightly forward.

_____   7.   In the stem-christie turn, the up-motion (unweighting) occurs midway through the turn.

_____   8.   As he increases his speed, the skier should decrease the amount of forward lean and leg flexion.

_____   9.   It is unwise for beginning skiers to wax their skis because "fast" skis are harder to control than "slow" skis.

_____   10.   The most important muscles for skiing are the extensors of the ankle, knee, and hip and the hip rotators.

_____   11.   It is considered discourteous to cover sitzmarks.

Sample multiple-choice questions about golf.   Directions: After each statement there are five choices, each preceded by a letter. In the space provided write the letter before the word or words which best complete the statement.

_____ 1.   Two strokes under a perfect score for a hole is called: (a) a bogie; (b) an honor; (c) a birdie; (d) an eagle; (e) par.

_____ 2.   Turf chopped up during a stroke is called a: (a) chop; (b) dormie; (c) slice; (d) divot; (e) hook.

_____ 3.   When on the green one should generally use a: (a) mashie; (b) putter; (c) midiron; (d) driver; (e) mashie niblick.

_____ 4.   A ball that curves to the right after it has been hit is called a: (a) hooked ball; (b) good ball; (c) sliced ball; (d) birdie; (e) divot.

_____ 5.   The area on which golf is played is called the: (a) link; (b) fairway; (c) teeing ground; (d) course; (e) rough.

Sample matching questions about folk dance and swimming.   Directions: Find the number in the right column that corresponds to each item in the left column and record the number in the blank.

1.   *Folk Dance:*

_____ Alunelul	1.	African
_____ Corrida	2.	American
_____ Cotton-eyed Joe	3.	Czechoslovakian
_____ D'Hammerschmiedsg'selln	4.	English
_____ Doudlebska Polka	5.	Estonian
_____ Gallopade	6.	German
_____ Hier Ek Weer	7.	Greek
_____ Hopak	8.	Irish
_____ Kalvelis	9.	Israeli

_____ Miserlau   10. Lithuanian

                                        11. Mexican

                                        12. Romanian

                                        13. Russian

2. *Swimming*:

_____ Flutter kick   1. Sidestroke

_____ Whip kick   2. Front crawl stroke

_____ Dolphin kick   3. Elementary backstroke

_____ Scissors kick   4. Butterfly stroke

_____ Fastest swimming stroke   5. Jellyfish float

_____ One kick per two strokes   6. Back crawl stroke

_____ Scissors and flutter kick   7. Single Trudgeon

_____ Tuck position   8. Trudgeon crawl

                                         9. Skulling

                                        10. Vertical float

Sample completion questions about tennis.   Directions: One or two blanks appear in each of the following sentences. Write the word in each blank that makes the statement correct.

1.   When one person has won one point and the other no points, the score is _____ _____.

2.   When both competitors have won three points, the score is _____.

3.   The _____ shot causes the ball to go high and deep into the opponent's court.

4.   Top spin on the ball will cause it to bounce _____ and _____.

5. The height of the net should be _____ feet at the center and _____ feet at the posts.

6. The _____ grip is the most common one.

7. To win a set, one competitor must win at least _____ games and hold a _____ game advantage.

8. When a high bouncing ball is returned with a swift overhead shot, the shot is called a _____.

Characteristics of
Different Types of Test Items

Each type of test question has certain characteristics which influence the usefulness of that type of question.

Essay. Essay questions have the following characteristics:

1. An essay test is easy to construct because a few briefly stated questions may cover extensive subject matter and require extensive responses from the student.

2. Essay questions are advantageous to students who express themselves well in writing.

3. They afford the students more freedom to explain what he knows and believes about the subject.

4. They tend to guide students toward learning the fundamental facts and larger concepts as opposed to specific facts and figures.

5. Their correction is time-consuming and it must be done by a person who thoroughly understands the content of the subject (usually the teacher).

True–False. True-false questions have the following characteristics:

1. A true–false test is more difficult to construct than an essay test because a relatively large number of questions are needed to cover the subject.

2. True–false questions encourage guessing when students are not sure of the answers.

3.   They are not good measures of major concepts because each question can deal with only a small amount of information. They tend to test trivial information.

4.   They are easy to correct and can be corrected by almost anyone who has the answer sheet.

Multiple-choice.   Multiple-choice questions have the following characteristics:

1.   A multiple-choice test is probably the most difficult to construct.

2.   Multiple-choice questions are more thought provoking than true–false questions.

3.   They require more than two choices of answers.

4.   They allow guessing on the part of the student.

5.   They are easy to correct and can be corrected by almost anyone who has the answer sheet.

6.   They are not good measures of large and fundamental concepts. They tend to test trivial information, but less so than true–false questions.

Matching.   Matching questions have the following characteristics:

1.   A matching test is fairly easy to construct.

2.   Matching questions tend to measure only recall rather than understanding.

3.   They can measure only certain kinds of information.

4.   They allow guessing on the part of the student.

5.   They can be corrected by almost anyone who has the answer sheet.

6.   They tend to measure trivial information.

7.   They can elicit a relatively large number of responses in a short test period.

Completion.   Completion questions have the following characteristics:

1.   A completion test is relatively easy to construct.

2.   Completion questions encourage memorization rather than understanding.

3.   They are simple to correct but should be corrected by a person who knows the various responses that are acceptable.

4.   They tend to measure trivial information.

In formulating test questions, the teacher might follow these suggestions:

1.   Avoid ambiguous questions. Example of an ambiguous true–false question: The maximum number of games in a set in tennis is six or more if one of the competitors does not have a two-game advantage.

2.   Avoid questions which are trivial and not pertinent to the unit of instruction. Example of a trivial completion question: The length of a tennis net is _____ feet.

3.   Avoid wordiness; state questions concisely and clearly. Example of a wordy true–false question: In wrestling it usually is not a very good idea, but sometimes it is beneficial to feint to the left then move to the right in order to pull the opponent out of position so you can take advantage of his error.

4.   Avoid trick questions. Example of a trick true–false question: In golf the club ordinarily used for teeing off is known as a driver.

5.   Avoid giveaway words such as *always, never, all* and *none.* Example of a giveaway true-false question: In basketball the players who warm up properly will *always* perform better than other players.

6.   Avoid terms that are too general. Example of a true–false question that is too general: In tennis there are *several* basic grips.

7.   Avoid stating questions negatively. Example of a negative true–false question: It is wrong for a free style swimmer not to breath on at least every second stroke.

8.   Avoid stating more than one concept in a question. Example of a true–false question involving more than one concept: In a swimming race the competitor should swim as fast as possible, conserve as much energy as possible, and use good swimming form.

Evaluation of Written Test Items

Each test item should be evaluated to determine contributing or noncontributing items; then noncontributing items should be discarded. An item is considered noncontributing if it is:

1.   Not highly discriminating; that is, if it does not distinguish between superior and inferior individuals on the trait being measured.

2.   Invalid; that is, if it does not really measure what it is supposed to measure.

3.   Unreliable; that is, if it does not consistently measure the same quality.

4.   Vague; that is, if it is difficult to interpret and easy to misinterpret so that it detracts from reliability.

The teacher should determine whether each item did what it was intended and, if so, how well it achieved its purpose. Each question in the test should be pertinent to the subject. Questions incidental to the subject or relatively unimportant should be omitted. The purpose of a question is to find out if the student knows the answer, not whether he can understand the question. Therefore questions should be stated in a clear and concise manner.

Motor Performance Tests

Athletic performance tests may be classified into two categories, standard tests and teacher-made tests. There are many standard performance tests, some of which are highly useful in instructional programs while others are useful only in research. Standard tests have been constructed to measure such traits as strength, power, agility, endurance, general athletic ability, and specific skills.

Frequently at the beginning, during, or at the completion of a unit of instruction the teacher may want to measure the performance levels of the students. Standard tests are often not suited to such use. Therefore the teacher will need to determine the specific skills included in the unit and establish a performance test to evaluate each student's mastery of the skills.

Construction and standardization of a performance test is an involved process. To develop such tests the teacher should:

1. Keep in mind the reason for giving the test, and identify the particular traits the test will measure, such as strength, power, or general athletic ability.

2. Select all test items that measure the specific qualities to be tested.

3. Eliminate items that are not feasible in terms of time, facilities, or cost.

4. Determine the validity and reliability of each of the remaining items. He can usually determine validity by administering the item to a representative group and then correlating the results with a selected criterion measure. He can determine reliability by the test-retest method.)

5. Make the final selection of items to be included, eliminating invalid, unreliable, or duplicate items.

6. Determine the order in which test items should be administered and the exact procedure to be followed in administering the items.

7. Establish final ratings of validity and reliability for the test as a whole. (He can establish the final validity rating by administering the test to a sample of the population for which it is designed, then correlating the results with the best criterion measure available. He can establish the final reliability rating by correlating the two sets of scores obtained by the test-retest method.)

8. Prepare written instructions explaining exactly how the test should be administered.

9. Prepare norms for the test.

For examples of standardized motor performance tests, see the tests described in Chapters 18, 19 and 20.

Construction of Teacher-Made Motor Performance Tests

Such tests should include skills that are frequently used in the sport and can accurately be measured. For example, a unit in basketball might have test items on shooting or accuracy, straight dribbling speed, dribbling speed over a zigzag course, or passing the ball repeatedly against a wall. After a unit of instruction on wrestling the teacher may test the students on their ability to perform certain holds, take downs, and escapes. At the end of a unit on tennis the teacher might conduct a tournament to determine the relative performance ability of the students.

Many skills commonly included in teacher-made tests can be scored by highly objective means, such as measures of speed, distance, and accuracy. However, performance of some skills must be judged subjectively. For instance, a teacher might subjectively judge a student on form in swimming, diving, gymnastics, and trampoline performance.

When subjective judgment is the basis for the score, a rating scale is often helpful. A five-point scale is used most frequently and consists of the following:

| Poor | Fair | Average | Good | Excellent |

The scale may then be converted to corresponding letter grades of F (poor), D, C, B, A (excellent). Or it may be converted to numbers on a 100-point scale (for example, 20, 40, 60, 80, 100), and the numbers may be added to other scores to form the basis for the letter grade.

If a more refined scoring system is desired, a ten-point scale may be used. On this scale the student is assigned a number between one and ten indicating his performance rating. One would signify very poor performance, five, average; and ten, outstanding.

Establishment of Norms

Standard tests often have a scale of scores that serve as a standard for comparison of any raw score on the test. These standards are called norms and are usually in the form of z scores, T scores, 6σ scores, or percentiles.

The use of a particular scale (z, T, 6σ, or percentile) is a matter of the examiner's preference since these scales furnish essentially the same information. The scales in Appendixes B, C, and D are examples of norms.

Norms provide a convenient way to find the relative status of any raw score and thereby greatly enhance the ability to interpret the score. To establish norms the test should be administered to a large, representative sample of the population for which the norms are to be developed, and a standard scale should be made to fit the scores from the sample. Chapter 7 on the interpretation of scores provides further information on norms.

Selected References

Barrow, Harold M., and McGee, Rosemary, *A Practical Approach to Measurement in Physical Education*. Philadelphia: Lea & Febiger, 1964, pp. 497–540.

Clarke, H. Harrison, *Application of Measurement to Health and Physical Education*, 4th ed. Englewood Cliffs, N.J.: Prentice-Hall, 1967, pp. 23–42.

Johnson, Barry L., and Nelson, Jack K., *Practical Measurements for Evaluation in Physical Education*. Minneapolis: Burgess Publishing Company, 1969, pp. 45–58.

McCloy, Charles H., and Young, Norma D., *Tests and Measurements in Health and Physical Education*, 3rd. ed. New York: Appleton-Century-Crofts, 1954, pp. 29–36.

Meyers, Carlton R., and Blesh, T. Erwin, *Measurement in Physical Education*. New York: The Ronald Press, 1962, pp. 78–101.

Scott, M. Gladys, and French, Esther, *Measurement and Evaluation in Physical Education*. Dubuque, Iowa: William C. Brown Company, 1959, pp. 10–42, 76–138.

23
Application of Test Results

Chapter 4 proposes a testing program which should be reviewed again at this point. Results of the tests in the program are useful in several ways: They can motivate students toward achievement; they can assist in evaluating the effectiveness of the program; and they can provide information for evaluating progress and establishing grades.

Motivation of Students

To perform well in school students must be motivated to achieve. Both written and motor performance tests can represent the goals that students want to attain. The results of such tests provide students with evidence of progress or lack of progress. The lack of such evidence detracts from motivation.

Students generally want to be more knowledgeable, fit, and skillful. They are stimulated by goals and want to demonstrate their achievements. Furthermore they want to see evidence that they are progressing and are satisfied by such evidence.

Program Evaluation

A student's progress is the best indication of a successful program. To determine progress the teacher must have clearly in mind the goals toward which the student should be progressing. Then the teacher should employ sound methods for evaluating progress.

One means that a teacher has for determining progress is periodic measurement of a student's achievement. Measures of achievement in tennis help to evaluate the effectiveness of the tennis phase of the program. Measures of achievement in gymnastics, swimming, basketball, and other sports help to evaluate the success of these phases of the program. When achievement is low and progress is slow, the teacher should look seriously at the program content and methods: Progress is closely related to a desire to progress, to course content (the extent to which the content is interesting, challenging, and suited to students' abilities), to teaching method, and to the teacher's competence.

Evaluation of Students
and Establishment of Marks

Every teacher should develop and use effective evaluation procedures and an accurate method of marking[1] students. A student's marks in school are important because they determine to some extent whether he will secure a good position, be admitted into college, win a scholarship, or gain prestige among his classmates. But perhaps more important, marks represent to the student and his parents an evaluation of his success in school. Because of the importance placed on marks an accurate system for determining and reporting marks must be adopted.

Purpose of Marking

Grades serve different purposes for students, teachers and guidance counselors, parents, and school administrators. A mark should inform the student how nearly he has met the standards on which the mark is based. It should clearly indicate to him how well he performed as contrasted to how well he might be expected to perform. If it is not accurate or justifiable and if it has a weak basis, then the mark loses its value to the student. It may even destroy the student's interest and incentive and result in a negative attitude toward the subject and the teacher.

Teachers and guidance personnel may use marks for guidance and counseling. If accurately determined, marks can help the teacher predict how successful a student might be in certain pursuits and may also help the teacher evaluate the effectiveness of his teaching.

Parents are usually eager to learn of their children's success in school and also desire to know the reason for the absence of success. Marks that are properly obtained, reported, and interpreted will furnish desired facts. As a result, guidance from home may help overcome deficiencies.

In the present school systems marks are essential to administrators, who interpret them as symbols of progress and indicators of achievement levels. Since marks become permanent records of achievement, they are also used as a basis for promotion and scholastic honor awards. It is essential, then, that marks be established on a solid, equally fair basis and that they be accurately reported and interpreted.

Criteria for Useful Marks

Marks should be valid. They must truly represent the quality and quantity of pupil achievement for which they purportedly stand.

Marks should be reliable. They must accurately and consistently represent the same results for each student.

---

[1] The term *marking* is preferred over the term *grading*.

Marks should be highly objective. Different teachers, given the same data on a student, should arrive at the same mark. This quality is dependent upon a clearly defined marking system.

Marks should be assigned on the basis of definite standards. The standards should not differ for each pupil nor should they fluctuate widely from one year to the next.

Marks should be capable of clear interpretation with regard to what they signify. If the significance of an A is not evident in terms of quality and quantity of achievement, then the grade lacks meaning.

Marks should be based on a system that allows for the most economical use of the teacher's time and effort. Since marking is only one of the teacher's many tasks, only a reasonable amount of time can be justified for it.

Marks should be timely. Final marks are recorded only at the end of semesters, but for purposes of incentive students should frequently be informed of their progress and present standing.

Basis for Determining Marks

Marks can be assigned on an absolute or a relative basis. An absolute mark is assigned solely on achievement, without regard for potential. A relative mark is assigned on achievement in reference to potential. Some authorities recommend that in physical education courses absolute marks be kept on record but that marks relative to the potential of the student be assigned as a final grade. They emphasize that a student who performs at his present potential, even though it may be low, should receive an A, while one who actually performs better but does not approach his potential should receive a lower mark.

On the other hand, many authorities take the stand that a student should be marked solely on his performance in class, without regard for his potential. On this basis those students who do the best in class will receive high marks even though they could have done better, and those students who perform poorly will receive low marks even though they performed near their potential.

There are sound arguments for both the absolute and relative methods of marking. The teachers in a particular school should decide what method is to be adopted, and then be consistent in the use of that method.

Marking is based on several factors and each factor should be weighted according to its importance. The following plan will serve as a guide.

The teacher determines the amount of weight given each factor. The score given for each factor is based on A = 5, B = 4, C = 3, D = 2, F = 1. To determine the points for each factor the teacher multiplies the score by the weight. The total points may be converted to a letter grade according to the following: 0–20 = F, 21–40 = D, 41–60 = C, 61–80 = B, 81–100 = A.

	Weight	Score	Points	Points Possible
Motor Fitness	5	4	20	25
Skill in the Activities	5	4	20	25
Knowledge of the Activities	3	3	9	15
Attendance	2	5	10	10
Uniform (dress) and grooming	1	2	2	5
Posture	1	4	4	5
Attitude	1	3	3	5
Character	2	3	6	10
			Total 74	100
			Final Grade = C+	

Valid and reliable tests can accurately measure such factors as motor fitness, skill, and knowledge. However, because of the difficulties in measuring attitudes and character, there is some disagreement as to whether these are valid factors on which to mark. Nevertheless some teachers insist that these outcomes are so vital to a good program that they must be considered in marking. Since there are no valid and objective measures of character and attitudes which are practical for class use, whatever weight these factors carry in marking must be based on subjective judgments.

In addition to the previously discussed criteria, marking should be based on reasonable, acceptable educational practices and on sound concepts and objectives. So they will not be misled, students should be aware of the basis for determining marks.

Methods of Reporting Marks

The following methods of reporting marks are used:

Five Letter Method. This is the most commonly used system. It consists of A, excellent; B, good; C, average; D, poor; and F, very poor or failing.

Pass or Fail Method. In this system a standard of acceptability is established. If the student performs up to the standard, he passes. If he performs below the standard, he fails. Sometimes *satisfactory* or *unsatisfactory* are terms used in place of *pass* or *fail*.

Percent Method. In this method the student is given a percentage score as a mark, with 100 percent representing excellent performance in the class. Percentages are frequently converted to letter grades in order to make them more meaningful. Usually it is assumed that 90–100 percent = A; 80–89 percent = B; 70–79 percent = C; 60–69 percent = D; below 60 percent = F.

Descriptive Statement Method. This method, which is becoming more popular in secondary schools, consists of a short paragraph explaining precisely the student's status and stating the student's strengths and weaknesses in the subject.

Whatever method of reporting is used, it should add dignity to the program, and it should be interpretable and meaningful to the student and his parents.

Selected References

Aschenbrenner, Robert A., A Study of the Reliability of One Type of Discrimination Index for Test Items. Unpublished master's thesis, State University of Iowa, 1949.

Barrow, Harold M., and McGee, Rosemary, *A Practical Approach to Measurement in Physical Education*. Philadelphia: Lea & Febiger, 1964, pp. 497–540.

Clarke, H. Harrison, *Application of Measurement to Health and Physical Education*, 4th ed. Englewood Cliffs, N.J.: Prentice-Hall, 1967, pp. 23–42.

Davis, Frederick B., "Item-Analysis Data: Their Computation, Interpretation and Use in Test Construction." Harvard Education Papers #2, Graduate School of Education, Harvard University, 1946, 42 pp.

Flanagan, John C., "General Considerations in the Selection of Test Items and a Short Method of Estimating the Product-Moment Coefficient from Data at the Tails of the Distribution." *Journal of Educational Psychology*, 1939, *30*, 674.

Johnson, Barry L., and Nelson, Jack K., *Practical Measurements for Evaluation in Physical Education*. Minneapolis: Burgess Publishing Company, 1969, pp. 45–58.

McCloy, Charles H., and Young, Norma D., *Tests and Measurements in Health and Physical Education*, 3rd ed. New York: Appleton-Century-Crofts, 1954, pp. 29–36.

Meyers, Carlton R., and Blesh, T. Erwin, *Measurement in Physical Education*, New York: The Ronald Press, 1962, pp. 78–101.

Richardson, M. M., and Kuder, G. F., "The Calculation of Test Reliability Coefficients Based on the Method of Rational Equivalence." *Journal of Educational Psychology*, 1939, *30*, 681.

Richardson, M. M., and Kuder, G. F., "The Theory of the Estimation of Test Reliability." *Psychometrika*, 1937, *2*, 151.

Scott, M. Gladys, and French, Esther, *Measurement and Evaluation in Physical Education*. Dubuque, Iowa: Wm. C. Brown Company, 1959, pp. 10–42, 76–138.

Swineford, F. "Validity of Test Items." *Journal of Educational Psychology*, 1936, *27*, 68.

Votaw, D. F., "Graphical Determination of Probable Error in Validation of Test Items." *Journal of Educational Psychology*, 1933, *22*, 682–86.

Weiss, Raymond, and Scott, M. Gladys, *Research Methods in Health, Physical Education and Recreation*, 2nd ed. Washington, D.C.: American Association for Health, Physical Education and Recreation, 1959, ch. 8.

NINE
Supplementary
Material

The information in this section supplements and supports the other material in the text.

Glossary

Appendix A: Data for Problems

Appendix B: Achievement Scales for Girls and Women

DGWS Performance Test

Hyde Archery Test

Newton Motor Ability Test

Scott Motor Ability Test (High School Girls)

Scott Motor Ability Test (College Women)

Iowa–Brace Test

Leilich Basketball Test

Russell–Lange Volleyball Test

AAHPER Fitness Test (Girls)
    Flexed-Arm Hang
    Sit-ups
    Shuttle Run
    Standing Long Jump
    50-Yard Dash
    Softball Throw
    600-Yard Run–Walk

AAHPER Fitness Test (College Women)

Appendix C: Achievement Scales for Boys

Iowa–Brace Test

Lehsten Basketball Test

AAHPER Fitness Test Items
    Pull-Ups
    Sit-Ups
    Shuttle Run
    Standing Long Jump

50-Yard Dash
Softball Throw
600-Yard Run–Walk

Other Individual Performance Tests
Dips on Parallel Bars
Push-Ups
Rope Climb
Vertical Jump
Shot Put—12 pound
100-Yard Run
440-Yard Run

Appendix D: Achievement Scales for College Men

Harvard Step Test

Stroup Basketball Test

JCR Test

Larson Motor Ability Test

AAHPER Fitness Test (Pull-Ups, Sit-Ups, Shuttle Run, Standing Long Jump, 50-Yard Dash, Softball Throw, 600-Yard Run–Walk)

Other Individual Performance Tests
Dips on Parallel Bars
Push-Ups
Rope Climb
Vertical Jump
Shot Put—12 pound
100-Yard Run
440-Yard Run

Appendix E: Table of Squares and Square Roots

Glossary

The physical educator is faced with the problem of choosing terms with clear meanings and relationships. The clarity of a term depends upon the choice of words used in defining it. The importance of terminology in the areas of statistics and measurement necessitates the use of simple words with clear meanings.

The terms in this glossary have been selected and defined in the context of their use in this book.

Ability. Development that has occurred within the limitations of capacity; represented by the highest performance record or achievement score attained within a recent period of time.

Abscissa. Horizontal axis in the coordinate system.

Accomplishment. An individual's best level of achievement.

Accuracy. Freedom from errors.

Achievement. Evaluation of a person's performance record based on the performance records of a group of like persons.

A.D. Average deviation.

Agility. Ability to move quickly and change position and direction rapidly.

Anteroposterior posture. Posture as seen from a side view.

Anthropometry. Science of measurement of people relating to structure; measurement of body dimensions—lengths, widths, depths, and circumferences.

Aptitude. Talent or potential indicating probability of success in a line of endeavor.

AR. Abbreviation for arbitrary reference.

Athletic ability. Ability to perform in physical education activities (athletics).

Attitude. Readiness to act in a particular way; an expression of different degrees of acceptance or rejection.

Average deviation. Average of the amount that scores deviate from the mean of the distribution.

Badge test. Test in which a badge is given for a standard performance; not an appropriate name for a test.

Balance. Ability to keep the center of gravity over the base of support; ability to maintain equilibrium.

Bar graph. Type of histogram shown horizontally.

Battery of tests. Number of tests given to a person or group of persons usually within a short period of time.

Bimodal. A distribution of scores with two modes. A curve with the two high points of equal height.

Calipers. Instrument used to measure body dimensions.

Capacity. Limits (potential) determined by heredity and other factors within which ability may be developed.

Cf. Abbreviation for cumulative frequencies.

Chest expansion. Difference in girth of chest with one measurement taken after full expiration and one taken following a full inspiration.

Chronological age. Age in years, months, and days from time of birth.

Circulorespiratory endurance. Ability to sustain activity over a period of time; the efficiency with which the cardiovascular and respiratory systems work.

Coefficient of correlation. Numerical expression of relationship of two or more variables, varying between minus 1 and plus 1.

Coefficient of reliability. Numerical expression of relationship between scores obtained from two applications of the *same* test to the *same* students by the *same* examiner, separated by a short interval of time; in most cases, .90 is considered relatively high.

Coefficient of validity. Numerical expression of relationship between test scores and criterion scores by which the validity of the test is being judged.

Comparable measures. Measures expressed in terms of the same unit and with reference to the same zero point.

Conduct. Overt behavior that is measured as performance.

Continuous series. Series of data capable of any degree of subdivision (tenths or hundredths of a second).

Control group. Group not subjected to experimental procedures.

Correlation. Relationship between two series of measures of the same individuals.

CR. Abbreviation for critical ratio.

Criterion. Law, fact, or standard by which the validity of some factor is to be determined.

Critical ratio. Obtained difference between two measures divided by the standard error of the difference.

Crude score. Raw score; original score obtained.

Curvilinear correlation. Relationship between two sets of scores expressed by a curved line.

Data. Facts or scores that are used as sources of information.

Decathlon test. Test consisting of ten events.

Decils. Points that divide the total number of cases in a frequency distribution into 10 equal parts; 10th, 20th, 30th, etc., percentiles.

Development. Improvement in function or behavior.

Discrete series. Series of data that cannot be subdivided without destroying the unit (such as basketballs or people).

Divergency. Extreme deviation from a range of normality; an anomaly that may be structural (six fingers on one hand) or functional (pneumonia).

Dynamic strength. Strength exhibited in motion.

Dynamometer. Instrument used to measure muscular strength.

Endurance. Ability to postpone fatigue.

Evaluation. Process of determining the value of something using numbers or words.

Examination. Appraisal of present status in any respect; means used to make the appraisal.

Experimental group. Group subjected to the experimental procedures.

f. Abbreviation for frequencies.

Flexibility. Range of movement with reference to joints in a body.

Frequency distribution. Scores listed in order of their size with the number of occurrence indicated opposite each score.

Frequency polygon. Line graph of a frequency distribution.

GA. Abbreviation for guessed average.

General ability test. A test that includes ability in art, music, physical education, and other fields.

General athletic ability. Ability exhibited in a considerable number of athletic activities.

General endurance. Ability to continue performance in a variety of activities.

General motor ability. Ability to perform effectively in a variety of motor activities.

Graph. Pictorial illustration of a frequency distribution.

Growth. Increase in size.

Health. Freedom from disease; condition that enables the body organs to function efficiently; quality of functioning of the human organism.

Histogram. Frequency distribution represented in a series of adjacent columns.

Impulsive traits. Traits involving feelings; interests, attitudes, emotions, and ideals.

Initial test. Test given at the beginning of an experimental period or period of time.

Interpretive traits. Ideas, concepts, comprehension, knowledge, and judgments.

Interquartile range. Distance between the 25th and 75th percentiles in a distribution of scores.

Knowledge. Facts; information.

Mark. Rating given a pupil.

Maturation. Degree of completion as a result of growth and development.

Mean (M). Arithmetic average; sum of the measures divided by the number of measures.

Measurement. Process of objective, precise evaluation; process by which a person tries to find the degree to which a trait is possessed by another person.

Measures of central tendency. Central points on a scale of scores.

Measures of variability. Distances along the scale of scores.

Median (Mdn). Point on the scale above and below which half the scores occur.

Mode. Point on the scale at which the most frequencies occur.

Motor ability. Developed ability to perform a variety of motor activities.

Motor capacity. The limits (potential) determined by heredity and other factors within which motor ability may be developed.

Multimodal. A distribution with more than two modes.

Muscular endurance. Ability of the muscles to continue repeated contractions.

Muscular power. Ability to use muscular force in one concentrated or explosive effort.

Muscular strength. Ability to exert muscular force against resistance.

Native ability. Native implies potential or capacity and should not be used in connection with ability which is developed as a result of activity.

Native capacity. Capacity determined by heredity which places limits on the structure and function of the human organism.

Neuromuscular development. Development of strength and skill (nerve–muscle coordinations).

Norm. Average or typical value (score) of a particular performance in a homogeneous population.

Normal curve. Bell-shaped curve with the mean, median, and mode equal, and with the curve fitting all other specifications of a normal curve as described in Chapter 6.

Objective. Goal, aim, or purpose; accurate test scores. (In an objective test different examiners use the same instrument to measure the same trait and obtain the same scores.)

Objectivity. Quality of dependence on factual evidence or established truth rather than on personal opinion or judgment.

Ogive curve. Cumulative frequency curve with a percentile scale added.

Ordinate. Vertical axis in the coordinate system.

Parameter. True statistic of the total population; True mean or true variance.

Pentathlon test. Test consisting of five events.

Performance. What a person does as distinguished from what his potential is.

Physique. Structural organization and body proportions; external appearance of the body.

Posture. Relative alignment and position of body segments.

Power. Rate at which work is performed; amount of work performed divided by the time taken to perform the work; the product of force and velocity.

PR. Abbreviation for percentile rank.

Proficiency. Less desirable term used to mean *efficiency* in performance.

Progress. Improvement indicated by the difference in scores obtained on two identical tests with an interval of time between the tests.

Pulse test. Test indicating the reaction of the human pulse to activity or other conditions.

Quality scale. Scale composed of a set of samples arranged in order of merit.

Questionnaire. Series of questions used in the collection of data only when there is not a more reliable technique to obtain the needed data.

Random sample. Representative sample that has been selected without bias from the total group.

Range. Difference between extreme scores.

Rank correlation. Method of finding relationship by computing the correlation between ranks rather than between exact scores.

Raw score. Original obtained score; crude score.

Rectilinear correlation. Relationship between two sets of scores expressed by a straight line.

Reliability of a test. The amount of agreement between the results secured from two applications of the *same* test to the *same* students by the *same* examiner (with a short interval of time between the tests).

SD (σ or sigma). Abbreviation for standard deviation.

Semi-interquartile range. Half the distance between the 25th and 75th percentiles.

SI. Abbreviation for the step interval used in a frequency distribution. In connection with Rogers strength test, *SI* means strength index.

Sigma difference. Standard deviation of a distribution of obtained differences.

Six sigma scale. A statistical scale (standard scale) covering 100 points (0–100) in six standard deviations. The mean of the scale is always 50, and the standard deviation is 16.67.

Skewed distribution. Condition whereby the mean, median, and mode are at different points and the balance of the curve is thrown to the left or to the right.

Skill. Ability to coordinate effectively the actions of the different muscles used in a body movement; neuromuscular functions.

Standard. Statement of the performance that students should reach at a certain time; standards may or may not be the same as norms.

Standard deviation. Square root of the average of the squared deviations in a distribution of scores; most reliable measure of variability.

Standard error. Standard deviation of the sample distribution of any measure (a mean, a sigma, or other such measure).

Standard score. Score expressed in terms of standard deviation units from the mean of the scores. Examples are z scores, *T* scores, and 6σ scores.

Standardized test. A test with satisfactory content for which norms and standard instructions have been established and which may be scored with a high degree of objectivity.

Static strength. Strength exhibited without overt motion.

Statistical method. Method of research based on the collection and interpretation of numerical data.

Strength. Ability of the muscles to exert force against resistance. (Strength is lessened by inadequate nutrition or inadequate exercise.)

Subjective. Dependence on personal judgment of truth rather than factual evidence or established truth.

Technique. Method or way of performing; technical form or skill.

Test. Device or procedure used to measure performance or ability.

T-scale. Statistical scale (standard scale) proposed by McCall and named in honor of Terman and Thorndike, consisting of 100 units and extending from five standard deviations below the mean to five standard deviations above the mean with the mean score always 50 on the scale, and the standard deviation of the scale is 10.

T score. Standard score based on a 10 standard deviation scale with the mean at 50.

Undistributed scores. Scores that fail to distinguish between degrees of student performances.

Unimodal. A distribution which has only one mode.

Validity of a test. Accurate measurement of that which the test is claimed to measure.

Variability of scores. Extent of differences in magnitude.

Variance. Average of the squared deviations taken from the mean of the distribution of scores.

Weighting scores. Assigning of values to be carried by each of a number of scores when determining a total or average score.

Work capacity. Potential for doing work.

z-scale. A statistical scale (standard scale) with the mean of the scale equalling zero and the standard deviation equalling one.

z scores. Standard scores based on a six standard deviation scale with the mean at zero.

Appendix A:
Data for Problems

Data I

The number of Sit-ups in 30 seconds Performed by
50 High School Girls

13	20	9	15	16
7	17	17	18	11
10	16	19	17	17
11	14	17	13	15
19	21	14	12	13
15	16	11	14	18
17	17	17	18	21
15	19	17	18	16
13	17	61	20	14
18	19	8	17	18

Data II

Scores Made by 75 High School Boys on the right Grip Test,
Measured to the Nearest Pound

100	94	106	64	97
95	86	139	121	133
94	124	96	100	107
99	103	103	96	99
85	76	91	104	110
101	125	111	113	117
75	102	92	93	120
60	88	80	123	105
102	127	104	97	138
110	113	90	89	118
98	128	100	114	65
115	101	63	102	109
109	78	114	79	80
95	112	99	108	125
110	90	89	129	79

Data III

Data on Five Different Factors for 25 Junior High School Boys

Case	Height (inches)	Weight (pounds)	Leg Strength (pounds)	High Jump (inches)	100-yard Run (Seconds)	Long Jump (inches)
1	65	126	560	55	12.4	199
2	66	156	720	58	10.7	196
3	68	143	616	59	10.3	193
4	67	125	592	55	12.3	197
5	69	132	472	57	13.0	168
6	66	121	513	52	13.0	166
7	62	97	460	49	12.4	176
8	69	147	614	42	10.1	199
9	68	145	520	58	12.8	187
10	60	124	480	51	13.7	149
11	63	111	470	54	12.6	177
12	63	100	450	41	12.9	174
13	69	145	736	58	12.4	214
14	58	61	372	45	15.6	112
15	64	112	510	53	12.6	185
16	70	136	615	61	12.5	177
17	68	138	662	58	12.9	196
18	67	137	640	56	12.5	170
19	70	143	687	59	13.6	166
20	67	129	532	53	13.5	167
21	65	118	510	55	14.0	177
22	60	90	470	45	14.8	141
23	68	157	767	56	12.0	204
24	68	150	620	59	13.0	187
25	68	127	540	60	15.8	185

Range =

Mean =

Data IV

Squares for Data III

Case	Height	Weight	Leg Strength	High Jump	100-yard Run	Long Jump
1	4225	15876	313600	3025	153.76	37601
2	4356	24336	518400	3364	114.49	38416
3	4624	20446	379456	3481	106.09	37249
4	4489	15625	350464	3025	151.29	38809
5	4761	17424	222784	3249	169.00	28224
6	4356	14641	263169	2704	169.00	27556
7	3844	9409	211600	2401	153.76	30976
8	4761	21609	376996	1764	102.01	39601
9	4624	21025	270400	3364	163.84	34969
10	3600	15376	230400	2601	187.69	22201
11	3969	12321	220900	2916	158.76	31329
12	3969	10000	202500	1681	166.41	30276
13	4761	21025	541696	3364	153.76	45796
14	2601	3721	138384	2025	243.36	12544
15	4096	12544	260100	2809	158.76	34225
16	4900	18496	378225	3721	156.25	31329
17	4624	19044	438244	3364	166.41	38416
18	4489	18769	409600	3136	156.25	28900
19	4900	20449	471969	3481	184.76	27556
20	4489	16641	283024	2809	182.25	27889
21	4225	13924	260100	3025	196.00	31329
22	3600	8100	220900	2025	219.04	19881
23	4624	24649	588289	3136	144.00	41616
24	4624	22500	384400	3481	169.00	34969
25	4624	16129	291600	3600	249.64	34225
ΣX^2	108135	414082	8601282	73551	4175.78	807882

Sigma =

Appendix B:
Achievement Scales for Girls and Women

Achievement Scales for DGWS Physical Performance Test*

Scale Score	Standing Broad Jump	Basket- ball Throw	Potato Race	Pull- Ups	Push- Ups	Sit- Ups	10- Second Squat Thrust	30- Second Squat Thrust	Score
100	7-9	78	8.4	47	61	65	9-1	24	100
95	7-7	75	8.6	45	58	61	9	23	95
90	7-4	72	8.8	42	54	57	8-3	22	90
85	7-2	68	9.0	39	51	54	8-1	21	85
80	6-11	65	9.4	37	47	50	8	20	80
75	6-9	62	9.6	34	43	46	7-3	19	75
70	6-7	59	10.0	32	39	43	7-1	18-2	70
65	6-4	56	10.2	29	36	39	7	18	65
60	6-2	53	10.4	26	32	36	6-2	17	60
55	6-0	50	10.6	24	28	33	6-1	16	55
50	5-9	46	11.0	21	25	29	6	15	50
45	5-7	43	11.2	18	21	25	5-2	14-2	45
40	5-5	40	11.6	16	17	22	5-1	14	40
35	5-2	37	11.8	13	13	18	4-3	13	35
30	5-0	34	12.0	10	10	15	4-2	12	30
25	4-9	31	12.4	8	6	11	4	11	25
20	4-7	27	12.6	5	2	7	3-3	10	20
15	4-4	24	13.0	3	1	3	3-2	9	15
10	4-2	21	13.2	1	0	1	3	8-2	10
5	4-0	18	13.4	0	0	0	2-3	7-2	5
0	3-9	15	13.6	0	0	0	2-2	7	0

* Eleanore Metheny, Chairman, "Physical Performance Levels for High School Girls," *Journal of Health and Physical Education*, June 1945. p. 309. Reprinted by permission of the AAHPER

Achievement Scales in Archery for Women*

Scale	First Columbia Total Score (Target Score)	Final Columbia Record (Target score)			
		Total Score	50 yards	40 yards	30 yards
100	436	466	150	176	194
99	430	460	148	174	192
98	424	455	146	171	190
97	418	449	143	169	187
96	412	443	141	167	185
95	406	438	139	164	183
94	400	432	137	162	181
93	394	426	135	160	179
92	388	420	132	157	176
91	382	415	130	155	174
90	376	409	128	153	172
89	370	403	126	150	170
88	364	398	124	148	168
87	358	392	121	146	165
86	352	386	119	143	163
85	346	381	117	141	161
84	340	375	115	139	159
83	334	369	113	136	157
82	328	363	110	134	154
81	322	358	108	132	152
80	316	352	106	129	150
79	310	346	104	127	148
78	304	341	102	125	146
77	298	335	99	122	143
76	292	329	97	120	141
75	286	324	95	118	139
74	280	318	93	115	137
73	274	312	91	113	135
72	268	306	88	111	132
71	262	301	86	108	130
70	256	295	84	106	128
69	250	289	82	104	126
68	244	284	80	101	124
67	238	278	77	99	121
66	232	272	75	97	119
65	226	267	73	94	117
64	220	261	71	92	115
63	214	255	69	90	113
62	208	249	66	87	110
61	202	244	64	85	108

* Edith I. Hyde, "An Achievement Scale in Archery," *Research Quarterly*, 1937, **7** (2), 109. Reprinted by permission of the AAHPER.

Achievement Scales for the Newton Motor Ability Test*

Point Score	Hurdles	Broad Jump	Scramble	Point Score	Hurdles	Broad Jump	Scramble
100	7.2	83.0	10.4	50	10.9	61.5	16.7
99	7.3	82.5	10.6	49		61.0	16.8
98	7.4	82.0	10.7	48	11.0	60.5	16.9
97			10.8	47	11.1	60.0	17.1
96	7.5	81.5	10.9	46	11.2	59.5	17.2
95	7.6	81.0	11.0	45		59.0	17.3
94	7.7	80.5	11.2	44	11.3		17.4
93		80.0	11.3	43	11.4	58.5	17.6
92	7.8	79.5	11.4	42	11.5	58.0	17.7
91	7.9	79.0	11.6	41		57.5	17.8
90		78.5	11.7	40	11.6	57.0	17.9
89	8.0		11.8	39	11.7	56.5	18.1
88	8.1	78.0	11.9	38		56.0	18.2
87	8.2	77.5	12.0	37	11.8		18.3
86		77.0	12.2	36	11.9	55.5	18.4
85	8.3	76.5	12.3	35	12.0	55.0	18.6
84	8.4	76.0	12.4	34		54.5	18.7
83	8.5	75.5	12.6	33	12.1	54.0	18.8
82		75.0	12.7	32	12.2	53.5	18.9
81	8.6		12.8	31	12.3	53.0	19.1
80	8.7	74.5	12.9	30			19.2
79	8.8	74.0	13.0	29	12.4	52.5	19.3
78		73.5	13.2	28	12.5	52.0	19.4
77	8.9	73.0	13.3	27		51.5	19.6
76	9.0	72.5	13.4	26	12.6	51.0	19.7
75		72.0	13.6	25	12.7	50.5	19.8
74	9.1		13.7	24	12.8	50.0	19.9
73	9.2	71.5	13.8	23			20.1
72	9.3	71.0	13.9	22	12.9	49.5	20.2
71		70.5	14.0	21	13.0	49.0	20.3
70	9.4	70.0	14.2	20	13.1	48.5	20.4
69	9.5	69.5	14.3	19		48.0	20.6
68	9.6	69.0	14.4	18	31.2	47.5	20.7
67			14.6	17	13.3	47.0	20.8
66	9.7	68.5	14.7	16	13.4		20.9
65	9.8	68.0	14.8	15		46.5	21.1
64		67.5	14.9	14	13.5	46.0	21.2
63	9.9	67.0	15.0	13	13.6	45.5	21.3
62	10.0	66.5	15.2	12		45.0	21.4
61	10.1	66.0	15.3	11	13.7	44.5	21.6
60			15.4	10	13.8	44.0	21.7
59	10.2	65.5	15.6	9	13.9	43.5	21.8
58	10.3	65.0	15.7	8		43.0	21.9
57	10.4	64.5	15.8	7	14.0		22.1
56		64.0	15.9	6	14.1	42.5	22.2
55	10.5	63.5	16.0	5	14.2	42.0	22.3
54	10.6	63.0	16.2	4		41.5	22.4
53		62.5	16.3	3	14.3	41.0	22.6
52	10.7		16.4	2	14.4	40.5	22.7
51	10.8	62.0	16.6	1			22.8

* Powell, Elizabeth, and Howe, Eugene C., Motor Ability Tests for High School Girls. *Research Quarterly* 1939, *10*, 81–88. Reprinted by permission of the AAHPER.

T-Scales for High School Girls on Scott Motor Ability Test**

T Score	Wall Pass (410)*	Basketball Throw (Feet) (310)*	Broad Jump (Inches) (287)*	4-Second Dash (Yards) (398)*	Obstacle Race (Seconds) (374)*	T Score
80	16	71				80
79			96			79
78						78
77	15	68	94	27		77
76		66			18.5–18.9	76
75		65				75
74		64	92			74
73	14	63				73
72		61				72
71		59	90	26		71
70		55	88		19.0–19.4	70
69	13	54				69
68		52	86	25		68
67		51			19.5–19.9	67
66		50				66
65		49				65
64		48	84	24	20.0–20.4	64
63	12	47				63
62		46	82		20.5–20.9	62
61			80			61
60		45		23		60
59		44	78		21.0–21.4	59
58	11	43				58
57		42	76		21.5–21.9	57
56		41				56
55		40	74	22		55
54					22.0–22.4	54
53		39				53
52	10		72			52
51		37			22.5–22.9	51
50		36		21		50
49		35	70			49
48			68		23.0–23.4	48
47		34	66			47
46	9	33			23.5–23.9	46
45		32	64	20		45
44		31			24.0–24.4	44
43			62			43
42		30			24.5–24.9	42
41	8	29	60	19		41
40		28				40
39			58		25.0–25.4	39
38		27	56			38
37	7		54		25.5–25.9	37
36		26			26.0–26.4	36
35			52	18	26.5–26.9	35

T Score	Wall Pass (410)*	Basketball Throw (Feet) (310)*	Broad Jump (Inches) (287)*	4-second Dash (Yards) (398)*	Obstacle Race (Seconds) (374)*	T Score
34		25	50		27.0–27.4	34
33						33
32		24	47		27.5–27.9	32
31	6	23				31
30			44		28.0–28.4	30
29		22		17	28.5–28.9	29
28					29.0–29.4	28
27		21			29.5–29.9	27
26			40		30.0–30.4	26
25	5	20				25
24				16	30.5–31.9	24
23		19	36		31.5–32.4	23
22				15	32.5–34.9	22
21		16				21
20	4			14	35.0–36.0	20

* Indicates the number of subjects on which the scale is based.
** Scott, M. Gladys, and French, Esther, *Measurement and Evaluation in Physical Education*. Dubuque, Iowa:William C. Brown Company, 1959. Reprinted by permission of the publisher.

T-Scales for College Women on Scott Motor Ability Test*

T Score	Basketball Throw	Passes	Broad Jump	Obstacle Race	T Score
85	75	18	86	17.5–17.9	85
84					84
83	71	17		18.0–18.4	83
82					82
81		16	85		81
80	70	15			80
79	69			18.5–18.9	79
78	68	14	84		78
77	67		83		77
76	66				76
75	65		82	19.0–19.4	75
74	64		81		74
73	62		80		73
72	61	13	79	19.5–19.9	72
71	59				71
70	58		78	20.0–20.4	70
69	57		77		69
68	56		76		68
67	55		75	20.5–20.9	67
66	54	12	74		66
65	52				65
64	51		73	21.0–21.4	64
63	50		72		63
62	48		71	21.5–21.9	62
61	47				61
60	46		70		60
59	45	11	69	22.0–22.4	59
58	44		68		58
57	43		67	22.5–22.9	57
56	42				56
55	41		66	23.0–23.4	55
54	40		65		54
53	39		64	23.5–23.9	53
52	38	10	63		52
51	37			24.0–24.4	51
50	36		62		50
49	35		61	24.5–24.9	49
48			60		48
47	34		59	25.0–25.4	47
46	33		58		46
45	32	9	57	25.5–25.9	45
44	31				44
43			56	26.0–26.4	43
42	30		55		42
41			54	26.5–26.9	41
40	29		53	27.0–27.4	40
39	28	8	52		39
38				27.5–27.9	38
37	27		51	28.0–28.4	37
36	26		50		36

T Score	Basketball Throw	Passes	Broad Jump	Obstacle Race	T Score
35			49	28.5–28.9	35
34	25		48	29.0–29.4	34
33			47	29.5–29.9	33
32		7	46	30.0–30.4	32
31			45	30.5–30.9	31
30	24		44	31.0–31.4	30
29			43	31.5–31.9	29
28	23		42	32.0–32.4	28
27	21		41	32.5–32.9	27
26		6	40	33.0–33.4	26
25	20		39	33.5–33.9	25
24			38	34.0–34.4	24
23		5	37	34.5–34.9	23
22			36		22
21	19			35.0–35.4	21
20					20
19			35	35.5–35.9	19
18					18
17	18	4			17
16					16
15					15
14				43.5–43.9	14
13			30	44.5–44.9	13

* Scott, M. Gladys, and French, Esther, *Measurement and Evaluation in Physical Education.* Dubuque, Iowa: William C. Brown Company, 1959. Reprinted by permission of the publisher.

T-Scales for Iowa–Brace Test*

Test Score Points	Girls		
	Elementary	Jr. High	Sr. High
20	67	64	71
19	65	61	66
18	62	58	63
17	60	56	60
16	58	53	57
15	56	50	55
14	54	47	53
13	52	45	51
12	50	43	49
11	48	41	47
10	45	39	45
9	42	37	43
8	‚39	35	41
7	36	32	39
6	33	30	37
5	30	26	34
4	28	—	32
3	25	—	30
2	24	—	28
1	—	—	—

* From *Tests and Measurements in Health and Physical Education*, Third Edition, by Charles Harold McCloy and Norma Dorothy Young. Copyright © 1954. Reprinted by permission of Appleton-Century-Crofts, Educational Division, Meredith Corporation.

Achievement Scales for Leilich Basketball Test for College Women
(Nonphysical Education Majors)*

T Score	½-Minute Shooting	Bounce and Shoot		Push-Pass	T Score
		Accuracy	Speed		
80	15			137	80
75	14		41	130	75
70	12		46	123	70
65	9	19	52	117	65
60	8	17	58	110	60
55	6	15	64	103	55
50	5	13	70	96	50
45	4	11	76	90	45
40		9	82	83	40
35	3	7	88	76	35
30	2	5	94	70	30
25		3	100	63	25
20	1	1	106	56	20

* Miller, Wilma K., "Achievement Levels in Basketball Skills for Women Physical Education Majors," *Research Quarterly*, 1954, *25*, 450-55. Reprinted by permission of the AAHPER.

Achievement Scales for Leilich Basketball Test for College Women
(Physical Education Majors)*

Percentile	½-Minute Shooting	Balance and Shoot		Push-Pass	Percentile
		Speed	Accuracy		
100	18	50	20	125	100
95	14	56		115	95
90	13	58	17	110	90
85	12	60		108	85
80			16	105	80
75	11	61		104	75
70		63	15	103	70
65	10	64		101	65
60		66	14	100	60
55	9	67		99	55
50		68	13	97	50
45	8	70		95	45
40		71	12	94	40
35	7	72	11	92	35
30		74	10	91	30
25	6	76		89	25
20		79	9	86	20
15	5	81	8	83	15
10	4	86	6	79	10
5	3	89	4	73	5
1	1			44	1

* Miller, Wilma K., "Achievement Levels in Basketball Skills for Women Physical Education Majors," *Research Quarterly*, 1954, *25*, 450–55. Reprinted by permission of the AAHPER.

Classification of Raw Scores in Leilich Test*
(Physical Education Majors)

Classification	$\frac{1}{2}$-Minute Shoot	B & S Speed	B & S Accuracy	Push-Pass
Superior	16 and above	47 and below	21 and above	122 and above
Good	12–15	48–61	16–20	106–121
Average	7–11	62–77	10–15	89–105
Fair	3–6	78–91	6–9	72–88
Poor	2 and below	92 and above	5 and below	71 and below
	N1812	N 1645	N 1645	N 1646
	M 9.11	M 69.69	M 12.95	M 96.66
	SD 3.50	SD 12.00	SD 4.12	SD 13.47

* Miller, Wilma K., "Achievement Levels in Basketball Skills for Women Physical Education Majors," *Research Quarterly*, 1954, *25*, 450–55. Reprinted by permission of the AAHPER.

Achievement Scales for Russell–Lange Volleyball Test
for Junior High School Girls*

Scale Score	Repeated Volley	Serve	Scale Score
100	51	45	100
95	48	42	95
90	45	39	90
85	42	36	85
80	39	34	80
75	36	31	75
70	33	28	70
65	30	25	65
60	27	22	60
55	24	19	55
50	22	16	50
45	19	15	45
40	17	13	40
35	15	11	35
30	13	10	30
25	11	8	25
20	8	6	20
15	6	5	15
10	4	3	10
5	2	1	5

*Based on scores from 1301 junior high school girls in Massachusetts and California. Reprinted by permission of the AAHPER.

Achievement Scales for Russell–Lange Volleyball Test
For Senior High School Girls*

T Score	Repeated Volley	Serve	T Score
75	25	42	75
70	22	34	70
65	19	31	65
60	16	27	60
55	13	22	55
50	11	14	50
45	10	9	45
40	8	6	40
35	6	4	35
30	4	2	30
25	3		25
20	2		20

* Based on the performance of 120 high school girls.
   Scott, M. Gladys, and French, Esther, *Measurement and Evaluation in Physical Education*. Dubuque, Iowa: William C. Brown Company, 1959, pp. 232–33. Reprinted by permission of the publisher.

Flexed-Arm Hang for Girls*
Percentile Scores Based on Age/Test Scores in Seconds

Percentile				Age					Percentile
	10	11	12	13	14	15	16	17	
100th	66	79	64	80	60	74	74	76	100th
95th	31	35	30	30	30	33	37	31	95th
90th	24	25	23	21	22	22	26	25	90th
85th	21	20	19	18	19	18	19	19	85th
80th	18	17	15	15	16	16	16	16	80th
75th	15	16	13	13	13	14	14	14	75th
70th	13	13	11	12	11	13	12	12	70th
65th	11	11	10	10	10	11	10	11	65th
60th	10	10	8	9	9	10	9	10	60th
55th	9	9	8	8	8	8	8	8	55th
50th	7	8	6	7	7	8	7	8	50th
45th	6	6	6	6	6	6	6	7	45th
40th	6	5	5	5	5	6	5	6	40th
35th	5	4	4	4	4	4	4	4	35th
30th	4	4	3	3	3	3	3	4	30th
25th	3	3	2	2	2	2	2	3	25th
20th	2	2	1	2	1	1	1	2	20th
15th	2	1	0	1	1	0	1	0	15th
10th	1	0	0	0	0	0	0	0	10th
5th	0	0	0	0	0	0	0	0	5th
0	0	0	0	0	0	0	0	0	0

*Reprinted by permission of the AAHPER.

Flexed-Arm Hang for Girls*
Percentile Scores Based on Neilson and Cozens, Classification Index/
Test Scores in Seconds

| Percentile | Classification Index | | | | | | | | | Percentile |
	A	B	C	D	E	F	G	H	HSG	
100th	72	70	80	64	61	61	64	40	76	100th
95th	39	35	35	28	31	30	17	17	34	95th
90th	29	27	27	22	23	21	13	14	25	90th
85th	24	22	23	18	20	18	11	11	20	85th
80th	21	19	20	15	17	14	11	9	17	80th
75th	18	17	18	13	14	13	9	7	14	75th
70th	16	15	16	11	12	11	8	6	13	70th
65th	14	13	14	10	11	10	7	5	11	65th
60th	12	11	12	9	9	9	6	4	10	60th
55th	11	10	10	8	8	8	5	2	8	55th
50th	10	8	9	7	7	7	4	2	8	50th
45th	9	7	8	6	6	6	3	2	6	45th
40th	8	6	7	6	5	5	2	1	6	40th
35th	7	6	6	5	4	4	2	1	4	35th
30th	6	5	5	4	3	3	1	1	4	30th
25th	5	4	4	3	3	2	0	0	2	25th
20th	4	4	3	2	2	1	0	0	2	20th
15th	3	2	2	1	1	0	0	0	1	15th
10th	2	2	1	0	0	0	0	0	0	10th
5th	1	0	0	0	0	0	0	0	0	5th
0	0	0	0	0	0	0	0	0	0	0

* Reprinted by permission of the AAHPER.

Sit-Up for Girls*
Percentile Scores Based on Age/Test Scores in Number of Sit-Ups

				Age					
Percentile	10	11	12	13	14	15	16	17	Percentile
100th	50	50	50	50	50	50	50	50	100th
95th	50	50	50	50	50	50	50	50	95th
90th	50	50	50	50	50	50	50	50	90th
85th	50	50	50	50	50	50	50	50	85th
80th	50	50	50	50	49	42	41	45	80th
75th	50	50	50	50	42	39	38	40	75th
70th	50	50	50	45	37	35	34	35	70th
65th	42	40	40	40	35	31	31	32	65th
60th	39	37	39	38	34	30	30	30	60th
55th	33	34	35	35	31	29	28	29	55th
50th	31	30	32	31	30	26	26	27	50th
45th	30	29	30	30	27	25	25	25	45th
40th	26	26	26	27	25	24	24	23	40th
35th	24	25	25	25	23	21	22	21	35th
30th	21	22	22	22	21	20	20	20	30th
25th	20	20	20	20	20	19	18	18	25th
20th	16	19	18	19	18	16	16	16	20th
15th	14	16	16	15	16	14	14	15	15th
10th	11	12	13	12	13	11	11	12	10th
5th	8	10	7	10	10	8	7	9	5th
0	0	0	0	0	0	0	0	0	0

* Reprinted by permission of the AAHPER.

Sit-Up for Girls*
Percentile Scores Based on Neilson and Cozens' Classification Index/
Test Scores in Number of Sit-Ups

| Percentile | Classification Index | | | | | | | | | Percentile |
	A	B	C	D	E	F	G	H	HSG	
100th	50	50	50	50	50	50	50	50	50	100th
95th	50	50	50	50	50	50	50	50	50	95th
90th	50	50	50	50	50	50	50	50	50	90th
85th	50	50	50	50	50	50	49	48	50	85th
80th	50	50	50	50	50	50	43	43	41	80th
75th	50	50	50	50	50	49	38	39	38	75th
70th	46	50	50	47	47	44	35	35	35	70th
65th	40	46	50	40	40	40	32	34	32	65th
60th	38	40	45	37	37	36	30	30	30	60th
55th	34	35	40	33	34	34	29	29	29	55th
50th	31	32	35	31	31	31	25	27	26	50th
45th	30	30	31	30	29	30	25	25	25	45th
40th	26	27	30	27	26	27	22	23	24	40th
35th	24	26	25	25	24	25	20	21	21	35th
30th	22	22	23	22	21	23	20	20	20	30th
25th	20	20	20	20	20	21	17	18	18	25th
20th	17	18	18	18	19	20	15	15	16	20th
15th	15	16	16	16	15	16	13	14	14	15th
10th	10	13	11	13	13	13	10	12	12	10th
5th	8	9	8	10	9	10	8	9	8	5th
0	1	2	0	0	0	0	1	3	0	0

* Reprinted by permission of the AAHPER.

Shuttle Run for Girls*
Percentile Scores Based on Age/Test Scores in Seconds and Tenths

Percentile	Age								Percentile
	10	11	12	13	14	15	16	17	
100th	8.5	8.8	9.0	8.3	9.0	8.0	8.3	9.0	100th
95th	10.0	10.0	10.0	10.0	10.0	10.0	10.0	10.0	95th
90th	10.5	10.2	10.2	10.2	10.3	10.3	10.2	10.3	90th
85th	10.8	10.6	10.5	10.5	10.4	10.5	10.4	10.4	85th
80th	11.0	10.9	10.8	10.6	10.5	10.7	10.6	10.5	80th
75th	11.0	11.0	10.9	10.8	10.6	10.9	10.8	10.6	75th
70th	11.1	11.0	11.0	11.0	10.8	11.0	10.9	10.8	70th
65th	11.4	11.2	11.2	11.0	10.9	11.0	11.0	11.0	65th
60th	11.5	11.4	11.3	11.1	11.0	11.1	11.0	11.0	60th
55th	11.8	11.6	11.5	11.3	11.1	11.2	11.2	11.1	55th
50th	11.9	11.7	11.6	11.4	11.3	11.3	11.2	11.2	50th
45th	12.0	11.8	11.8	11.6	11.4	11.5	11.4	11.4	45th
40th	12.0	12.0	11.9	11.8	11.5	11.6	11.5	11.5	40th
35th	12.1	12.0	12.0	12.0	11.7	11.8	11.8	11.6	35th
30th	12.4	12.1	12.1	12.0	12.0	11.9	12.0	11.8	30th
25th	12.6	12.4	12.3	12.2	12.0	12.0	12.0	12.0	25th
20th	12.8	12.6	12.5	12.5	12.3	12.3	12.2	12.0	20th
15th	13.0	13.0	12.9	13.0	12.6	12.5	12.5	12.3	15th
10th	13.1	13.4	13.2	13.3	13.1	13.0	13.0	13.0	10th
5th	14.0	14.1	13.9	14.0	13.9	13.5	13.9	13.8	5th
0	16.6	18.5	19.8	18.5	17.6	16.0	17.6	20.0	0

* Reprinted by permission of the AAHPER.

Shuttle Run for Girls*
Percentile Scores Based on Neilson and Cozens' Classification Index/
Test Scores in Seconds and Tenths

Percentile	Classification Index									Percentile
	A	B	C	D	E	F	G	H	HSG	
100th	8.5	8.8	9.0	8.9	9.0	9.0	8.3	9.3	8.0	100th
95th	9.5	10.0	10.0	9.9	10.0	10.0	10.1	10.1	10.0	95th
90th	10.2	10.5	10.2	10.2	10.2	10.2	10.3	10.5	10.2	90th
85th	10.7	10.8	10.5	10.5	10.5	10.5	10.5	10.6	10.4	85th
80th	11.0	11.0	10.8	10.8	10.6	10.5	10.6	10.8	10.6	80th
75th	11.0	11.0	11.0	11.0	10.8	10.7	10.8	10.9	10.8	75th
70th	11.1	11.2	11.0	11.0	11.0	10.9	11.0	11.0	10.9	70th
65th	11.3	11.4	11.2	11.1	11.0	11.0	11.0	11.1	11.0	65th
60th	11.5	11.6	11.4	11.3	11.1	11.0	11.2	11.3	11.0	60th
55th	11.6	11.7	11.5	11.4	11.3	11.2	11.3	11.5	11.1	55th
50th	11.8	11.8	11.5	11.6	11.5	11.4	11.5	11.6	11.3	50th
45th	12.0	11.9	11.7	11.8	11.7	11.5	11.7	11.8	11.4	45th
40th	12.0	12.0	11.9	12.0	12.0	11.7	11.8	12.0	11.5	40th
35th	12.2	12.0	12.0	12.0	12.0	11.9	12.0	12.2	11.7	35th
30th	12.5	12.2	12.0	12.1	12.1	12.0	12.0	12.4	11.8	30th
25th	12.6	12.4	12.2	12.3	12.3	12.2	12.3	12.5	12.0	25th
20th	12.9	12.5	12.5	12.6	12.5	12.5	12.5	13.0	12.1	20th
15th	13.0	12.9	12.7	12.9	12.9	13.0	12.9	13.0	12.5	15th
10th	13.5	13.1	13.0	13.3	13.2	13.5	13.3	13.5	13.0	10th
5th	14.4	14.0	13.8	14.0	14.0	14.0	14.0	14.0	13.6	5th
0	16.2	19.8	17.0	16.0	17.6	18.5	17.0	17.3	20.0	0

* Reprinted by permission of the AAHPER.

Standing Long Jump for Girls*
Percentile Scores Based on Age/Test scores in Feet and Inches

				Age					
Percentile	10	11	12	13	14	15	16	17	Percentile
100th	7′ 0″	7′ 10″	8′ 2″	7′ 6″	7′ 4″	7′ 8″	7′ 5″	7′ 8″	100th
95th	5′ 8″	6′ 2″	6′ 3″	6′ 3″	6′ 4″	6′ 6″	6′ 7″	6′ 8″	95th
90th	5′ 6″	5′ 10″	6′ 0″	6′ 0″	6′ 2″	6′ 3″	6′ 4″	6′ 4″	90th
85th	5′ 4″	5′ 8″	5′ 9″	5′ 10″	6′ 0″	6′ 1″	6′ 2″	6′ 2″	85th
80th	5′ 2″	5′ 6″	5′ 8″	5′ 8″	5′ 10″	6′ 0″	6′ 0″	6′ 0″	80th
75th	5′ 1″	5′ 4″	5′ 6″	5′ 6″	5′ 9″	5′ 10″	5′ 10″	5′ 11″	75th
70th	5′ 0″	‛5′ 3″	5′ 5″	5′ 5″	5′ 7″	5′ 9″	5′ 8″	5′ 10″	70th
65th	5′ 0″	5′ 2″	5′ 4″	5′ 4″	5′ 6″	5′ 7″	5′ 7″	5′ 9″	65th
60th	4′ 10″	5′ 0″	5′ 2″	5′ 3″	5′ 5″	5′ 6″	5′ 6″	5′ 7″	60th
55th	4′ 9″	5′ 0″	5′ 1″	5′ 2″	5′ 4″	5′ 5″	5′ 5″	5′ 6″	55th
50th	4′ 7″	4′ 10″	5′ 0″	5′ 0″	5′ 3″	5′ 4″	5′ 4″	5′ 5″	50th
45th	4′ 6″	4′ 9″	4′ 11″	5′ 0″	5′ 1″	5′ 3″	5′ 3″	5′ 3″	45th
40th	4′ 5″	4′ 8″	4′ 9″	4′ 10″	5′ 0″	5′ 1″	5′ 2″	5′ 2″	40th
35th	4′ 4″	4′ 7″	4′ 8″	4′ 8″	5′ 0″	5′ 0″	5′ 0″	5′ 0″	35th
30th	4′ 3″	4′ 6″	4′ 7″	4′ 6″	4′ 9″	4′ 10″	4′ 11″	5′ 0″	30th
25th	4′ 2″	4′ 4″	4′ 5″	4′ 6″	4′ 8″	4′ 8″	4′ 10″	4′ 10″	25th
20th	4′ 0″	4′ 3″	4′ 4″	4′ 4″	4′ 6″	4′ 7″	4′ 8″	4′ 9″	20th
15th	3′ 11″	4′ 1″	4′ 2″	4′ 2″	4′ 3″	4′ 6″	4′ 6″	4′ 7″	15th
10th	3′ 9″	3′ 11″	4′ 0″	4′ 0″	4′ 1″	4′ 4″	4′ 4″	4′ 5″	10th
5th	3′ 6″	3′ 9″	3′ 8″	3′ 9″	3′ 10″	4′ 0″	4′ 0″	4′ 2″	5th
0	2′ 8″	2′ 11″	2′ 11″	2′ 11″	3′ 0″	2′ 11″	3′ 2″	3′ 0″	0

* Reprinted by permission of the AAHPER.

Standing Long Jump for Girls*
Percentile Scores Based on Neilson and Cozens' Classification Index/
Test Scores in Feet and Inches

	Classification Index									
Percentile	A	B	C	D	E	F	G	H	HSG	Percentile
100th	7′ 0″	7′ 10″	7′ 10″	7′ 0″	7′ 10″	8′ 2″	7′ 4″	7′ 4″	7′ 8″	100th
95th	5′ 8″	6′ 0″	6′ 2″	6′ 1″	6′ 4″	6′ 3″	6′ 3″	6′ 5″	6′ 7″	95th
90th	5′ 5″	5′ 8″	5′ 11″	5′ 11″	6′ 0″	6′ 1″	6′ 0″	6′ 2″	6′ 4″	90th
85th	5′ 3″	5′ 6″	5′ 8″	5′ 8″	5′ 10″	5′ 11″	5′ 9″	5′ 11″	6′ 1″	85th
80th	5′ 2″	5′ 4″	5′ 7″	5′ 7″	5′ 8″	5′ 9″	5′ 7″	5′ 8″	6′ 0″	80th
75th	5′ 1″	5′ 3″	5′ 5″	5′ 5″	5′ 7″	5′ 7″	5′ 6″	5′ 7″	5′ 10″	75th
70th	5′ 0″	5′ 2″	5′ 4″	5′ 4″	5′ 6″	5′ 6″	5′ 5″	5′ 6″	5′ 9″	70th
65th	4′ 11″	5′ 1″	5′ 2″	5′ 3″	5′ 4″	5′ 4″	5′ 4″	5′ 4″	5′ 8″	65th
60th	4′ 9″	5′ 0″	5′ 1″	5′ 2″	5′ 2″	5′ 3″	5′ 3″	5′ 3″	5′ 7″	60th
55th	4′ 8″	4′ 11″	5′ 0″	5′ 1″	5′ 1″	5′ 2″	5′ 2″	5′ 1″	5′ 6″	55th
50th	4′ 7″	4′ 10″	4′ 11″	5′ 0″	5′ 0″	5′ 1″	5′ 0″	5′ 0″	5′ 4″	50th
45th	4′ 6″	4′ 8″	4′ 10″	4′ 11″	4′ 11″	5′ 0″	5′ 0″	4′ 9″	5′ 3″	45th
40th	4′ 5″	4′ 7″	4′ 9″	4′ 9″	4′ 10″	4′ 11″	4′ 10″	4′ 9″	5′ 2″	40th
35th	4′ 4″	4′ 6″	4′ 8″	4′ 8″	4′ 8″	4′ 9″	4′ 9″	4′ 8″	5′ 0″	35th
30th	4′ 4″	4′ 5″	4′ 6″	4′ 7″	4′ 7″	4′ 7″	4′ 7″	4′ 6″	4′ 11″	30th
25th	4′ 2″	4′ 4″	4′ 5″	4′ 5″	4′ 6″	4′ 6″	4′ 6″	4′ 5″	4′ 10″	25th
20th	4′ 0″	4′ 2″	4′ 3″	4′ 4″	4′ 4″	4′ 4″	4′ 5″	4′ 4″	4′ 8″	20th
15th	3′ 10″	4′ 0″	4′ 2″	4′ 2″	4′ 2″	4′ 2″	4′ 2″	4′ 2″	4′ 6″	15th
10th	3′ 9″	3′ 11″	4′ 0″	4′ 0″	4′ 0″	4′ 0″	4′ 0″	4′ 0″	4′ 4″	10th
5th	3′ 6″	3′ 7″	3′ 7″	3′ 11″	3′ 8″	3′ 9″	3′ 9″	3′ 7″	4′ 0″	5th
0	3′ 1″	2′ 8″	3′ 0″	2′ 11″	2′ 11″	2′ 11″	3′ 1″	2′ 11″	3′ 0″	0

* Reprinted by permission of the AAHPER.

50-Yard Dash for Girls*
Percentile Scores Based on Age/Test Scores in Seconds and Tenths

Percentile	Age								Percentile
	10	11	12	13	14	15	16	17	
100th	6.0	6.0	5.9	6.0	6.0	6.4	6.0	6.4	100th
95th	7.0	7.0	7.0	7.0	7.0	7.1	7.0	7.1	95th
90th	7.3	7.4	7.3	7.3	7.2	7.3	7.3	7.3	90th
85th	7.5	7.6	7.5	7.5	7.4	7.5	7.5	7.5	85th
80th	7.7	7.7	7.6	7.6	7.5	7.6	7.5	7.6	80th
75th	7.9	7.9	7.8	7.7	7.6	7.7	7.7	7.8	75th
70th	8.0	8.0	7.9	7.8	7.7	7.8	7.9	7.9	70th
65th	8.1	8.0	8.0	7.9	7.8	7.9	8.0	8.0	65th
60th	8.2	8.1	8.0	8.0	7.9	8.0	8.0	8.0	60th
55th	8.4	8.2	8.1	8.0	8.0	8.0	8.1	8.1	55th
50th	8.5	8.4	8.2	8.1	8.0	8.1	8.3	8.2	50th
45th	8.6	8.5	8.3	8.2	8.2	8.2	8.4	8.3	45th
40th	8.8	8.5	8.4	8.4	8.3	8.3	8.5	8.5	40th
35th	8.9	8.6	8.5	8.5	8.5	8.4	8.6	8.6	35th
30th	9.0	8.8	8.7	8.6	8.6	8.6	8.8	8.8	30th
25th	9.0	9.0	8.9	8.8	8.9	8.8	9.0	9.0	25th
20th	9.2	9.0	9.0	9.0	9.0	9.0	9.0	9.0	20th
15th	9.4	9.2	9.2	9.2	9.2	9.0	9.2	9.1	15th
10th	9.6	9.6	9.5	9.5	9.5	9.5	9.9	9.5	10th
5th	10.0	10.0	10.0	10.2	10.4	10.0	10.5	10.4	5th
0	14.0	13.0	13.0	15.7	16.0	18.0	17.0	12.0	0

* Reprinted by permission of the AAHPER.

50-Yard Dash for Girls*
Percentile Scores Based on Neilson and Cozens' Classification Index/
Test Scores in Seconds and Tenths

	Classification Index									
Percentile	A	B	C	D	E	F	G	H	HSG	Percentile
100th	6.5	6.0	6.0	6.0	6.0	5.9	6.0	6.0	6.0	100th
95th	7.0	7.0	7.0	7.2	7.0	7.0	7.3	7.2	7.0	95th
90th	7.4	7.5	7.3	7.4	7.2	7.2	7.5	7.4	7.2	90th
85th	7.6	7.6	7.5	7.6	7.5	7.4	7.6	7.5	7.4	85th
80th	7.8	7.8	7.7	7.7	7.6	7.5	7.8	7.6	7.6	80th
75th	8.0	7.9	7.8	7.9	7.7	7.6	7.8	7.8	7.7	75th
70th	8.0	8.0	7.9	7.9	7.8	7.8	7.9	7.9	7.8	70th
65th	8.2	8.0	8.0	8.0	7.9	7.9	8.0	8.0	7.9	65th
60th	8.3	8.2	8.0	8.0	8.0	7.9	8.0	8.1	8.0	60th
55th	8.5	8.3	8.2	8.1	8.1	8.0	8.1	8.2	8.0	55th
50th	8.5	8.4	8.3	8.2	8.2	8.1	8.3	8.2	8.1	50th
45th	8.7	8.5	8.4	8.3	8.3	8.3	8.4	8.4	8.3	45th
40th	8.8	8.6	8.5	8.4	8.4	8.4	8.4	8.5	8.4	40th
35th	9.0	8.8	8.6	8.5	8.5	8.5	8.6	8.6	8.5	35th
30th	9.0	8.9	8.8	8.7	8.6	8.7	8.8	8.8	8.7	30th
25th	9.0	9.0	9.0	8.9	8.8	8.9	9.0	9.0	8.9	25th
20th	9.2	9.1	9.1	9.0	9.0	9.0	9.1	9.2	9.0	20th
15th	9.6	9.2	9.2	9.1	9.2	9.4	9.3	9.4	9.1	15th
10th	10.0	9.5	9.5	9.5	9.5	9.7	9.7	9.6	9.5	10th
5th	10.0	10.0	9.8	10.0	10.0	10.5	10.4	10.0	10.3	5th
0	11.5	11.6	11.3	12.0	14.0	15.7	13.0	11.0	18.0	0

* Reprinted by permission of the AAHPER.

Softball Throw for Girls*
Percentile Scores Based on Age/Test Scores in Feet

Percentile	Age								Percentile
	10	11	12	13	14	15	16	17	
100th	167	141	159	150	156	165	175	183	100th
95th	84	95	103	111	114	120	123	120	95th
90th	76	86	96	102	103	110	113	108	90th
85th	71	81	90	94	100	105	104	102	85th
80th	69	77	85	90	95	100	98	98	80th
75th	65	74	80	86	90	95	92	93	75th
70th	60	71	76	82	87	90	89	90	70th
65th	57	66	74	79	84	87	85	87	65th
60th	54	64	70	75	80	84	81	82	60th
55th	52	62	67	73	78	82	78	80	55th
50th	50	59	64	70	75	78	75	75	50th
45th	48	57	61	68	72	75	74	74	45th
40th	46	55	59	65	70	73	71	71	40th
35th	45	52	57	63	68	69	69	69	35th
30th	42	50	54	60	65	66	66	66	30th
25th	40	46	50	57	61	64	63	62	25th
20th	37	44	48	53	59	60	60	58	20th
15th	34	40	45	49	54	58	55	52	15th
10th	30	37	41	45	50	51	50	48	10th
5th	21	32	37	36	45	45	45	40	5th
0	8	13	20	20	25	12	8	20	0

* Reprinted by permission of the AAHPER.

Softball Throw for Girls*
Percentile Scores Based on Neilson and Cozens' Classification Index/
Test Scores in Feet

| Percentile | Classification Index | | | | | | | | | Percentile |
	A	B	C	D	E	F	G	H	HSG	
100th	167	136	133	135	141	159	143	168	183	100th
95th	78	85	90	101	106	111	111	120	121	95th
90th	71	77	85	93	99	102	102	112	110	90th
85th	66	73	80	87	92	97	100	104	103	85th
80th	63	69	76	81	87	92	92	102	98	80th
75th	58	65	73	78	84	88	90	99	93	75th
70th	55	62	71	74	80	85	87	92	90	70th
65th	52	60	68	71	76	81	85	85	86	65th
60th	51	57	65	69	74	78	81	82	82	60th
55th	50	55	61	65	70	75	78	80	80	55th
50th	48	51	59	63	67	72	75	77	75	50th
45th	46	50	57	60	64	70	73	75	74	45th
40th	45	47	54	58	61	67	70	72	71	40th
35th	42	45	52	57	60	65	67	70	69	35th
30th	40	43	49	54	56	61	65	66	66	30th
25th	38	41	46	50	53	58	60	63	63	25th
20th	34	39	44	46	50	54	58	60	60	20th
15th	32	36	40	44	47	50	53	57	55	15th
10th	30	30	37	40	43	46	48	51	50	10th
5th	19	26	32	35	39	38	44	44	45	5th
0	8	10	18	18	21	20	20	21	8	0

* Reprinted by permission of the AAHPER.

600-Yard Run–Walk for Girls*
Percentile Scores Based on Age/Test Scores in Minutes and Seconds

Percentile	10	11	12	13	14	15	16	17	Percentile
100th	1′ 42″	1′ 40″	1′ 39″	1′ 40″	1′ 45″	1′ 40″	1′ 50″	1′ 54″	100th
95th	2′ 5″	2′ 13″	2′ 14″	2′ 12″	2′ 9″	2′ 9″	2′ 10″	2′ 11″	95th
90th	2′ 15″	2′ 19″	2′ 20″	2′ 19″	2′ 18″	2′ 18″	2′ 17″	2′ 22″	90th
85th	2′ 20″	2′ 24″	2′ 24″	2′ 25″	2′ 22″	2′ 23″	2′ 23″	2′ 27″	85th
80th	2′ 26″	2′ 28″	2′ 27″	2′ 29″	2′ 25″	2′ 26″	2′ 26″	2′ 31″	80th
75th	2′ 30″	2′ 32″	2′ 31″	2′ 33″	2′ 30″	2′ 28″	2′ 31″	2′ 34″	75th
70th	2′ 34″	2′ 36″	2′ 35″	2′ 37″	2′ 34″	2′ 34″	2′ 36″	2′ 37″	70th
65th	2′ 37″	2′ 39″	2′ 39″	2′ 40″	2′ 37″	2′ 36″	2′ 39″	2′ 42″	65th
60th	2′ 41″	2′ 43″	2′ 42″	2′ 44″	2′ 41″	2′ 40″	2′ 42″	2′ 46″	60th
55th	2′ 45″	2′ 47″	2′ 45″	2′ 47″	2′ 44″	2′ 43″	2′ 45″	2′ 49″	55th
50th	2′ 48″	2′ 49″	2′ 49″	2′ 52″	2′ 46″	2′ 46″	2′ 49″	2′ 51″	50th
45th	2′ 50″	2′ 53″	2′ 55″	2′ 56″	2′ 51″	2′ 49″	2′ 53″	2′ 57″	45th
40th	2′ 55″	2′ 59″	2′ 58″	3′ 0″	2′ 55″	2′ 52″	2′ 56″	3′ 0″	40th
35th	2′ 59″	3′ 4″	3′ 3″	3′ 3″	3′ 0″	2′ 56″	2′ 59″	3′ 5″	35th
30th	3′ 3″	3′ 10″	3′ 7″	3′ 9″	3′ 6″	3′ 0″	3′ 1″	3′ 10″	30th
25th	3′ 8″	3′ 15″	3′ 11″	3′ 15″	3′ 12″	3′ 5″	3′ 7″	3′ 16″	25th
20th	3′ 13″	3′ 22″	3′ 18″	3′ 20″	3′ 19″	3′ 10″	3′ 12″	3′ 22″	20th
15th	3′ 18″	3′ 30″	3′ 24″	3′ 30″	3′ 30″	3′ 18″	3′ 19″	3′ 29″	15th
10th	3′ 27″	3′ 41″	3′ 40″	3′ 49″	3′ 48″	3′ 28″	3′ 30″	3′ 41″	10th
5th	3′ 45″	3′ 59″	4′ 0″	4′ 11″	4′ 8″	3′ 56″	3′ 45″	3′ 56″	5th
0	4′ 47″	4′ 53″	5′ 10″	5′ 10″	5′ 50″	5′ 10″	5′ 52″	6′ 40″	0

* Reprinted by permission of the AAHPER.

600-Yard Run–Walk for Girls*
Percentile Scores Based on Neilson and Cozens' Classification Index/ Test Scores in Minutes and Seconds

Percentile	Classification Index									Percentile
	A	B	C	D	E	F	G	H	HSG	
100th	1′ 46″	1′ 42″	1′ 46″	1′ 39″	1′ 40″	1′ 50″	1′ 55″	2′ 4″	1′ 45″	100th
95th	2′ 4″	2′ 10″	2′ 11″	2′ 10″	2′ 11″	2′ 13″	2′ 13″	2′ 19″	2′ 10″	95th
90th	2′ 15″	2′ 16″	2′ 17″	2′ 17″	2′ 19″	2′ 18″	2′ 22″	2′ 25″	2′ 18″	90th
85th	2′ 22″	2′ 22″	2′ 22″	2′ 23″	2′ 24″	2′ 25″	2′ 25″	2′ 30″	2′ 24″	85th
80th	2′ 25″	2′ 26″	2′ 26″	2′ 26″	2′ 27″	2′ 29″	2′ 30″	2′ 33″	2′ 27″	80th
75th	2′ 30″	2′ 30″	2′ 29″	2′ 30″	2′ 32″	2′ 33″	2′ 35″	2′ 38″	2′ 32″	75th
70th	2′ 34″	2′ 33″	2′ 32″	2′ 33″	2′ 36″	2′ 37″	2′ 40″	2′ 41″	2′ 35″	70th
65th	2′ 36″	2′ 36″	2′ 36″	2′ 37″	2′ 40″	2′ 40″	2′ 44″	2′ 46″	2′ 38″	65th
60th	2′ 41″	2′ 39″	2′ 39″	2′ 40″	2′ 43″	2′ 43″	2′ 47″	2′ 50″	2′ 42″	60th
55th	2′ 45″	2′ 43″	2′ 43″	2′ 45″	2′ 46″	2′ 47″	2′ 50″	2′ 55″	2′ 45″	55th
50th	2′ 47″	2′ 47″	2′ 45″	2′ 48″	2′ 50″	2′ 50″	2′ 54″	2′ 59″	2′ 48″	50th
45th	2′ 51″	2′ 49″	2′ 49″	2′ 51″	2′ 55″	2′ 55″	2′ 59″	3′ 4″	2′ 52″	45th
40th	2′ 56″	2′ 51″	2′ 53″	2′ 55″	3′ 0″	2′ 59″	3′ 3″	3′ 10″	2′ 55″	40th
35th	3′ 0″	2′ 55″	2′ 59″	3′ 0″	3′ 2″	3′ 2″	3′ 6″	3′ 13″	3′ 0″	35th
30th	3′ 5″	3′ 1″	3′ 3″	3′ 7″	3′ 6″	3′ 9″	3′ 12″	3′ 16″	3′ 3″	30th
25th	3′ 9″	3′ 7″	3′ 11″	3′ 11″	3′ 12″	3′ 13″	3′ 17″	3′ 21″	3′ 9″	25th
20th	3′ 13″	3′ 13″	3′ 18″	3′ 16″	3′ 17″	3′ 18″	3′ 25″	3′ 29″	3′ 15″	20th
15th	3′ 18″	3′ 20″	3′ 25″	3′ 24″	3′ 25″	3′ 26″	3′ 43″	3′ 39″	3′ 24″	15th
10th	3′ 30″	3′ 30″	3′ 40″	3′ 38″	3′ 45″	3′ 40″	3′ 52″	3′ 48″	3′ 35″	10th
5th	3′ 45″	3′ 49″	3′ 59″	3′ 59″	4′ 4″	4′ 0″	4′ 7″	4′ 11″	3′ 56″	5th
0	4′ 30″	4′ 47″	5′ 0″	4′ 53″	5′ 10″	5′ 10″	5′ 50″	5′ 30″	6′ 40″	0

* Reprinted by permission of the AAHPER.

AAHPER Fitness Test*
Percentile Scores for College Women

Percentile	Modified Pull-Up	Sit-Up	Shuttle Run	Standing Broad Jump	50-Yard Dash	Softball Throw	600-Yard Run–Walk
100th	40	50	7.5	7′ 10″	5.4	184	1:49
95th	39	43	10.2	6′ 6″	7.3	115	2:19
90th	38	35	10.5	6′ 3″	7.6	103	2:27
85th	33	31	10.7	6′ 1″	7.7	96	2:32
80th	30	29	10.9	5′ 11″	7.8	90	2:37
75th	28	27	11.0	5′ 10″	7.9	86	2:41
70th	26	25	11.1	5′ 8″	8.0	82	2:44
65th	24	24	11.2	5′ 7″	8.1	79	2:48
60th	22	22	11.3	5′ 6″	8.2	76	2:51
55th	21	21	11.5	5′ 5″	8.3	73	2:54
50th	20	20	11.6	5′ 4″	8.4	70	2:58
45th	18	19	11.7	5′ 3″	8.6	67	3:01
40th	17	18	11.9	5′ 2″	8.7	65	3:05
35th	16	16	12.0	5′ 0″	8.8	62	3:08
30th	15	15	12.1	4′ 11″	9.0	59	3:13
25th	13	14	12.2	4′ 10″	9.1	57	3:18
20th	12	13	12.4	4′ 8″	9.2	54	3:23
15th	11	11	12.6	4′ 7″	9.4	51	3:29
10th	9	9	12.9	4′ 5″	9.7	47	3:38
5th	7	7	13.4	4′ 1″	10.1	42	3:53
0	0	0	17.3	2′ 3″	13.7	5	5:29

* Reprinted by permission of the AAHPER.

Appendix C:
Achievement Scales for Boys

T-Scale for Iowa–Brace Test*

Test Score Points	Boys		
	Elementary	Jr. High	Sr. High
20	69	66	71
19	66	63	65
18	63	60	60
17	60	57	56
16	57	54	53
15	54	51	50
14	51	48	47
13	48	45	44
12	45	42	41
11	43	39	38
10	41	36	35
9	39	34	33
8	37	32	31
7	35	30	29
6	33	28	—
5	31	26	—
4	29	24	—
3	27	22	—
2	25	20	—
1	23	19	—

* From *Tests and Measurements in Health and Physical Education,* Third Edition, by Charles Harold McCloy and Norma Dorothy Young. Copyright © 1954. Reprinted by permission of Appleton-Century-Crofts, Educational Division, Meredith Corporation.

Achievement Scales for Lehsten Basketball Test*

Scale Score	Baskets Per Minute	Vertical Jump	40-foot Dash	Wall Bounce	Dodging Run	Scale Score	
100			2.0	18	16.0	100	
99	41				16.1	99	
98				17	16.2	98	
97	40				16.3	97	
96					16.4	96	
95	39				16.5	95	
94					16.6	94	
93	38				16.7	93	
92					16.8	92	
91	37				16.9	91	
90			2.1		17.0	90	A
89	36	25.0		16	17.1	89	
88					17.2	88	
87	35				17.3	87	
86		24.5			17.4	86	
85	34				17.5	85	
84	33	24.0			17.6	84	
83					17.7	83	
82	32				17.8	82	
81		23.5		15	17.9	81	
80	31		2.2		18.0	80	
79					18.1	79	
78	30	23.0			18.2	78	
77					18.3	77	
76	29				18.4	76	
75					18.5	75	
74	28	22.5			18.6	74	
73					18.7	73	
72	27	22.0		14	18.8	72	
71					18.9	71	
70	26		2.3		19.0	70	B
69		21.5			19.2	69	
68	25				19.3	68	
67					19.4	67	
66	24	21.0			19.5	66	
65					19.6	65	
64	23				19.7	64	
63		20.5		13	19.8	63	
62	22				19.9	62	
61		20.0			20.0	61	
60	21		2.4		20.1	60	

A (left side rows 90–80), B (left side rows 79–60)

	Scale Score	Baskets Per Minute	Vertical Jump	40-foot Dash	Wall Bounce	Dodging Run	Scale Score	
C	59		19.5			20.2	59	C
	58	20				20.3	58	
	57					20.4	57	
	56	19				20.5	56	
	55		19.0		12	20.6	55	
	54	18				20.7	54	
	53					20.8	53	
	52	17	18.5			20.9	52	
	51					21.0	51	
	50	16		2.5		21.1	50	
	49		18.0			21.2	49	
	48	15				21.3	48	
	47					21.4	47	
	46	14	17.5		11	21.5	46	
	45					21.6	45	
	44	13				21.7	44	
	43		17.0			21.8	43	
	42	12				21.9	42	
	41					22.0	41	
	40	11	16.5	2.6		22.1	40	
D	39					22.2	39	D
	38	10				22.3	38	
	37		16.0		10	22.4	37	
	36	9				22.5	36	
	35					22.6	35	
	34	8	15.5			22.7	34	
	33	7				22.8	33	
	32					22.9	32	
	31	6	15.0			23.0	31	
	30			2.7		23.1	30	
	29	5	14.5		9	23.2	29	
	28					23.3	28	
	27	4				23.4	27	
	26		14.0			23.5	26	
	25	3				23.6	25	
	24					23.7	24	
	23	2	13.5			23.8	23	
	22					23.9	22	
	21	1				24.0	21	
	20		13.0	2.8	8	24.1	20	

	Scale Score	Baskets Per Minute	Vertical Jump	40-foot Dash	Wall Bounce	Dodging Run	Scale Score	
	19					24.3	19	
	18					24.4	18	
	17		12.5			24.5	17	
	16					24.6	16	
	15					24.7	15	
	14		12.0			24.8	14	
	13					24.9	13	
	12					25.0	12	
	11		11.5		7	25.1	11	
F	10			2.9		25.2	10	F
	9		11.0			23.3	9	
	8					25.4	8	
	7					25.5	7	
	6		10.5			25.6	6	
	5					25.7	5	
	4					25.8	4	
	3				6	25.9	3	
	2		10.0			26.0	2	
	1			3.0		26.1	1	

* Lehsten, Nelson G., "A Measure of Basketball Skills in High School Boys," *The Physical Educator*, 1948, 5: 103–109. Reprinted by permission.

Pull-Up for Boys*
Percentile Scores Based on Age/Test Scores in Numbers of Pull-Ups

Percen-tile	Age								Percen-tile
	10	11	12	13	14	15	16	17	
100th	16	20	15	24	20	25	25	32	100th
95th	8	8	9	10	12	13	14	16	95th
90th	7	7	7	9	10	11	13	14	90th
85th	6	6	6	8	10	10	12	12	85th
80th	5	5	5	7	8	10	11	12	80th
75th	4	4	5	6	8	9	10	10	75th
70th	4	4	4	5	7	8	10	10	70th
65th	3	3	3	5	6	7	9	10	65th
60th	3	3	3	4	6	7	9	9	60th
55th	3	2	3	4	5	6	8	8	55th
50th	2	2	2	3	5	6	7	8	50th
45th	2	2	2	3	4	5	6	7	45th
40th	1	1	1	2	4	5	6	7	40th
35th	1	1	1	2	3	4	5	6	35th
30th	1	1	1	1	3	4	5	5	30th
25th	0	0	0	1	2	3	4	5	25th
20th	0	0	0	0	2	3	4	4	20th
15th	0	0	0	0	1	2	3	4	15th
10th	0	0	0	0	0	1	2	2	10th
5th	0	0	0	0	0	0	0	1	5th
0	0	0	0	0	0	0	0	0	0

* Reprinted by permission of the AAHPER.

Pull-Up for High School Boys*
Percentile Scores Based on Neilson and Cozens' Classification Index/ Test Scores in Number of Pull-Ups

Percentile	Classification Index			Percentile
	C	B	A	
100th	20	25	32	100th
95th	14	16	15	95th
90th	12	14	12	90th
85th	10	12	12	85th
80th	10	12	10	80th
75th	9	11	10	75th
70th	8	10	9	70th
65th	7	10	9	65th
60th	7	9	8	60th
55th	6	9	7	55th
50th	5	8	7	50th
45th	5	7	6	45th
40th	4	7	6	40th
35th	4	6	5	35th
30th	4	6	5	30th
25th	3	5	4	25th
20th	3	4	3	20th
15th	2	4	2	15th
10th	1	3	1	10th
5th	0	2	0	5th
0	0	0	0	0

* Reprinted by permission of the AAHPER.

Sit-Up for Boys*
Percentile Scores Based on Age/Test Scores in Number of Sit-Ups

Percentile	Age								Percentile
	10	11	12	13	14	15	16	17	
100th	100	100	100	100	100	100	100	100	100th
95th	100	100	100	100	100	100	100	100	95th
90th	100	100	100	100	100	100	100	100	90th
85th	100	100	100	100	100	100	100	100	85th
80th	76	89	100	100	100	100	100	100	80th
75th	65	73	93	100	100	100	100	100	75th
70th	57	60	75	99	100	100	100	100	70th
65th	51	55	70	90	99	100	99	99	65th
60th	50	50	59	75	99	99	99	85	60th
55th	49	50	52	70	77	90	85	77	55th
50th	41	46	50	60	70	80	76	70	50th
45th	37	40	49	53	62	70	70	62	45th
40th	34	35	42	50	60	61	63	57	40th
35th	30	31	40	50	52	54	56	51	35th
30th	28	30	35	41	50	50	50	50	30th
25th	25	26	30	38	45	49	50	45	25th
20th	23	23	28	35	40	42	42	40	20th
15th	20	20	25	30	36	39	38	35	15th
10th	15	17	20	25	30	33	34	30	10th
5th	11	12	15	20	24	27	28	23	5th
0	1	0	0	1	6	5	10	8	0

* Reprinted by permission of the AAHPER.

Sit-Up for High School Boys*
Percentile Scores Based on Neilson and Cozens' Classification Index/
Test Scores in Number of Sit-Ups

Percentile	Classification Index			Percentile
	C	B	A	
100th	100	100	100	100th
95th	100	100	100	95th
90th	100	100	100	90th
85th	100	100	100	85th
80th	100	100	100	80th
75th	100	100	100	75th
70th	100	100	100	70th
65th	100	100	99	65th
60th	100	99	91	60th
55th	91	97	80	55th
50th	75	83	74	50th
45th	65	71	67	45th
40th	60	65	60	40th
35th	55	55	55	35th
30th	50	50	50	30th
25th	45	48	49	25th
20th	39	42	41	20th
15th	35	39	37	15th
10th	31	34	32	10th
5th	26	26	26	5th
0	8	8	5	0

* Reprinted by permission of the AAHPER.

Shuttle Run for Boys*
Percentile Scores Based on Age/Test Scores in Seconds and Tenths

					Age				
Percentile	10	11	12	13	14	15	16	17	Percentile
100th	9.0	9.0	8.5	8.0	8.3	8.0	8.1	8.0	100th
95th	10.0	10.0	9.8	9.5	9.3	9.1	9.0	8.9	95th
90th	10.2	10.1	10.0	9.8	9.5	9.3	9.1	9.0	90th
85th	10.4	10.3	10.0	9.9	9.6	9.4	9.2	9.1	85th
80th	10.5	10.4	10.2	10.0	9.8	9.5	9.3	9.2	80th
75th	10.7	10.5	10.3	10.1	9.9	9.6	9.5	9.3	75th
70th	10.8	10.7	10.5	10.2	9.9	9.7	9.5	9.4	70th
65th	10.9	10.8	10.6	10.3	10.0	9.8	9.6	9.5	65th
60th	11.0	10.9	10.7	10.4	10.0	9.8	9.7	9.6	60th
55th	11.0	11.0	10.9	10.5	10.2	9.9	9.8	9.7	55th
50th	11.2	11.1	11.0	10.6	10.2	10.0	9.9	9.8	50th
45th	11.4	11.2	11.0	10.8	10.3	10.0	10.0	9.9	45th
40th	11.5	11.3	11.1	10.9	10.5	10.1	10.0	10.0	40th
35th	11.6	11.4	11.3	11.0	10.5	10.2	10.1	10.0	35th
30th	11.8	11.6	11.5	11.1	10.7	10.3	10.2	10.1	30th
25th	12.0	11.8	11.6	11.3	10.9	10.5	10.4	10.4	25th
20th	12.0	12.0	11.9	11.5	11.0	10.6	10.5	10.6	20th
15th	12.2	12.1	12.0	11.8	11.2	10.9	10.8	10.9	15th
10th	12.6	12.4	12.4	12.0	11.5	11.1	11.1	11.2	10th
5th	13.1	13.0	13.0	12.5	12.0	11.7	11.5	11.7	5th
0	15.0	20.0	22.0	16.0	16.0	16.6	16.7	14.0	0

* Reprinted by permission of the AAHPER.

Shuttle Run for High School Boys*
Percentile Scores Based on Neilson and Cozens' Classification Index/
Test Scores in Seconds and Tenths

| Percentile | Classification Index | | | Percentile |
	C	B	A	
100th	8.3	8.0	8.0	100th
95th	9.2	9.0	9.0	95th
90th	9.4	9.1	9.0	90th
85th	9.6	9.2	9.2	85th
80th	9.7	9.3	9.3	80th
75th	9.8	9.5	9.4	75th
70th	9.9	9.5	9.5	70th
65th	9.9	9.6	9.6	65th
60th	10.0	9.7	9.6	60th
55th	10.0	9.8	9.7	55th
50th	10.1	9.9	9.8	50th
45th	10.2	10.0	10.0	45th
40th	10.2	10.0	10.0	40th
35th	10.4	10.1	10.1	35th
30th	10.5	10.2	10.2	30th
25th	10.6	10.3	10.4	25th
20th	10.9	10.5	10.6	20th
15th	11.0	10.8	10.9	15th
10th	11.2	11.1	11.1	10th
5th	11.7	11.4	11.5	5th
0	15.0	15.0	16.6	0

* Reprinted by permission of the AAHPER.

Standing Long Jump for Boys*
Percentile Scores Based on Age/Test Scores in Feet and Inches

Percentile	Age 10	11	12	13	14	15	16	17	Percentile
100th	6′ 8″	10′ 0″	7′ 10″	8′ 9″	8′ 11″	9′ 2″	9′ 1″	9′ 8″	100th
95th	6′ 1″	6′ 3″	6′ 6″	7′ 2″	7′ 9″	8′ 0″	8′ 5″	8′ 6″	95th
90th	5′ 10″	6′ 0″	6′ 4″	6′ 11″	7′ 5″	7′ 9″	8′ 1″	8′ 3″	90th
85th	5′ 8″	5′ 10″	6′ 2″	6′ 9″	7′ 3″	7′ 6″	7′ 11″	8′ 1″	85th
80th	5′ 7″	5′ 9″	6′ 1″	6′ 7″	7′ 0″	7′ 6″	7′ 9″	8′ 0″	80th
75th	5′ 6″	5′ 7″	6′ 0″	6′ 5″	6′ 11″	7′ 4″	7′ 7″	7′ 10″	75th
70th	5′ 5″	5′ 6″	5′ 11″	6′ 3″	6′ 9″	7′ 2″	7′ 6″	7′ 8″	70th
65th	5′ 4″	5′ 6″	5′ 9″	6′ 1″	6′ 8″	7′ 1″	7′ 5″	7′ 7″	65th
60th	5′ 2″	5′ 4″	5′ 8″	6′ 0″	6′ 7″	7′ 0″	7′ 4″	7′ 6″	60th
55th	5′ 1″	5′ 3″	5′ 7″	5′ 11″	6′ 6″	6′ 11″	7′ 3″	7′ 5″	55th
50th	5′ 0″	5′ 2″	5′ 6″	5′ 10″	6′ 4″	6′ 9″	7′ 1″	7′ 3″	50th
45th	5′ 0″	5′ 1″	5′ 5″	5′ 9″	6′ 3″	6′ 8″	7′ 0″	7′ 2″	45th
40th	4′ 10″	5′ 0″	5′ 4″	5′ 7″	6′ 1″	6′ 6″	6′ 11″	7′ 0″	40th
35th	4′ 10″	4′ 11″	5′ 2″	5′ 6″	6′ 0″	6′ 6″	6′ 9″	6′ 11″	35th
30th	4′ 8″	4′ 10″	5′ 1″	5′ 5″	5′ 10″	6′ 4″	6′ 7″	6′ 10″	30th
25th	4′ 6″	4′ 8″	5′ 0″	5′ 3″	5′ 8″	6′ 3″	6′ 6″	6′ 8″	25th
20th	4′ 5″	4′ 7″	4′ 10″	5′ 2″	5′ 6″	6′ 1″	6′ 4″	6′ 6″	20th
15th	4′ 4″	4′ 5″	4′ 8″	5′ 0″	5′ 4″	5′ 10″	6′ 1″	6′ 4″	15th
10th	4′ 3″	4′ 2″	4′ 5″	4′ 9″	5′ 2″	5′ 7″	5′ 11″	6′ 0″	10th
5th	4′ 0″	4′ 0″	4′ 2″	4′ 5″	4′ 11″	5′ 4″	5′ 6″	5′ 8″	5th
0	2′ 10″	1′ 8″	3′ 0″	2′ 9″	3′ 8″	2′ 10″	2′ 2″	3′ 7″	0

* Reprinted by permission of the AAHPER.

Standing Long Jump for High School Boys*
Percentile Scores Based on Neilson and Cozens' Classification Index/
Test Scores in Feet and Inches

Percentile	C	B	A	Percentile
		Classification Index		
100th	8′ 11″	8′ 10″	9′ 8″	100th
95th	7′ 9″	8′ 2″	8′ 6″	95th
90th	7′ 6″	7′ 11″	8′ 3″	90th
85th	7′ 5″	7′ 9″	8′ 0″	85th
80th	7′ 3″	7′ 7″	7′ 11″	80th
75th	7′ 0″	7′ 6″	7′ 9″	75th
70th	6′ 10″	7′ 5″	7′ 7″	70th
65th	6′ 9″	7′ 3″	7′ 6″	65th
60th	6′ 8″	7′ 1″	7′ 5″	60th
55th	6′ 6″	7′ 0″	7′ 4″	55th
50th	6′ 5″	7′ 0″	7′ 3″	50th
45th	6′ 3″	6′ 10″	7′ 1″	45th
40th	6′ 2″	6′ 9″	7′ 0″	40th
35th	6′ 0″	6′ 7″	6′ 11″	35th
30th	5′ 10″	6′ 6″	6′ 9″	30th
25th	5′ 8″	6′ 5″	6′ 7″	25th
20th	5′ 6″	6′ 4″	6′ 6″	20th
15th	5′ 3″	6′ 1″	6′ 3″	15th
10th	5′ 0″	5′ 10″	6′ 0″	10th
5th	4′ 10″	5′ 5″	5′ 7″	5th
0	2′ 10″	4′ 6″	3′ 7″	0

* Reprinted by permission of the AAHPER.

50-Yard Dash for Boys*
Percentile Scores Based on Age/Test Scores in Seconds and Tenths

Percentile	10	11	12	13	14	15	16	17	Percentile
					Age				
100th	6.0	6.0	6.0	5.8	5.8	5.6	5.6	5.6	100th
95th	7.0	7.0	6.8	6.5	6.3	6.1	6.0	6.0	95th
90th	7.1	7.2	7.0	6.7	6.4	6.2	6.1	6.0	90th
85th	7.4	7.4	7.0	6.9	6.6	6.4	6.2	6.1	85th
80th	7.5	7.5	7.2	7.0	6.7	6.5	6.3	6.2	80th
75th	7.6	7.6	7.3	7.0	6.8	6.5	6.3	6.3	75th
70th	7.8	7.7	7.5	7.1	6.9	6.6	6.4	6.3	70th
65th	8.0	7.8	7.5	7.2	7.0	6.7	6.5	6.4	65th
60th	8.0	7.8	7.6	7.3	7.0	6,7	6.5	6.5	60th
55th	8.1	8.0	7.8	7.4	7.0	6.8	6.6	6.5	55th
50th	8.2	8.0	7.8	7.5	7.1	6.9	6.7	6.6	50th
45th	8.3	8.0	7.9	7.5	7.2	7.0	6.7	6.7	45th
40th	8.5	8.1	8.0	7.6	7.2	7.0	6.8	6.7	40th
35th	8.5	8.3	8.0	7.7	7.3	7.1	6.9	6.8	35th
30th	8.7	8.4	8.2	7.9	7.5	7.1	6.9	6.9	30th
25th	8.8	8.5	8.3	8.0	7.6	7.2	7.0	7.0	25th
20th	9.0	8.7	8.4	8.0	7.8	7.3	7.1	7.0	20th
15th	9.1	9.0	8.6	8.2	8.0	7.5	7.2	7.1	15th
10th	9.5	9.1	8.9	8.4	8.1	7.7	7.5	7.3	10th
5th	10.0	9.5	9.2	8.9	8.6	8.1	7.8	7.7	5th
0	12.0	11.9	12.0	11.1	11.6	12.0	8.6	10.6	0

* Reprinted by permission of the AAHPER.

50-Yard Dash for High School Boys*
Percentile Scores Based on Neilson and Cozens' Classification Index/
Test Scores in Seconds and Tenths

| Percentile | Classification Index | | | Percentile |
	C	B	A	
100th	6.0	5.6	5.6	100th
95th	6.3	6.0	6.0	95th
90th	6.4	6.1	6.1	90th
85th	6.5	6.2	6.2	85th
80th	6.6	6.3	6.2	80th
75th	6.7	6.4	6.3	75th
70th	6.9	6.5	6.4	70th
65th	7.0	6.5	6.4	65th
60th	7.0	6.5	6.5	60th
55th	7.1	6.6	6.6	55th
50th	7.1	6.7	6.6	50th
45th	7.2	6.8	6.7	45th
40th	7.3	6.8	6.8	40th
35th	7.4	6.9	6.8	35th
30th	7.5	7.0	6.9	30th
25th	7.6	7.1	7.0	25th
20th	7.8	7.2	7.0	20th
15th	8.0	7.3	7.2	15th
10th	8.1	7.5	7.3	10th
5th	8.6	7.9	7.7	5th
0	10.4	10.0	10.6	0

* Reprinted by permission of the AAHPER.

Softball Throw for Boys*
Percentile Scores Based on Age/Test Scores in Feet

Percentile				Age					Percentile
	10	11	12	13	14	15	16	17	
100th	175	205	207	245	246	250	271	291	100th
95th	138	151	165	195	208	221	238	249	95th
90th	127	141	156	183	195	210	222	235	90th
85th	122	136	150	175	187	204	213	226	85th
80th	118	129	145	168	181	198	207	218	80th
75th	114	126	141	163	176	192	201	213	75th
70th	109	121	136	157	172	189	197	207	70th
65th	105	119	133	152	168	184	194	203	65th
60th	102	115	129	147	165	180	189	198	60th
55th	98	113	124	142	160	175	185	195	55th
50th	96	111	120	140	155	171	180	190	50th
45th	93	108	119	135	150	167	175	185	45th
40th	91	105	115	131	146	165	172	180	40th
35th	89	101	112	128	141	160	168	176	35th
30th	84	98	110	125	138	156	165	171	30th
25th	81	94	106	120	133	152	160	163	25th
20th	78	90	103	115	127	147	153	155	20th
15th	73	85	97	110	122	141	147	150	15th
10th	69	78	92	101	112	135	141	141	10th
5th	60	70	76	88	102	123	127	117	5th
0	35	14	25	50	31	60	30	31	0

* Reprinted by permission of the AAHPER.

Softball Throw for High School Boys*
Percentile Scores Based on Neilson and Cozens' Classification Index/
Test Scores in Feet

| Percentile | Classification Index | | | Percentile |
	C	B	A	
100th	209	270	291	100th
95th	199	225	246	95th
90th	185	215	231	90th
85th	180	207	222	85th
80th	174	201	216	80th
75th	171	196	210	75th
70th	166	192	206	70th
65th	164	188	201	65th
60th	159	182	196	60th
55th	156	179	192	55th
50th	152	174	187	50th
45th	148	170	183	45th
40th	145	167	180	40th
35th	143	165	175	35th
30th	140	157	170	30th
25th	127	150	165	25th
20th	123	147	159	20th
15th	111	139	153	15th
10th	105	130	145	10th
5th	88	109	129	5th
0	43	31	30	0

* Reprinted by permission of the AAHPER.

600-Yard Run–Walk for Boys*
Percentile Scores Based on Age/Test Scores in Minutes and Seconds

	Age								
Percentile	10	11	12	13	14	15	16	17	Percentile
100th	1′ 30″	1′ 27″	1′ 31″	1′ 29″	1′ 25″	1′ 26″	1′ 24″	1′ 23″	100th
95th	1′ 58″	1′ 59″	1′ 52″	1′ 46″	1′ 37″	1′ 34″	1′ 32″	1′ 31″	95th
90th	2′ 9″	2′ 3″	2′ 0″	1′ 50″	1′ 42″	1′ 38″	1′ 35″	1′ 34″	90th
85th	2′ 12″	2′ 8″	2′ 2″	1′ 53″	1′ 46″	1′ 40″	1′ 37″	1′ 36″	85th
80th	2′ 15″	2′ 11″	2′ 5″	1′ 55″	1′ 48″	1′ 42″	1′ 39″	1′ 38″	80th
75th	2′ 18″	2′ 14″	2′ 9″	1′ 59″	1′ 51″	1′ 44″	1′ 40″	1′ 40″	75th
70th	2′ 20″	2′ 16″	2′ 11″	2′ 1″	1′ 53″	1′ 46″	1′ 43″	1′ 42″	70th
65th	2′ 23″	2′ 19″	2′ 13″	2′ 3″	1′ 55″	1′ 47″	1′ 45″	1′ 44″	65th
60th	2′ 26″	2′ 21″	2′ 15″	2′ 5″	1′ 57″	1′ 49″	1′ 47″	1′ 45″	60th
55th	2′ 30″	2′ 24″	2′ 18″	2′ 7″	1′ 59″	1′ 51″	1′ 49″	1′ 48″	55th
50th	2′ 33″	2′ 27″	2′ 21″	2′ 10″	2′ 1″	1′ 54″	1′ 51″	1′ 50″	50th
45th	2′ 36″	2′ 30″	2′ 24″	2′ 12″	2′ 3″	1′ 55″	1′ 53″	1′ 52″	45th
40th	2′ 40″	2′ 33″	2′ 26″	2′ 15″	2′ 5″	1′ 58″	1′ 56″	1′ 54″	40th
35th	2′ 43″	2′ 36″	2′ 30″	2′ 17″	2′ 9″	2′ 0″	1′ 58″	1′ 57″	35th
30th	2′ 45″	2′ 39″	2′ 34″	2′ 22″	2′ 11″	2′ 3″	2′ 1″	2′ 0″	30th
25th	2′ 49″	2′ 42″	2′ 39″	2′ 25″	2′ 14″	2′ 7″	2′ 5″	2′ 4″	25th
20th	2′ 55″	2′ 48″	2′ 47″	2′ 30″	2′ 19″	2′ 13″	2′ 9″	2′ 9″	20th
15th	3′ 1″	2′ 55″	2′ 57″	2′ 35″	2′ 25″	2′ 20″	2′ 14″	2′ 16″	15th
10th	3′ 8″	3′ 9″	3′ 8″	2′ 45″	2′ 33″	2′ 32″	2′ 22″	2′ 26″	10th
5th	3′ 23″	3′ 30″	3′ 32″	3′ 3″	2′ 47″	2′ 50″	2′ 37″	2′ 40″	5th
0	4′ 58″	5′ 6″	4′ 55″	5′ 14″	5′ 10″	4′ 10″	4′ 9″	4′ 45″	0

* Reprinted by permission of the AAHPER.

600-Yard Run–Walk for High School Boys*
Percentile Scores Based on Neilson and Cozens' Classification Index/
Test Scores in Minutes and Seconds

| Percentile | Classification Index | | | Percentile |
	C	B	A	
100th	1′ 29″	1′ 25″	1′ 23″	100th
95th	1′ 40″	1′ 32″	1′ 31″	95th
90th	1′ 41″	1′ 35″	1′ 34″	90th
85th	1′ 44″	1′ 37″	1′ 36″	85th
80th	1′ 46″	1′ 39″	1′ 38″	80th
75th	1′ 50″	1′ 41″	1′ 40″	75th
70th	1′ 52″	1′ 43″	1′ 42″	70th
65th	1′ 53″	1′ 45″	1′ 44″	65th
60th	1′ 55″	1′ 47″	1′ 45″	60th
55th	1′ 57″	1′ 49″	1′ 47″	55th
50th	1′ 58″	1′ 51″	1′ 49″	50th
45th	2′ 1″	1′ 53″	1′ 51″	45th
40th	2′ 3″	1′ 55″	1′ 54″	40th
35th	2′ 5″	1′ 58″	1′ 57″	35th
30th	2′ 8″	2′ 1″	2′ 0″	30th
25th	2′ 12″	2′ 5″	2′ 3″	25th
20th	2′ 16″	2′ 9″	2′ 8″	20th
15th	2′ 22″	2′ 15″	2′ 14″	15th
10th	2′ 34″	2′ 25″	2′ 22″	10th
5th	2′ 45″	2′ 37″	2′ 39″	5th
0	3′ 12″	4′ 34″	4′ 45″	0

* Reprinted by permission of the AAHPER.

Dips on Parallel Bars (High School Boys)*
Scores Based on Neilson and Cozens' Classification Index/Number of Dips

Score	F	E	D	C	B	A	Score
100			17	19	22	25	100
98					21	24	98
96			16	18		23	96
94					20		94
92			15	17		22	92
90					19	21	90
88			14	16	18		88
86			13	15		20	86
84					17	19	84
82			12	14			82
80					16	18	80
78			11	13	15	17	78
76							76
74			10	12	14	16	74
72						15	72
70			9	11	13		70
68					12	14	68
66			8	10		13	66
64				9	11		64
62	Dip not desirable for class F	Dip not desirable for class E	7			12	62
60			6	8	10	11	60
58					9		58
56			5	7		10	56
54					8	9	54
52			4	6			52
50					7	8	50
48				5			48
46			3				46
44					6	7	44
42							42
40			2	4			40
38					5	6	38
36							36
34			1	3			34
32					4	5	32
30							30
28				2			28
26					3	4	26
24							24
22				1			22
20					2	3	20
18							18
16							16
14					1	2	14
12							12
10							10
8						1	8
6							6
4							4
2							2
0							0

* Revised from scales prepared by Frederick W. Cozens, Martin Trieb, and N. P. Neilson. Used by permission of N. P. Neilson.

Push-Ups (High School Boys)*
Scores Based on Neilson and Cozens' Classification Index/ Number of Push-Ups

Score	F	E	D	C	B	A	Score
100	44	44	45	46	48	50	100
98	43	43	44	45	46	48	98
96	41	42	43	44	45	47	96
94	40	41	41	43	44	46	94
92	39	40	40	41	43	45	92
90	38	38	39	40	42	44	90
88	37	37	38	39	40	42	88
86	35	36	37	38	39	41	86
84	34	35	35	37	38	40	84
82	33	34	34	35	37	39	82
80	32	32	33	34	36	38	80
78	31	31	32	33	34	36	78
76	29	30	31	32	33	35	76
74	28	29	29	31	32	34	74
72	27	28	28	29	31	33	72
70	26	26	27	28	30	32	70
68	25	25	26	27	28	30	68
66	23	24	25	26	27	29	66
64	22	23	23	25	26	28	64
62	21	22	22	23	25	27	62
60	20	20	21	22	24	26	60
58	19	19	20	21	22	24	58
56	17	18	19	20	21	23	56
54	16	17	17	19	20	22	54
52	15	16	16	17	19	21	52
50	14		15		18	20	50
48		14		16	17	19	48
46	13		14				46
44		13		15	16	18	44
42	12		13	14			42
40	11	12			15	17	40
38		11	12	13			38
36	10				14	16	36
34		10	11	12			34
32	9		10		13	15	32
30		9		11		14	30
28	8		9		12		28
26		8		10	11	13	26
24	7		8	9			24
22	6	7			10	12	22
20		6	7	8			20
18	5				9	11	18
16		5	6	7			16
14	4				8	10	14
12		4	5	6		9	12
10	3		4		7		10
8		3		5	6	8	8
6	2		3				6
4		2		4	5	7	4
2	1		2	3			2
0							0

* Revised from scales prepared by Frederick W. Cozens, Martin Trieb, and N. P. Neilson. Used by permission of N. P. Neilson.

Rope Climb—20 Feet (High School Boys)
Scores Based on Neilson and Cozens' Classification Index/
Time in Seconds

Score	F	E	D	C	B	A	Score
100	8.0	7.5	7.2	6.8	6.0	5.1	100
98	8.4	7.8	7.5	7.1	6.3	5.4	98
96	8.7	8.2	7.9	7.4	6.6	5.7	96
94	9.1	8.5	8.2	7.8	6.9	6.0	94
92	9.4	8.9	8.5	8.1	7.2	6.3	92
90	9.8	9.2	8.9	8.4	7.6	6.6	90
88	10.2	9.6	9.2	8.7	7.9	6.9	88
86	10.5	9.9	9.6	9.1	8.2	7.2	86
84	10.9	10.3	9.9	9.4	8.5	7.5	84
82	11.2	10.6	10.2	9.7	8.8	7.8	82
80	11.6	11.0	10.6	10.0	9.1	8.1	80
78	12.0	11.3	10.9	10.4	9.4	8.4	78
76	12.3	11.7	11.2	10.7	9.7	8.7	76
74	12.7	12.0	11.6	11.0	10.1	9.0	74
72	13.0	12.4	11.9	11.3	10.4	9.3	72
70	13.4	12.7	12.2	11.7	10.7	9.6	70
68	13.8	13.1	12.6	12.0	11.0	9.9	68
66	14.1	13.4	12.9	12.2	11.3	10.2	66
64	14.5	13.8	13.2	12.6	11.6	10.5	64
62	14.8	14.1	13.6	13.0	11.9	10.8	62
60	15.2	14.5	13.9	13.3	12.2	11.1	60
58	15.6	14.8	14.3	13.6	12.6	11.4	58
56	15.9	15.2	14.6	13.9	12.9	11.7	56
54	16.3	15.5	14.9	14.3	13.2	12.0	54
52	16.6	15.9	15.3	14.6	13.5	12.3	52
50	17.0	16.2	15.6	14.9	13.8	12.6	50
48	17.4	16.5	15.9	15.2	14.1	12.9	48
46	17.7	16.9	16.3	15.5	14.4	13.2	46
44	18.1	17.2	16.6	15.9	14.7	13.5	44
42	18.4	17.6	16.9	16.2	15.0	13.8	42
40	18.8	17.9	17.3	16.5	15.4	14.1	40
38	19.2	18.3	17.6	16.8	15.7	14.4	38
36	19.5	18.6	18.0	17.2	16.0	14.7	36
34	19.9	19.0	18.3	17.5	16.3	15.0	34
32	20.2	19.3	18.6	17.8	16.6	15.3	32
30	20.6	19.7	19.0	18.1	16.9	15.6	30
28	21.0	20.0	19.3	18.5	17.2	15.9	28
26	21.3	20.4	19.6	18.8	17.5	16.2	26
24	21.7	20.7	20.0	19.1	17.9	16.5	24
22	22.0	21.1	20.3	19.4	18.2	16.8	22
20	22.4	21.4	20.6	19.8	18.5	17.1	20
18	22.8	21.8	21.0	20.1	18.8	17.4	18
16	23.1	22.1	21.3	20.4	19.1	17.7	16
14	23.5	22.5	21.6	20.7	19.4	18.0	14
12	23.8	22.8	22.0	21.1	19.7	18.3	12
10	24.2	23.2	22.3	21.4	20.0	18.6	10
8	24.6	23.5	22.7	21.7	20.4	18.9	8
6	24.9	23.9	23.0	22.0	20.7	19.2	6
4	25.3	24.2	23.3	22.4	21.0	19.5	4
2	25.6	24.6	23.7	22.7	21.3	19.8	2
0							0

* Revised from scales prepared by Frederick W. Cozens, Martin Trieb, and N. P. Neilson. Used by permission of N. P. Neilson.

Vertical Jump—Jump and Reach (High School Boys)
Scores Based on Neilson and Cozens' Classification Index/Height in Inches

Score	F	E	D	C	B	A	Score
100	21	21½	22	22½	23½	24½	100
98					23	24	98
96	20½	21	21½	22			96
94	20	20½	21	21½	22½	23½	94
92					22	23	92
90	19½	20	20½	21			90
88	19	19½	20	20½	21½	22½	88
86					21	22	86
84	18½	19	19½	20			84
82	18	18½	19	19½	20½	21½	82
80					20	21	80
78	17½	18	18½	19			78
76	17	17½	18	18½	19½	20½	76
74					19	20	74
72	16½	17	17½	18			72
70	16	16½	17	17½	18½	19½	70
68					18	19	68
66	15½	16	16½	17			66
64	15	15½	16	16½	17½	18½	64
62					17	18	62
60	14½	15	15½	16			60
58	14	14½	15	15½	16½	17½	58
56					16	17	56
54	13½	14	14½	15			54
52	13	13½	14	14½	15½	16½	52
50					15	16	50
48	12½	13	13½	14			48
46	12	12½	13	13½	14½	15½	46
44					14	15	44
42	11½	12	12½	13			42
40	11	11½	12	12½	13½	14½	40
38					13	14	38
36	10½	11	11½	12			36
34	10	10½	11	11½	12½	13½	34
32					12	13	32
30	9½	10	10½	11			30
28	9	9½	10	10½	11½	12½	28
26					11	12	26
24	8½	9	9½	10			24
22	8	8½	9	9½	10½	11½	22
20					10	11	20
18	7½	8	8½	9			18
16	7	7½	8	8½	9½	10½	16
14					9	10	14
12	6½	7	7½	8			12
10	6	6½	7	7½	8½	9½	10
8					8	9	8
6	5½	6	6½	7			6
4	5	5½	6	6½	7½	8½	4
2							2
0							0

* Revised from scales prepared by Frederick W. Cozens, Martin Trieb, and N. P. Neilson. Used by permission of N. P. Neilson.

Shot Put—12 Pound (High School Boys)
Scores Based on Neilson and Cozens' Classification Index/
Distance in Feet and Inches

Score	F	E	D	C	B	A	Score
100			33-11	36-5	38-5	41-8	100
98			33-6	36-0	38-0	41-1	98
96			33-0	35-6	37-6	40-7	96
94			32-7	35-0	37-0	40-1	94
92			32-1	34-6	36-8	39-6	92
90			31-8	34-1	36-1	39-0	90
88			31-2	33-7	35-7	38-6	88
86			30-9	33-1	35-1	37-11	86
84			30-3	32-7	34-7	37-5	84
82			29-10	32-2	34-2	36-11	82
80			29-4	31-8	33-8	36-4	80
78			28-11	31-2	33-2	35-10	78
76			28-5	30-8	32-8	35-4	76
74			28-0	30-3	32-3	34-9	74
72			27-6	29-9	31-9	34-3	72
70			27-0	29-3	31-3	33-9	70
68			26-7	28-9	30-9	33-2	68
66			26-1	28-3	30-3	32-8	66
64			25-8	27-10	29-10	32-2	64
62			25-2	27-4	29-4	31-7	62
60			24-9	26-10	28-10	31-1	60
58			24-3	26-4	28-4	30-7	58
56	12 lb. shot not used for Class F	12 lb. shot not used for Class E	23-10	25-11	27-11	30-0	56
54			23-4	25-5	27-5	29-6	54
52			22-11	24-11	26-11	29-0	52
50			22-5	24-5	26-5	28-6	50
48			22-0	24-0	26-0	27-11	48
46			21-6	23-6	25-6	27-5	46
44			21-1	23-0	25-0	26-11	44
42			20-7	22-6	24-6	26-4	42
40			20-2	22-1	24-1	25-10	40
38			19-8	21-7	23-7	25-4	38
36			19-3	21-1	23-1	24-9	36
34			18-9	20-7	22-7	24-3	34
32			18-4	20-2	22-2	23-9	32
30			17-10	19-8	21-8	23-2	30
28			17-5	19-2	21-2	22-8	28
26			16-11	18-8	20-8	22-2	26
24			16-6	18-3	20-3	21-7	24
22			16-0	17-9	19-9	21-1	22
20			15-6	17-3	19-3	20-7	20
18			15-1	16-9	18-9	20-0	18
16			14-7	16-3	18-3	19-6	16
14			14-2	15-10	17-10	19-0	14
12			13-8	15-4	17-4	18-5	12
10			13-3	14-10	16-10	17-11	10
8			12-9	14-4	16-4	17-5	8
6			12-4	13-11	15-11	16-10	6
4			11-10	13-5	15-5	16-4	4
2			11-5	12-11	14-11	15-10	2
0							0

* Revised from scales prepared by Frederick W. Cozens, Martin Trieb, and N. P. Neilson. Used by permission of N. P. Neilson.

100-Yard Run (High School Boys)
Scores Based on Neilson and Cozens' Classification Index/
Time in Seconds

Score	F	E	D	C	B	A	Score
100	12.1	11.5	11.0	10.7	10.4	10.3	100
98	12.2	11.6	11.1	10.8	10.5	10.4	98
96	12.3	11.7	11.2	10.9	10.6	10.5	96
94	12.4	11.8	11.3	11.0	10.7	10.6	94
92			11.4		10.8		92
90	12.5	11.9	11.5	11.1	10.9	10.7	90
88	12.6	12.0	11.6	11.2	11.0	10.8	88
86	12.7	12.1	11.7	11.3	11.1	10.9	86
84	12.8	12.2		11.4		11.0	84
82	12.9	12.3	11.8	11.5	11.2	11.1	82
80	13.0	12.4	11.9	11.6	11.3	11.2	80
78	13.1	12.5	12.0	11.7	11.4	11.3	78
76	13.2	12.6	12.1	11.8	11.5	11.4	76
74	13.3	12.7	12.2	11.9	11.6	11.5	74
72			12.3		11.7		72
70	13.4	12.8	12.4	12.0	11.8	11.6	70
68	13.5	12.9	12.5	12.1	11.9	11.7	68
66	13.6	13.0	12.6	12.2	12.0	11.8	66
64	13.7	13.1		12.3		11.9	64
62	13.8	13.2	12.7	12.4	12.1	12.0	62
60	13.9	13.3	12.8	12.5	12.2	12.1	60
58	14.0	13.4	12.9	12.6	12.3	12.2	58
56	14.1	13.5	13.0	12.7	12.4	12.3	56
54	14.2	13.6	13.1	12.8	12.5	12.4	54
52			13.2		12.6		52
50	14.3	13.7	13.3	12.9	12.7	12.5	50
48	14.4	13.8	13.4	13.0	12.8	12.6	48
46	14.5	13.9	13.5	13.1	12.9	12.7	46
44	14.6	14.0		13.2		12.8	44
42	14.7	14.1	13.6	13.3	13.0	12.9	42
40	14.8	14.2	13.7	13.4	13.1	13.0	40
38	14.9	14.3	13.8	13.5	13.2	13.1	38
36	15.0	14.4	13.9	13.6	13.3	13.2	36
34	15.1	14.5	14.0	13.7	13.4	13.3	34
32			14.1		13.5		32
30	15.2	14.6	14.2	13.8	13.6	13.4	30
28	15.3	14.7	14.3	13.9	13.7	13.5	28
26	15.4	14.8	14.4	14.0	13.8	13.6	26
24	15.5	14.9		14.1		13.7	24
22	15.6	15.0	14.5	14.2	13.9	13.8	22
20	15.7	15.1	14.6	14.3	14.0	13.9	20
18	15.8	15.2	14.7	14.4	14.1	14.0	18
16	15.9	15.3	14.8	14.5	14.2	14.1	16
14	16.0	15.4	14.9	14.6	14.3	14.2	14
12			15.0		14.4		12
10	16.1	15.5	15.1	14.7	14.5	14.3	10
8	16.2	15.6	15.2	14.8	14.6	14.4	8
6	16.3	15.7	15.3	14.9	14.7	14.5	6
4	16.4	15.8		15.0		14.6	4
2	16.5	15.9	15.4	15.1	14.8	14.7	2
0							0

* Revised from scales prepared by Frederick W. Cozens, Martin Trieb, and N. P. Neilson. Used by permission of N. P. Neilson.

440-Yard Run (High School Boys)
Scores Based on Neilson and Cozens' Classification Index/
Time in Seconds

Score	F	E	D	C	B	A	Score
100	61.3	59.1	57.0	54.9	53.2	51.5	100
98	61.9	59.8	57.7	55.6	53.9	52.1	98
96	62.6	60.4	58.3	56.2	54.5	52.8	96
94	63.3	61.1	59.0	56.9	55.2	53.4	94
92	63.9	61.7	59.6	57.5	55.8	54.1	92
90	64.5	62.4	60.3	58.2	56.5	54.7	90
88	65.2	63.0	60.9	58.8	57.1	55.4	88
86	65.8	63.7	61.6	59.5	57.8	56.0	86
84	66.5	64.3	62.2	60.1	58.4	56.7	84
82	67.1	65.0	62.9	60.8	59.1	57.3	82
80	67.8	65.6	63.5	61.4	59.7	58.0	80
78	68.4	66.3	64.2	62.1	60.4	58.6	78
76	69.1	66.9	64.8	62.7	61.0	59.3	76
74	69.7	67.6	65.5	63.4	61.7	59.9	74
72	70.4	68.2	66.1	64.0	62.3	60.6	72
70	71.0	68.9	66.8	64.7	63.0	61.2	70
68	71.7	69.5	67.4	65.3	63.6	61.9	68
66	72.3	70.2	68.1	66.0	64.3	62.5	66
64	73.0	70.8	68.7	66.6	64.9	63.2	64
62	73.6	71.5	69.4	67.3	65.6	63.8	62
60	74.3	72.1	70.0	67.9	66.2	64.5	60
58	74.9	72.8	70.7	68.6	66.9	65.1	58
56	75.6	73.4	71.3	69.2	67.5	65.8	56
54	76.2	74.1	72.0	69.9	68.2	66.4	54
52	76.9	74.7	72.6	70.5	68.8	67.1	52
50	77.5	75.4	73.3	71.2	69.5	67.7	50
48	78.2	76.0	73.9	71.8	70.1	68.4	48
46	78.8	76.7	74.6	72.5	70.8	69.0	46
44	79.5	77.3	75.2	73.1	71.4	69.7	44
42	80.1	78.0	75.9	73.8	72.1	70.3	42
40	80.8	78.6	76.5	74.4	72.7	71.0	40
38	81.4	79.3	77.2	75.1	73.4	71.6	38
36	82.1	79.9	77.8	75.7	74.0	72.3	36
34	82.7	80.6	78.5	76.4	74.7	72.9	34
32	83.4	81.2	79.1	77.0	75.3	73.6	32
30	84.0	81.9	79.8	77.7	76.0	74.2	30
28	84.7	82.5	80.4	78.3	76.6	74.9	28
26	85.3	83.2	81.1	79.0	77.3	75.5	26
24	86.0	83.8	81.7	79.6	77.9	76.2	24
22	86.6	84.5	82.4	80.3	78.6	76.8	22
20	87.3	85.1	83.0	80.9	79.2	77.5	20
18	87.9	85.8	83.7	81.6	79.9	78.1	18
16	88.6	86.4	84.3	82.2	80.5	78.8	16
14	89.2	87.1	85.0	82.9	81.2	79.4	14
12	89.9	87.7	85.6	83.5	81.8	80.1	12
10	90.5	88.4	86.3	84.2	82.5	80.7	10
8	91.2	89.0	86.9	84.8	83.1	81.4	8
6	91.8	89.7	87.6	85.5	83.8	82.0	6
4	92.5	90.3	88.2	86.1	84.4	82.7	4
2	93.1	91.0	88.9	86.8	85.1	83.3	2
0							0

* Revised from scales prepared by Frederick W. Cozens, Martin Trieb, and N. P. Neilson. Used by permission of N. P. Neilson.

Appendix D:
Achievement Scales for College Men

Achievement Scales for the Harvard Step Test*

Duration of Effort (Minutes)	Total Heart Beats 1½ Minutes in Recovery											
	40–44	45–49	50–54	55–59	60–64	65–69	70–74	75–79	80–84	85–89	90–94	95–99
	Score (Arbitrary Units)											
$0 - \frac{1}{2}$	6	6	5	5	4	4	4	4	3	3	3	3
$\frac{1}{2}$–1	19	17	16	14	13	12	11	11	10	9	9	8
$1 -1\frac{1}{2}$	32	29	26	24	22	20	19	18	17	16	15	14
$1\frac{1}{2}$–2	45	41	38	34	31	29	27	25	23	22	21	20
$2 -2\frac{1}{2}$	58	52	47	43	40	36	34	32	30	28	27	25
$2\frac{1}{2}$–3	71	64	58	53	48	45	42	39	37	34	33	31
$3 -3\frac{1}{2}$	84	75	68	62	57	53	49	46	43	41	39	37
$3\frac{1}{2}$–4	97	87	79	72	66	61	57	53	50	47	45	42
$4 -4\frac{1}{2}$	110	98	89	82	75	70	65	61	57	54	51	48
$4\frac{1}{2}$–5	123	110	100	91	84	77	72	68	63	60	57	54
5	129	116	105	96	88	82	76	71	67	63	60	56

* From *Physiological Measurements of Metabolic Function in Man* by Consolazio, Johnson, and Pecora. Copyright 1963. Reprinted by permission of McGraw-Hill Book Company.

Achievement Scales for the Stroup Basketball Test*

Shooting	Passing	Dribbling	Scale Score	Shooting	Passing	Dribbling	Scale Score
6	53	27	51	24	78	42	76
7	55		52				77
8	56	28	53	25	79	43	78
9	57	29	54	26	80		79
	59	30	55	27	81	44	80
10	60	31	56		82		81
11	61		57	28		45	82
12	62	32	58	29	83		83
13	64	33	59		84	46	84
14	65	34	60	30	85		85
	66		61		86	47	86
15		35	62	31	87		87
16	67		63	32	88	48	88
	68	36	64		89	49	89
17	69		65	33	90	50	90
	70	37	66	34	91		91
			67	35	93	51	92
18			68	36	94		93
19	71	38	69	37	95	52	94
	72		70		97		95
20	73	39	71	38	98	53	96
21			72	39	99		97
	74	40	73	40	100	54	98
22	75		74	41	102	55	99
23	76	41	75	42	103	56	100
	77						

* Stroup, Francis, "Games Results as a Criterion for Validating Basketball Skill Tests." *Research Quarterly*, 1955, *26*, 353. Reprinted by permission of AAHPER

Achievement Scales for the JCR Test*

Jump	Chin	Run	Standard Score	Rating	Jump	Chin	Run	Standard Score	Rating
28	18	19	100		19	6	—	50	
—	—	—	99		—	—	—	49	
—	—	—	98		—	—	23.5	48	A
27	17	—	97		—	—	—	47	V
—	—	19.5	96		—	—	—	46	E
—	—	—	95		—	5	—	45	R
—	16	—	94		18	—	—	44	A
—	—	—	93	E	—	—	24	43	G
26	—	—	92		—	—	—	42	E
—	—	—	91	X	—	—	—	41	
—	15	20	90		—	—	—	40	
—	—	—	89	C	—	4	—	39	
—	—	—	88		17	—	24.5	38	
—	—	—	87	E	—	—	—	37	P
25	14	—	86		—	—	—	36	O
—	—	—	85	L	—	—	—	35	O
—	—	20.5	84		—	—	—	34	R
—	—	—	83	L	—	3	25	33	
—	13	—	82		16	—	—	32	
—	—	—	81	E	—	—	—	31	
24	—	—	80		—	—	—	30	
—	—	—	79	N	—	—	—	29	
—	12	21	78		—	—	25.5	28	
—	—	—	77	T	—	2	—	27	
—	—	—	76		15	—	—	26	
—	—	—	75		—	—	—	25	
23	11	—	74		—	—	26	24	V
—	—	—	73		—	—	—	23	
—	—	21.5	72		—	—	—	22	E
—	—	—	71		—	1	—	21	
—	10	—	70		14	—	26.5	20	R
—	—	—	69		—	—	—	19	
22	—	—	68	G	—	—	—	18	Y
—	—	—	67		—	—	—	17	
—	—	22	66	O	—	—	27	16	
—	9	—	65		—	—	—	15	P
—	—	—	64	O	13	—	—	14	
—	—	—	63		—	0	—	13	O
21	—	—	62	D	—	—	27.5	12	
—	—	—	61		—	—	—	11	O
—	8	22.5	60		—	—	—	10	
—	—	—	59		—	—	—	9	R
—	—	—	58	A	12	—	28	8	
—	—	—	57	V	—	—	—	7	
20	—	—	56	E	—	—	—	6	
—	7	—	55	R	—	—	—	5	
—	—	23	54	A	—	—	28.5	4	
—	—	—	53	G	11	—	—	3	
—	—	—	52	E	—	—	—	2	
—	—	—	51		—	—	29	1	
					10	—	29.5	0	

* Phillips, Bernath E., "The JCR Test." *Research Quarterly*, 1947, *18*, 12–29. Reprinted by permission of the AAHPER.

Achievement Scales for the Larson Motor Ability Test*
Indoor Test

Dodging Run (Wt. = 1.09)

Raw Score (Sec.)	T-Score	Wtd. T-Score
28.0	27	29
27.8	28.2	31
27.6	29.4	32
27.4	30.6	33
27.2	31.8	35
27.0	33	36
26.8	34	37
26.6	35	38
26.4	36	39
26.2	37	40
26.0	38	41
25.8	38.8	42
25.6	39.6	43
25.4	40.4	44
25.2	41.2	45
25.0	42	46
24.8	42.8	47
24.6	43.6	48
24.4	44.4	48
24.2	45.2	49
24.0	46	50
23.8	47.2	51
23.6	48.4	53
23.4	49.6	54
23.2	50.8	55
23.0	52	57
22.8	53.2	58
22.6	54.4	59
22.4	55.6	61
22.2	56.8	62
22.0	58	63
21.8	59.2	65
21.6	60.4	66
21.4	61.6	67
21.2	62.8	68
21.0	64	70
20.8	65.4	71
20.6	66.8	73
20.4	68.2	74
20.2	69.6	76
20.0	71	77
19.8	72.2	79
19.6	73.4	80
19.4	74.6	81
19.2	75.8	83
19.0	77	84

Bar Snap (Wt. = 4.05)

Raw Score (Ins.)	T-Score	Wtd. T-Score
102	80	324
101	79.3	321
100	78.7	319
99	78	316
98	77.3	313
97	76.7	311
96	76	308
95	75.5	306
94	75	304
93	74.5	302
92	74	300
91	73.5	298
90	73	296
89	72.5	294
88	72	292
87	71.5	290
86	71	288
85	70.5	286
84	70	284
83	69.5	281
82	69	279
81	68.5	277
80	68	275
79	67.5	273
78	67	271
77	66.5	269
76	66	267
75	65.5	265
74	65	263
73	64.5	261
72	64	259
71	63.3	256
70	62.7	254
69	62	251
68	61.3	248
67	60.7	246
66	60	240
65	59.3	240
64	58.7	238
63	58	235
62	57.3	232
61	56.7	230
60	56	227
59	55.3	224
58	54.7	222
57	54	219
56	53.3	216
55	52.7	213
54	52	210
53	51.2	207
52	50.3	204
51	49.5	200
50	48.7	197
49	47.8	194
48	47	190
47	46	186
46	45	182
45	44	178
44	43	174
43	42	170
42	41	166
41	39.7	161
40	38.3	155
39	37	150
38	35.7	145
37	34.3	139
36	33	134
35	31.5	128
34	30	122
33	28.5	115
32	27	109
31	25.5	103
30	24	97

Dipping (Wt. = 1.60)

Raw Score	T-Score	Wtd. T-Score
23	80	128
22	78	125
21	76	122
20	73	117
19	71	114
18	70	112
17	69	110
16	67	107
15	64	102
14	62	99
13	60	96
12	58	93
11	56	90
10	54	86
9	52	83
8	50	80
7	47	75
6	45	72
5	43	69
4	41	66
3	38	61
2	35	56
1	30	48
0	24	38

Chinning (Wt. = 2.73)

Raw Score	T-Score	Wtd. T-Score
23	80	218
22	78	213
21	77	210
20	76	207
19	75	205
18	73	199
17	71	194
16	69	188
15	67	183
14	65	177
13	63	172
12	60	164
11	58	158
10	55	150
9	52	142
8	50	137
7	48	131
6	45	123
5	42	115
4	40	109
3	37	101
2	34	93
1	30	84
0	27	74

Vertical Jump (Wt. = 1.00)

Raw Score (Ins.)	T-Score	Wtd. T-Score
26.0	78	78
25.5	76	76
25.0	74	74
24.5	72	72
24.0	70	70
23.5	68	68
23.0	66	66
22.5	64	64
22.0	62	62
21.5	60.5	61
21.0	59	59
20.5	57.5	58
20.0	56	56
19.5	54	54
19.0	52	52
18.5	50.5	51
18.0	49	49
17.5	47	47
17.0	45	45
16.5	43.5	44
16.0	42	42
15.5	40	40
15.0	38	38
14.5	36.5	37
14.0	35	35
13.5	33	33
13.0	31	31
12.5	29	29
12.0	27	27
11.5	25.5	26
11.0	24	24

Outdoor Test

Baseball Throw (Wt. = 2.23)

Raw Score (Ft.)	T-Score	Wtd. T-Score
270	80	178
268	79.6	178
266	79.2	177
264	78.8	176
262	78.4	175
260	78	174
258	77.8	173
256	77.6	173
254	77.4	173
252	77.2	172
250	77	172
248	76	169
246	75	167
244	74	165
242	73	163
240	72	161
238	71.2	159
236	70.4	157
234	69.6	155
232	68.8	153
230	68	152
228	67.2	150
226	66.4	148
224	65.6	146
222	64.8	145
220	64	143
218	63.2	141
216	62.4	139
214	61.6	137
212	60.8	136
210	60	134
208	59.6	133
206	59.2	132
204	58.8	131
202	58.4	130
200	58.0	129
198	57.4	128
196	56.8	127
194	56.2	125
192	55.6	124
190	55	123
188	54.2	121
186	53.4	119
184	52.6	117
182	51.8	116
180	51	114
178	50.2	112
176	49.4	110
174	48.6	108
172	47.8	107
170	47	105
168	46.4	103
166	45.8	102
164	45.2	101
162	44.6	99
160	44	98
158	43.4	97
156	42.8	95
154	42.2	94
152	41.6	93
150	41	91
148	40.4	90
146	39.8	89
144	39.2	87
142	38.6	86
140	38	85
138	37.4	83
136	36.8	82
134	36.2	81
132	35.6	79
130	35	78
128	34.4	77
126	33.8	75
124	33.2	74
122	32.6	73
120	32	71
118	31.6	70
116	31.2	70
114	30.8	69
112	30.4	68
110	30	67
108	29.6	66
106	29.2	65
104	28.8	64
102	28.4	63
100	28	62
98	27.4	61
96	26.8	60
94	26.2	58
92	25.6	57
90	25	56
88	24.8	55
86	24.6	55
84	24.4	54
82	24.2	54
80	24	54
78	23	51
76	22	49
74	21	47
72	20	45
70	19	42

Chinning (Wt. = 3.66)

Raw Score	T-Score	Wtd. T-Score
23	80	293
22	78	285
21	77	282
20	76	278
19	75	275
18	73	267
17	71	260
16	69	253
15	67	245
14	65	238
13	63	231
12	60	220
11	58	212
10	55	201
9	52	190
8	50	183
7	48	176
6	45	165
5	42	154
4	40	146
3	37	135
2	34	124
1	32	117
0	27	99

Bar Snap (Wt. = 4.91)

Raw Score (Ins.)	T-Score	Wtd. T-Score
102	80	393
101	79.3	389
100	78.7	386
99	78	383
98	77.3	380
97	76.7	377
96	76.1	373
95	75.5	371
94	75	368
93	74.5	366
92	74	363
91	73.5	361
90	73	358
89	72.5	356
88	72	354
87	71.5	351
86	71	349
85	70.5	346
84	70	344
83	69.5	341
82	69	339
81	68.5	336
80	68	334
79	67.5	331
78	67	329
77	66.5	327
76	66	324
75	65.5	322
74	65	319
73	64.5	317
72	64	314
71	63.3	311
70	62.7	308
69	62	304
68	61.3	301
67	60.7	298
66	60	295
65	59.3	291
64	58.7	288
63	58	285
62	57.3	281
61	56.7	278
60	56	275
59	55.3	272
58	54.7	269
57	54	265
56	53.3	262
55	52.7	259
54	52	255
53	51.2	251
52	50.3	247
51	49.5	243
50	48.7	239
49	47.8	235
48	47	231
47	46	226
46	45	221
45	44	216
44	43	211
43	42	206
42	41	201
41	39.7	195
40	38.3	188
39	37	182
38	35.7	175
37	34.3	168
36	33	162
35	31.5	155
34	30	147
33	28.5	140
32	27	133
31	25.5	125
30	24	118

Vertical Jump (Wt. = 1.00)

Raw Score (Ins.)	T-Score	Wtd. T-Score
26.0	78	78
25.5	76	76
25.0	74	74
24.5	72	72
24.0	70	70
23.5	68	68
23.0	66	66
22.5	64	64
22.0	62	62
21.5	60.5	61
21.0	59	59
20.5	57.5	58
20.0	56	56
19.5	54	54
19.0	52	52
18.5	50.5	51
18.0	49	49
17.5	47	47
17.0	45	45
16.5	43.5	44
16.0	42	42
15.5	40	40
15.0	38	38
14.5	36.5	37
14.0	35	35
13.5	33	33
13.0	31	31
12.5	29	29
12.0	27	27
11.5	25.5	26
11.0	24	24

* Larson, L. A., "A Factor Analysis of Motor Ability Variables and Tests, with Tests for College Men," *Research Quarterly*, 1941, 12, 499-517. Reprinted by permission of the AAHPER.

AAHPER Fitness Test*
Percentile Scores for College Men

Percentile	Pull-Up	Sit-Up	Shuttle Run	Standing Long Jump	50-Yard Dash	Softball Throw	600-Yard Run–Walk
100th	20	100	8.3	9' 6"	5.5	315	1:12
95th	12	99	9.0	8' 5"	6.1	239	1:35
90th	10	97	9.1	8' 2"	6.2	226	1:38
85th	10	79	9.1	7' 11"	6.3	217	1:40
80th	9	68	9.2	7' 10"	6.4	211	1:42
75th	8	61	9.4	7' 8"	6.5	206	1:44
70th	8	58	9.5	7' 7"	6.5	200	1:45
65th	7	52	9.5	7' 6"	6.6	196	1:47
60th	7	51	9.6	7' 5"	6.6	192	1:49
55th	6	50	9.6	7' 4"	6.7	188	1:50
50th	6	47	9.7	7' 3"	6.8	184	1:52
45th	5	44	9.8	7' 1"	6.8	180	1:53
40th	5	41	9.9	7' 0"	6.9	176	1:55
35th	4	38	10.0	6' 11"	7.0	171	1:57
30th	4	36	10.0	6' 10"	7.0	166	1:59
25th	3	34	10.1	6' 9"	7.1	161	2:01
20th	3	31	10.2	6' 7"	7.1	156	2:05
15th	2	29	10.4	6' 5"	7.2	150	2:09
10th	1	26	10.6	6' 2"	7.5	140	2:15
5th	0	22	11.1	5' 10"	7.7	125	2:25
0	0	0	13.9	4' 2"	9.1	55	3:43

* Reprinted by permission of the AAHPER.

Dip on Parallel Bars (College Men)*
Scores Based on Cozens' Height–Weight Divisions/Number of Dips

Score	Tall Slender	Tall Medium	Tall Heavy	Medium Slender	Medium Medium	Medium Heavy	Short Slender	Short Medium	Short Heavy	Score
100		23	22	23	24	23		25	24	100
98	21	22	21	22	23		23			98
96	20					22	22	24	23	96
94		21	20	21	22				22	94
92	19					21	21	23		92
90		20	19	20	21	20		22	21	90
88	18	19	18	19	20		20			88
86	17					19	19	21	20	86
84		18	17	18	19				19	84
82	16	17		17		18	18	20		82
80	15		16		18	17		19	18	80
78		16	15	16	17		17			78
76	14				16	16	16	18	17	76
74		15	14	15		15		17	16	74
72	13	14		14			15			72
70	12		13		15	14		16	15	70
68		13	12	13	14		14			68
66	11				13	13	13	15	14	66
64		12	11	12		12		14	13	64
62	10	11		11			12			62
60	9		10		12	11		13	12	60
58		10	9	10	11		11			58
56	8					10	10	12		56
54		9	8	9	10	9		11	10	54
52	7	8	7	8	9		9			52
50	6					8		10	9	50
48		7	6	7	8		8		8	48
46	5					7	7	9		46
44		6	5	6	7	6	6	8	7	44
42	4	5	4	5	6					42
40	3					5	5	7	6	40
38		4	3	4	5				5	38
36	2	3		3		4	4	6		36
34	1		2		4	3		5	4	34
32		2	1	2	3		3			32
30						2	2	4	3	30
28		1		1	2	1		3	2	28
26							1			26
24					1			2	1	24
22										22
20								1		20
18										18
16										16
14										14
12										12
10										10
8										8
6										6
4										4
2										2
0										0

* Revised from scales prepared by Frederick W. Cozens. Used by permission of Lea & Febiger Publishing Company.

Push-Ups (College Men)*
Scores Based on Cozens' Height–Weight Divisions/Number of Push-Ups

Score	Tall Slender	Tall Medium	Tall Heavy	Medium Slender	Medium Medium	Medium Heavy	Short Slender	Short Medium	Short Heavy	Score
100	43	44	48	46	47	49	46	49	50	100
98	42	43	47	45	46	48	45	48	49	98
96	41		46	44	45	47	44	47	48	96
94	40	42	45	43	44	46	43	46	47	94
92	39	41	44	42	43	45	42	45	46	92
90	38	40	43	41	42	44	41	44	45	90
88	37	39	42	40	41	43	40	43	44	88
86		38	41		40	42		42	43	86
84	36	37	40	39	39	41	39	41	42	84
82	35	36	39	38	38	40	38	40	41	82
80	34	35	38	37	37	39	37	39	40	80
78	33	34	37	36	36	38	36	38	39	78
76	32	33	36	35	35	37	35	37	38	76
74	31	32	35	34	34	36	34	36	37	74
72	30	31	34	33		35	33		36	72
70	29	30	33	32	33	34	32	35	35	70
68	28	29	32	31	32	33	31	34	34	68
66	27	28	31	30	31	32	30	33	33	66
64	26	27	30	29	30	31	29	32	32	64
62	25	26	29	28	29	30	28	31	31	62
60	24	25	28	27	28	29	27	30	30	60
58	23	24	27	26	27	28	26	29	29	58
56	22	23		25	26	27	25	28		56
54	21	22	26	24	25	26	24	27	28	54
52	20	21	25	23	24		23	26	27	52
50	19	20	24	22	23	25	22	25	26	50
48	18	19	23	21	22	24	21	24	25	48
46	17		22	20	21	23	20	23	24	46
44	16	18	21	19	20	22	19	22	23	44
42	15	17	20	18	19	21	18	21	22	42
40	14	16	19	17	18	20	17	20	21	40
38	13	15	18	16	17	19	16	19	20	38
36		14	17		16	18		18	19	36
34	12	13	16	15	15	17	15	17	18	34
32	11	12	15	14	14	16	14	16	17	32
30	10	11	14	13	13	15	13	15	16	30
28	9	10	13	12	12	14	12	14	15	28
26	8	9	12	11	11	13	11	13	14	26
24	7	8	11	10	10	12	10	12	13	24
22	6	7	10	9		11	9		12	22
20	5	6	9	8	9	10	8	11	11	20
18	4	5	8	7	8	9	7	10	10	18
16	3	4	7	6	7	8	6	9	9	16
14	2	3	6	5	6	7	5	8	8	14
12	1	2	5	4	5	6	4	7	7	12
10		1	4	3	4	5	3	6	6	10
8			3	2	3	4	2	5	5	8
6				1	2	3	1	4		6
4			2		1	2		3	4	4
2			1					2	3	2
0										0

* Revised from scales prepared by Frederick W. Cozens. Used by permission of Lea & Febiger Publishing Company.

Rope Climb—20 Feet (College Men)*
Scores Based on Cozens' Height–Weight Division/Time in Seconds

Score	Tall Slender	Tall Medium	Tall Heavy	Medium Slender	Medium Medium	Medium Heavy	Short Slender	Short Medium	Short Heavy	Score
100	6.9	5.5	4.8	4.8	5.9	7.3	6.4	6.7	5.3	100
98	7.2	5.8	5.0	5.1	6.2	7.6	6.7	7.0	5.5	98
96	7.5	6.1	5.3	5.4	6.5	7.9	6.9	7.2	5.8	96
94	7.8	6.4	5.6	5.7	6.8	8.2	7.2	7.5	6.1	94
92	8.1	6.7	5.9	6.0	7.1	8.5	7.5	7.8	6.4	92
90	8.3	7.0	6.2	6.3	7.4	8.8	7.8	8.1	6.7	90
88	8.6	7.2	6.5	6.6	7.7	9.1	8.1	8.4	7.0	88
86	8.9	7.5	6.8	6.9	8.0	9.3	8.4	8.7	7.3	86
84	9.2	7.8	7.1	7.1	8.2	9.6	8.7	9.0	7.6	84
82	9.5	8.1	7.3	7.4	8.5	9.9	9.0	9.3	7.8	82
80	9.8	8.4	7.6	7.7	8.8	10.2	9.3	9.6	8.1	80
78	10.1	8.7	7.9	8.0	9.1	10.5	9.5	9.8	8.4	78
76	10.4	9.0	8.2	8.3	9.4	10.8	9.8	10.1	8.7	76
74	10.6	9.3	8.5	8.6	9.7	11.1	10.1	10.4	9.0	74
72	10.9	9.6	8.8	8.9	10.0	11.4	10.4	10.7	9.3	72
70	11.2	9.8	9.1	9.2	10.3	11.7	10.7	11.0	9.6	70
68	11.5	10.1	9.4	9.4	10.5	11.9	11.0	11.3	9.9	68
66	11.8	10.4	9.6	9.7	10.8	12.2	11.3	11.6	10.1	66
64	12.0	10.7	9.9	10.0	11.1	12.5	11.6	11.9	10.4	64
62	12.3	11.0	10.2	10.3	11.4	12.8	11.8	12.1	10.7	62
60	12.6	11.3	10.5	10.6	11.7	13.1	12.1	12.4	11.0	60
58	12.9	11.6	10.8	10.9	12.0	13.4	12.4	12.7	11.3	58
56	13.2	11.9	11.1	11.2	12.3	13.7	12.7	13.0	11.6	56
54	13.5	12.1	11.4	11.5	12.6	14.0	13.0	13.3	11.9	54
52	13.8	12.4	11.7	11.8	12.9	14.2	13.3	13.6	12.2	52
50	14.1	12.7	12.0	12.0	13.1	14.5	13.6	13.9	12.5	50
48	14.4	13.0	12.2	12.3	13.4	14.8	13.9	14.2	12.7	48
46	14.7	13.3	12.5	12.6	13.7	15.1	14.1	14.4	13.0	46
44	15.0	13.6	12.8	14.0	14.3	15.4	14.4	14.7	13.3	44
42	15.2	13.9	13.1	13.2	14.3	15.7	14.7	15.0	13.6	42
40	15.5	14.2	13.4	13.5	14.6	16.0	15.0	15.3	13.9	40
38	15.8	14.4	13.7	13.8	14.9	16.3	15.3	15.6	14.2	38
36	16.1	14.7	14.0	14.1	15.2	16.5	15.6	15.9	14.5	36
34	16.4	15.0	14.3	14.3	15.4	16.8	15.9	16.2	14.8	34
32	16.7	15.3	14.5	14.6	15.7	17.1	16.2	16.5	15.0	32
30	17.0	15.6	14.8	14.9	16.0	17.4	16.5	16.8	15.3	30
28	17.3	15.9	15.1	15.2	16.3	17.7	16.7	17.0	15.6	28
26	17.5	16.2	15.4	15.5	16.6	18.0	17.0	17.3	15.9	26
24	17.8	16.5	15.7	15.8	16.9	18.3	17.3	17.6	16.2	24
22	18.1	16.8	16.0	16.1	17.2	18.6	17.6	17.9	16.5	22
20	18.4	17.0	16.3	16.4	17.5	18.9	17.9	18.2	16.8	20
18	18.7	17.3	16.6	16.6	17.7	19.1	18.2	18.5	17.1	18
16	19.0	17.6	16.8	16.9	18.0	19.4	18.5	18.8	17.3	16
14	19.3	17.9	17.1	17.2	18.3	19.7	18.8	19.1	17.6	14
12	19.6	18.2	17.4	17.5	18.6	20.0	19.0	19.3	17.9	12
10	19.9	18.5	17.7	17.8	18.9	20.3	19.3	19.6	18.2	10
8	20.1	18.8	18.0	18.1	19.2	20.6	19.6	19.9	18.5	8
6	20.4	19.1	18.3	18.4	19.5	20.9	19.9	20.2	18.8	6
4	20.7	19.3	18.6	18.7	19.8	21.2	20.2	20.5	19.1	4
2	21.0	19.6	18.9	19.0	20.1	21.4	20.5	20.8	19.4	2
0										0

* Revised from scales prepared by Frederick W. Cozens. Used by permission of Lea & Febiger Publishing Company.

Vertical Jump—Jump and Reach (College Men)*
Scores Based on Cozens' Height–Weight Divisions/
Height to Nearest Half Inch

Score	Tall Slender	Tall Medium	Tall Heavy	Medium Slender	Medium Medium	Medium Heavy	Short Slender	Short Medium	Short Heavy	Score
100		28	29		27	27½	26½	26½		100
98	28	27½	28½	27½			26		27	98
96	27½			27	26½	27		26	26½	96
94		27	28		26	26½	25½	25½		94
92	27	26½	27½	26½			25		26	92
90	26½			26	25½	26		25	25½	90
88		26	27		25	25½	24½	24½		88
86	26	25½	26½	25½			24		25	86
84	25½			25	24½	25		24	24½	84
82		25	26		24	24½	23½	23½		82
80	25	24½	25½	24½			23		24	80
78	24½			24	23½	24		23	23½	78
76		24	25		23	23½	22½	22½		76
74	24	23½	24½	23½			22		23	74
72	23½			23	22½	23		22	22½	72
70		23	24		22	22½	21½	21½		70
68	23	22½	23½	22½			21		22	68
66	22½			22	21½	22		21	21½	66
64		22	23		21	21½	20½	20½		64
62	22	21½	22½	21½			20		21	62
60	21½			21	20½	21		20	20½	60
58		21	22		20	20½	19½	19½		58
56	21	20½	21½	20½			19		20	56
54	20½			20	19½	20		19	19½	54
52		20	21		19	19½	18½	18½		52
50	20	19½	20½	19½			18		19	50
48	19½			19	18½	19		18	18½	48
46		19	20		18	18½	17½	17½		46
44	19	18½	19½	18½			17		18	44
42	18½			18	17½	18		17	17½	42
40		18	19		17	17½	16½	16½		40
38	18	17½	18½	17½			16		17	38
36	17½			17	16½	17		16	16½	36
34		17	18		16	16½	15½	15½		34
32	17	16½	17½	16½			15		16	32
30	16½			16	15½	16		15	15½	30
28		16	17		15	15½	14½	14½		28
26	16	15½	16½	15½			14		15	26
24	15½			15	14½	15		14	14½	24
22		15	16		14	14½	13½	13½		22
20	15	14½	15½	14½			13		14	20
18	14½			14	13½	14		13	13½	18
16		14	15		13	13½	12½	12½		16
14	14	13½	14½	13½			12		13	14
12	13½			13	12½	13		12	12½	12
10		13	14		12	12½	11½	11½		10
8	13	12½	13½	12½			11		12	8
6	12½			12	11½	12		11	11½	6
4		12	13		11	11½	10½	10½		4
2	12	11½	12½	11½			10		11	2
0										0

* Revised from scales prepared by Frederick W. Cozens. Used by permission of Lea & Febiger Publishing Company.

Shot Put—12 Pound (College Men)*
Scores Based on Cozens' Height–Weight Divisions/
Distance in Feet and Inches

Score	Tall Slender	Tall Medium	Tall Heavy	Medium Slender	Medium Medium	Medium Heavy	Short Slender	Short Medium	Short Heavy	Score
100	40–3	42–10	46–1	39–10	41–11	43–6	38–1	40–1	41–7	100
98	39–9	42–5	45–8	39–5	41–6	43–0	37–8	39–7	41–2	98
96	39–4	42–0	45–2	38–11	41–0	42–7	37–2	39–2	40–9	96
94	38–10	41–6	44–9	38–6	40–7	42–1	36–9	38–9	40–3	94
92	38–5	41–1	44–3	38–0	40–2	41–8	36–3	38–3	39–10	92
90	38–0	40–7	43–10	37–7	39–8	41–3	35–10	37–10	39–4	90
88	37–6	40–2	43–5	37–2	39–3	40–9	35–5	37–4	38–11	88
86	37–1	39–9	42–11	36–8	38–9	40–4	34–11	36–11	38–6	86
84	36–7	39–3	42–6	36–3	38–4	39–10	34–6	36–6	38–0	84
82	36–2	38–10	42–0	35–9	37–11	39–5	34–0	36–0	37–7	82
80	35–9	38–4	41–7	35–4	37–5	39–0	33–7	35–7	37–1	80
78	35–3	37–11	41–2	34–11	37–0	38–6	33–2	35–1	36–8	78
76	34–10	37–6	40–8	34–5	36–6	38–1	32–8	34–8	36–3	76
74	34–4	37–0	40–3	34–0	36–1	37–7	32–3	34–3	35–9	74
72	33–11	36–7	39–9	33–6	35–8	37–2	31–9	33–9	35–4	72
70	33–6	36–1	39–4	33–1	35–2	36–9	31–4	33–4	34–10	70
68	33–0	35–8	38–11	32–8	34–9	36–3	30–11	32–10	34–5	68
66	32–7	35–3	38–5	32–2	34–3	35–10	30–5	32–5	34–0	66
64	32–1	34–9	38–0	31–9	33–10	35–4	30–0	32–0	33–6	64
62	31–8	34–4	37–6	31–3	33–5	34–11	29–6	31–6	33–1	62
60	31–3	33–10	37–1	30–10	32–11	34–6	29–1	31–1	32–7	60
58	30–9	33–5	36–8	30–5	32–6	34–0	28–8	30–7	32–2	58
56	30–4	33–0	36–2	29–11	32–0	33–7	28–2	30–2	31–9	56
54	29–10	32–6	35–9	29–6	31–7	33–1	27–9	29–9	31–3	54
52	29–5	32–1	35–3	29–0	31–2	32–8	27–3	29–3	30–10	52
50	29–0	31–7	34–10	28–7	30–8	32–3	26–10	28–10	30–4	50
48	28–6	31–2	34–5	28–2	30–3	31–9	26–5	28–4	29–11	48
46	28–1	30–9	33–11	27–8	29–9	31–4	25–11	27–11	29–6	46
44	27–7	30–3	33–6	27–3	29–4	30–10	25–6	27–6	29–0	44
42	27–2	29–10	33–0	26–9	28–11	30–5	25–0	27–0	28–7	42
40	26–9	29–4	32–7	26–4	28–5	30–0	24–7	26–7	28–1	40
38	26–3	28–11	32–2	25–11	28–0	29–6	24–2	26–1	27–8	38
36	25–10	28–6	31–8	25–5	27–6	29–1	23–8	25–8	27–3	36
34	25–4	28–0	31–3	25–0	27–1	28–7	23–3	25–3	26–9	34
32	24–11	27–7	30–9	24–6	26–8	28–2	22–9	24–9	26–4	32
30	24–6	27–1	30–4	24–1	26–2	27–9	22–4	24–4	25–10	30
28	24–0	26–8	29–11	23–8	25–9	27–3	21–11	23–10	25–5	28
26	23–7	26–3	29–5	23–2	25–3	26–10	21–5	23–5	25–0	26
24	23–1	25–9	29–0	22–9	24–10	26–4	21–0	23–0	24–6	24
22	22–8	25–4	28–6	22–3	24–5	25–11	20–6	22–6	24–1	22
20	22–3	24–10	28–1	21–10	23–11	25–6	20–1	22–1	23–7	20
18	21–9	24–5	27–8	21–5	23–6	25–0	19–8	21–7	23–2	18
16	21–4	24–0	27–2	20–11	23–0	24–7	19–2	21–2	22–9	16
14	20–10	23–6	26–9	20–6	22–7	24–1	18–9	20–9	22–3	14
12	20–5	23–1	26–3	20–0	22–2	23–8	18–3	20–3	21–10	12
10	20–0	22–7	25–10	19–7	21–8	23–3	17–10	19–10	21–4	10
8	19–6	22–2	25–5	19–2	21–3	22–9	17–5	19–4	20–11	8
6	19–1	21–9	24–11	18–8	20–9	22–4	16–11	18–11	20–6	6
4	18–7	21–3	24–6	18–3	20–4	21–10	16–6	18–6	20–0	4
2	18–2	20–10	24–0	17–9	19–11	21–5	16–0	18–0	19–7	2
0										0

* Revised from scales prepared by Frederick W. Cozens. Used by permission of Lea & Febiger Publishing Comapny.

100-Yard Run (College Men)*
Scores Based on Cozens' Height–Weight Divisions/Time in Seconds

Score	Tall Slender	Tall Medium	Tall Heavy	Medium Slender	Medium Medium	Medium Heavy	Short Slender	Short Medium	Short Heavy	Score
100		10.3			10.2	10.3	10.4		10.3	100
98	10.5		10.3	10.3		10.4		10.3	10.4	98
96	10.6	10.4	10.4	10.4	10.3		10.5	10.4		96
94	10.7	10.5		10.5	10.4	10.5	10.6	10.5	10.5	94
92		10.6	10.5			10.6	10.7		10.6	92
90	10.8		10.6	10.6	10.5	10.7		10.6		90
88	10.9	10.7	10.7	10.7	10.6	10.8		10.7	10.7	88
86		10.8		10.8	10.7	10.8	10.9	10.8	10.8	86
84	11.0		10.8			10.9			10.9	84
82	11.1	10.9	10.9	10.9	10.8		11.0	10.9		82
80	11.2	11.0		11.0	10.9	11.0	11.1	11.0	11.0	80
78		11.1	11.0			11.1	11.2		11.1	78
76	11.3		11.1	11.1	11.0	11.2		11.1		76
74	11.4	11.2	11.2	11.2	11.1		11.3	11.2	11.2	74
72		11.3		11.3	11.2	11.3	11.4	11.3	11.3	72
70	11.5		11.3			11.4	11.5		11.4	70
68	11.6	11.4	11.4	11.4	11.3			11.4		68
66	11.7	11.5		11.5	11.4	11.5	11.6	11.5	11.5	66
64		11.6	11.5			11.6	11.7	11.6	11.6	64
62	11.8		11.6	11.6	11.5	11.7		11.6	11.7	62
60	11.9	11.7	11.7	11.7	11.6		11.8	11.7		60
58		11.8		11.8	11.7		11.9	11.8	11.8	58
56	12.0		11.8			11.9	12.0		11.9	56
54	12.1	11.9	11.9	11.9	11.8	12.0		11.9		54
52	12.2	12.0	12.0	12.0	11.9		12.1	12.0	12.0	52
50		12.1			12.0	12.1	12.2		12.1	50
48	12.3		12.1	12.1		12.2		12.1	12.2	48
46	12.4	12.2	12.2	12.2	12.1		12.3	12.2		46
44	12.5	12.3		12.3	12.2	12.3	12.4	12.3	12.3	44
42		12.4	12.3			12.4	12.5		12.4	42
40	12.6		12.4	12.4	12.3	12.5		12.4		40
38	12.7	12.5	12.5	12.5	12.4		12.6	12.5	12.5	38
36		12.6		12.6	12.5	12.6	12.7	12.6	12.6	36
34	12.8		12.6			12.7			12.7	34
32	12.9	12.7	12.7	12.7	12.6		12.8	12.7		32
30	13.0	12.8		12.8	12.7	12.8	12.9	12.8	12.8	30
28		12.9	12.8			12.9	13.0		12.9	28
26	13.1		12.9	12.9	12.8	13.0		12.9		26
24	13.2	13.0	13.0	13.0	12.9		13.1	13.0	13.0	24
22		13.1		13.1	13.0	13.1	13.2	13.1	13.1	22
20	13.3		13.1			13.2	13.3		13.2	20
18	13.4	13.2	13.2	13.2	13.1			13.2		18
16	13.5	13.3		13.3	13.2	13.3	13.4	13.3	13.3	16
14		13.4	13.3			13.4	13.5		13.4	14
12	13.6		13.4	13.4	13.3	13.5		13.4	13.5	12
10	13.7	13.5	13.5	13.5	13.4		13.6	13.5		10
8		13.6		13.6	13.5	13.6	13.7	13.6	13.6	8
6	13.8		13.6			13.7	13.8		13.7	6
4	13.9	13.7	13.7	13.7	13.6	13.8		13.7		4
2	14.0	13.8	13.8	13.8	13.7		13.9	13.8	13.8	2
0										0

* Revised from scales prepared by Frederick W. Cozens. Used by permission of Lea & Febiger Publishing Company.

440-Yard Run (College Men)*
Scores Based on Cozens' Height–Weight Divisions/Time in Seconds

Score	Tall Slender	Tall Medium	Tall Heavy	Medium Slender	Medium Medium	Medium Heavy	Short Slender	Short Medium	Short Heavy	Score
100	54.0	51.9	53.3	55.2	52.3	53.4	55.6	53.1	54.7	100
98	54.7	52.6	53.9	55.8	53.0	54.1	56.3	53.8	55.4	98
96	55.4	53.2	54.6	56.5	53.6	54.8	57.0	54.5	56.0	96
94	56.0	53.9	55.3	57.2	54.3	55.4	57.6	55.1	56.7	94
92	56.7	54.6	55.9	57.8	55.0	56.1	58.3	55.8	57.4	92
90	57.4	55.2	56.6	58.5	55.6	56.8	59.0	56.5	58.0	90
88	58.0	55.9	57.3	59.2	56.3	57.4	59.6	57.1	58.7	88
86	58.7	56.6	57.9	59.8	57.0	58.1	60.3	57.8	59.4	86
84	59.4	57.2	58.6	60.5	57.6	58.8	61.0	58.5	60.0	84
82	60.0	57.9	59.3	61.2	58.3	59.4	61.6	59.1	60.7	82
80	60.7	58.6	59.9	61.8	59.0	60.1	62.3	59.8	61.4	80
78	61.4	59.2	60.6	62.5	59.6	60.8	63.0	60.5	62.0	78
76	62.0	59.9	61.3	63.2	60.3	61.4	63.6	61.1	62.7	76
74	62.7	60.6	61.9	63.8	61.0	62.1	64.3	61.8	63.4	74
72	63.4	61.2	62.6	64.5	61.6	62.8	65.0	62.5	64.0	72
70	64.0	61.9	63.3	65.2	62.3	63.4	65.6	63.1	64.7	70
68	64.7	62.6	63.9	65.8	63.0	64.1	66.3	63.8	65.4	68
66	65.4	63.2	64.6	66.5	63.6	64.8	67.0	64.5	66.0	66
64	66.0	63.9	65.3	67.2	64.3	65.4	67.6	65.1	66.7	64
62	66.7	64.6	65.9	67.8	65.0	66.1	68.3	65.8	67.4	62
60	67.4	65.2	66.6	68.5	65.6	66.8	69.0	66.5	68.0	60
58	68.0	65.9	67.3	69.2	66.3	67.4	69.6	67.1	68.7	58
56	68.7	66.6	67.9	69.8	67.0	68.1	70.3	67.8	69.4	56
54	69.4	67.2	68.6	70.5	67.6	68.8	71.0	68.5	70.0	54
52	70.0	67.9	69.3	71.2	68.3	69.4	71.6	69.1	70.7	52
50	70.7	68.6	69.9	71.8	69.0	70.1	72.3	69.8	71.4	50
48	71.4	69.2	70.6	72.5	69.6	70.8	73.0	70.5	72.0	48
46	72.0	69.9	71.3	73.2	70.3	71.4	73.6	71.1	72.7	46
44	72.7	70.6	71.9	73.8	71.0	72.1	74.3	71.8	73.4	44
42	73.4	71.2	72.6	74.5	71.6	72.8	75.0	72.5	74.0	42
40	74.0	71.9	73.3	75.2	72.3	73.4	75.6	73.1	74.7	40
38	74.7	72.6	73.9	75.8	73.0	74.1	76.3	73.8	75.4	38
36	75.4	73.2	74.6	76.5	73.6	74.8	77.0	74.5	76.0	36
34	76.0	73.9	75.3	77.2	74.3	75.4	77.6	75.1	76.7	34
32	76.7	74.6	75.9	77.8	75.0	76.1	78.3	75.8	77.4	32
30	77.4	75.2	76.6	78.5	75.6	76.8	79.0	76.5	78.0	30
28	78.0	75.9	77.3	79.2	76.3	77.4	79.6	77.1	78.7	28
26	78.7	76.6	77.9	79.8	77.0	78.1	80.3	77.8	79.4	26
24	79.4	77.2	78.6	80.5	77.6	78.8	81.0	78.5	80.0	24
22	80.0	77.9	79.3	81.2	78.3	79.4	81.6	79.1	80.7	22
20	80.7	78.6	79.9	81.8	79.0	80.1	82.3	79.8	81.4	20
18	81.4	79.2	80.6	82.5	79.6	80.8	83.0	80.5	82.0	18
16	82.0	79.9	81.3	83.2	80.3	81.4	83.6	81.1	82.7	16
14	82.7	80.6	81.9	83.8	81.0	82.1	84.3	81.8	83.4	14
12	83.4	81.2	82.6	84.5	81.6	82.8	85.0	82.5	84.0	12
10	84.0	81.9	83.3	85.2	82.3	83.4	85.6	83.1	84.7	10
8	84.7	82.6	83.9	85.8	83.0	84.1	86.3	83.8	85.4	8
6	85.4	83.2	84.6	86.5	83.6	84.8	87.0	84.5	86.0	6
4	86.0	83.9	85.3	87.2	84.3	85.4	87.6	85.1	86.7	4
2	86.7	84.6	85.9	87.8	85.0	86.1	88.3	85.8	87.4	2
0										0

* Revised from scales prepared by Frederick W. Cozens. Used by permission of Lea & Febiger Publishing Company.

Appendix E:
Table of Squares and Square Roots

Table of Squares and Square Roots of Numbers from 1 to 1000

Number	Square	Square Root	Number	Square	Square Root
1	1	1.000	41	16 81	6.403
2	4	1.414	42	17 64	6.481
3	9	1.732	43	18 49	6.557
4	16	2.000	44	19 36	6.633
5	25	2.236	45	20 25	6.708
6	36	2.449	46	21 16	6.782
7	49	2.646	47	22 09	6.856
8	64	2.828	48	23 04	6.928
9	81	3.000	49	24 01	7.000
10	1 00	3.162	50	25 00	7.071
11	1 21	3.317	51	26 01	7.141
12	1 44	3.464	52	27 04	7.211
13	1 69	3.606	53	28 09	7.280
14	1 96	3.742	54	29.16	7.348
15	2 25	3.873	55	30 25	7.416
16	2 56	4.000	56	31 36	7.483
17	2 89	4.123	57	32 49	7.550
18	3 24	4.243	58	33 64	7.616
19	3 61	4.359	59	34 81	7.681
20	4 00	4.472	60	36 00	7.746
21	4 41	4.583	61	37 21	7.810
22	4 84	4.690	62	38 44	7.874
23	5 29	4.796	63	39 69	7.937
24	5 76	4.899	64	40 96	8.000
25	6 25	5.000	65	42 25	8.062
26	6 76	5.099	66	43 56	8.124
27	7 29	5.196	67	44 89	8.184
28	7 84	5.292	68	46 24	8.246
29	8 41	5.385	69	47 61	8.307
30	9 00	5.477	70	49 00	8.367
31	9 61	5.568	71	50 41	8.426
32	10 24	5.657	72	51 84	8.485
33	10 89	5.745	73	53 29	8.544
34	11 56	5.831	74	54 76	8.602
35	12 25	5.916	75	56 25	8.660
36	12 96	6.000	76	57 76	8.718
37	13 69	6.083	77	59 29	8.775
38	14 44	6.164	78	60 84	8.832
39	15 21	6.245	79	62 41	8.888
40	16 00	6.325	80	64 00	8.944

Number	Square	Square Root	Number	Square	Square Root
81	65 61	9.000	136	1 84 96	11.662
82	67 24	9.055	137	1 87 69	11.705
83	68 89	9.110	138	1 90 44	11.747
84	70 56	9.165	139	1 93 21	11.790
85	72 25	9.220	140	1 96 00	11.832
86	73 96	9.274	141	1 98 81	11.874
87	75 69	9.327	142	2 01 64	11.916
88	77 44	9.381	143	2 04 49	11.958
89	79 21	9.434	144	2 07 36	12.000
90	81 00	9.487	145	2 10 25	12.042
91	82 81	9.539	146	2 13 16	12.083
92	84 64	9.592	147	2 16 09	12.124
93	86 49	9.644	148	2 19 04	12.166
94	88 36	9.695	149	2 22 01	12.207
95	90 25	9.747	150	2 25 00	12.247
96	92 16	9.798	151	2 28 01	12.288
97	94 09	9.849	152	2 31 04	12.329
98	96 04	9.899	153	2 34 09	12.369
99	98 01	9.950	154	2 37 16	12.410
100	1 00 00	10.000	155	2 40 25	12.450
101	1 02 01	10.050	156	2 43 36	12.490
102	1 04 04	10.100	157	2 46 49	12.530
103	1 06 09	10.149	158	2 49 64	12.570
104	1 08 16	10.198	159	2 52 81	12.610
105	1 10 25	10.247	160	2 56 00	12.649
106	1 12 36	10.296	161	2 59 21	12.689
107	1 14 49	10.344	162	2 62 44	12.728
108	1 16 64	10.392	163	2 65 69	12.767
109	1 18 81	10.440	164	2 68 96	12.806
110	1 21 00	10.488	165	2 72 25	12.845
111	1 23 21	10.536	166	2 75 56	12.884
112	1 25 44	10.583	167	2 78 89	12.923
113	1 27 69	10.630	168	2 82 24	12.961
114	1 29 96	10.677	169	2 85 61	13.000
115	1 32 25	10.724	170	2 89 00	13.038
116	1 34 56	10.770	171	2 92 41	13.077
117	1 36 89	10.817	172	2 95 84	13.115
118	1 39 24	10.863	173	2 99 29	13.153
119	1 41 61	10.909	174	3 02 76	13.191
120	1 44 00	10.954	175	3 06 25	13.229
121	1 46 41	11.000	176	3 09 76	13.266
122	1 48 84	11.045	177	3 13 29	13.304
123	1 51 29	11.091	178	3 16 84	13.342
124	1 53 76	11.136	179	3 20 41	13.379
125	1 56 25	11.180	180	3 24 00	13.416
126	1 58 76	11.225	181	3 27 61	13.454
127	1 61 29	11.269	182	3 31 24	13.491
128	1 63 84	11.314	183	3 34 89	13.528
129	1 66 41	11.358	184	3 38 56	13.565
130	1 69 00	11.402	185	3 42 25	13.601
131	1 71 61	11.446	186	3 45 96	13.638
132	1 74 24	11.489	187	3 49 69	13.675
133	1 76 89	11.533	188	3 53 44	13.711
134	1 79 56	11.576	189	3 57 21	13.748
135	1 82 25	11.619	190	3 61 00	13.784

Number	Square	Square Root	Number	Square	Square Root
191	3 64 81	13.820	246	6 05 16	15.684
192	3 68 64	13.856	247	6 10 09	15.716
193	3 72 49	13.892	248	6 15 04	15.748
194	3 76 36	13.928	249	6 20 01	15.780
195	3 80 25	13.964	250	6 25 00	15.811
196	3 84 16	14.000	251	6 30 01	15.843
197	3 88 09	14.036	252	6 35 04	15.875
198	3 92 04	14.071	253	6 40 09	15.906
199	3 96 01	14.107	254	6 45 16	15.937
200	4 00 00	14.142	255	6 50 25	15.969
201	4 04 01	14.177	256	6 55 36	16.000
202	4 08 04	14.213	257	6 60 49	16.031
203	4 12 09	14.248	258	6 65 64	16.062
204	4 16 16	14.283	259	6 70 81	16.093
205	4 20 25	14.318	260	6 76 00	16.125
206	4 24 36	14.353	261	6 81 21	16.155
207	4 28 49	14.387	262	6 86 44	16.186
208	4 32 64	14.422	263	6 91 69	16.217
209	4 36 81	14.457	264	6 96 96	16.248
210	4 41 00	14.491	265	7 02 25	16.279
211	4 45 21	14.526	266	7 07 56	16.310
212	4 49 44	14.560	267	7 12 89	16.340
213	4 53 69	14.595	268	7 18 24	16.371
214	4 57 96	14.629	269	7 23 61	16.401
215	4 62 25	14.663	270	7 29 00	16.432
216	4 66 56	14.697	271	7 34 41	16.462
217	4 70 89	14.731	272	7 39 84	16.492
218	4 75 24	14.765	273	7 45 29	16.523
219	4 79 61	14.799	274	7 50 76	16.553
220	4 84 00	14.832	275	7 56 25	16.583
221	4 88 41	14.866	276	7 61 76	16.613
222	4 92 84	14.900	277	7 67 29	16.643
223	4 97 29	14.933	278	7 72 84	16.673
224	5 01 76	14.967	279	7 78 41	16.703
225	5 06 25	15.000	280	7 84 00	16.733
226	5 10 76	15.033	281	7 89 61	16.763
227	5 15 29	15.067	282	7 95 24	16.793
228	5 19 84	15.100	283	8 00 89	16.823
229	5 24 41	15.133	284	8 06 56	16.852
230	5 29 00	15.166	285	8 12 25	16.882
231	5 33 61	15.199	286	8 17 96	16.912
232	5 38 24	15.232	287	8 23 69	16.941
233	5 42 89	15.264	288	8 29 44	16.971
234	5 47 56	15.297	289	8 35 21	17.000
235	5 52 25	15.330	290	8 41 00	17.029
236	5 56 96	15.362	291	8 46 81	17.059
237	5 61 69	15.395	292	8 52 64	17.088
238	5 66 44	15.427	293	8 58 40	17.117
239	5 71 21	15.460	294	8 64 36	17.146
240	5 76 00	15.492	295	8 70 25	17.176
241	5 80 81	15.524	296	8 76 16	17.205
242	5 85 64	15.556	297	8 82 09	17.234
243	5 90 49	15.588	298	8 88 04	17.263
244	5 95 36	15.620	299	8 94 01	17.292
245	6 00 25	15.652	300	9 00 00	17.321

Number	Square	Square Root	Number	Square	Square Root
301	9 06 01	17.349	356	12 67 36	18.868
302	9 12 04	17.378	357	12 74 49	18.894
303	9 18 09	17.407	358	12 81 64	18.921
304	9 24 16	17.436	359	12 88 81	18.947
305	9 30 25	17.464	360	12 96 00	18.974
306	9 36 36	17.493	361	13 03 21	19.000
307	9 42 49	17.521	362	13 10 44	19.026
308	9 48 64	17.550	363	13 17 69	19.053
309	9 54 81	17.578	364	13 24 96	19.079
310	9 61 00	17.607	365	13 32 25	19.105
311	9 67 21	17.635	366	13 39 56	19.131
312	9 73 44	17.664	367	13 46 89	19.157
313	9 79 69	17.692	368	13 54 24	19.183
314	9 85 96	17.720	369	13 61 61	19.209
315	9 92 25	17.748	370	13 69 00	19.235
316	9 98 56	17.776	371	13 76 41	19.261
317	10 04 89	17.804	372	13 83 84	19.287
318	10 11 24	17.833	373	13 91 29	19.313
319	10 17 61	17.861	374	13 98 76	19.339
320	10 24 00	17.889	375	14 06 25	19.363
321	10 30 41	17.916	376	14 13 76	19.391
322	10 36 84	17.944	377	14 21 29	19.416
323	10 43 29	17.972	378	14 28 84	19.442
324	10 49 76	18.000	379	14 36 41	19.468
325	10 56 25	18.028	380	14 44 00	19.494
326	10 62 76	18.055	381	14 51 61	19.519
327	10 69 29	18.083	382	14 59 24	19.545
328	10 75 84	18.111	383	14 66 89	19.570
329	10 82 41	18.138	384	14 74 56	19.596
330	10 89 00	18.166	385	14 82 25	19.621
331	10 95 61	18.193	386	14 89 96	19.647
332	11 02 24	18.221	387	14 97 69	19.672
333	11 08 89	18.248	388	15 05 44	19.698
334	11 15 56	18.276	389	15 13 21	19.723
335	11 22 25	18.303	390	15 21 00	19.748
336	11 28 96	18.330	391	15 28 81	19.774
337	11 35 69	18.358	392	15 36 64	19.799
338	11 42 44	18.385	393	15 44 49	19.824
339	11 49 21	18.412	394	15 52 36	19.849
340	11 56 00	18.439	395	15 60 25	19.875
341	11 62 81	18.466	396	15 68 16	19.900
342	11 69 64	18.493	397	15 76 09	19.925
343	11 76 49	18.520	398	15 84 04	19.950
344	11 83 36	18.547	399	15 92 01	19.975
345	11 90 25	18.574	400	16 00 00	20.000
346	11 97 16	18.601	401	16 08 01	20.025
347	12 04 09	18.628	402	16 16 04	20.050
348	12 11 04	18.655	403	16 24 09	20.075
349	12 18 01	18.682	404	16 32 16	20.100
350	12 25 00	18.708	405	16 40 25	20.125
351	12 32 01	18.735	406	16 48 36	20.149
352	12 39 04	18.762	407	16 56 49	20.174
353	12 46 09	18.788	408	16 64 64	20.199
354	12 53 16	18.815	409	16 72 81	20.224
355	12 60 25	18.841	410	16 81 00	20.248

Number	Square	Square Root	Number	Square	Square Root
411	16 89 21	20.273	466	21 71 56	21.587
412	16 97 44	20.298	467	21 80 89	21.610
413	17 05 69	20.322	468	21 90 24	21.633
414	17 13 96	20.347	469	21 99 61	21.656
415	17 22 25	20.372	470	22 09 00	21.679
416	17 30 56	20.396	471	22 18 41	21.703
417	17 38 89	20.421	472	22 27 84	21.726
418	17 47 24	20.445	473	22 37 29	21.749
419	17 55 61	20.469	474	22 46 76	21.772
420	17 64 00	20.494	475	22 56 25	21.794
421	17 72 41	20.518	476	22 65 76	21.817
422	17 80 84	20.543	477	22 75 29	21.840
423	17 89 29	20.567	478	22 84 84	21.863
424	17 97 76	20.591	479	22 94 41	21.886
425	18 06 25	20.616	480	23 04 00	21.909
426	18 14 76	20.640	481	23 13 61	21.932
427	18 23 29	20.664	482	23 23 24	21.954
428	18 31 84	20.688	483	23 32 89	21.977
429	18 40 41	20.712	484	23 42 56	22.000
430	18 49 00	20.736	485	23 52 25	22.023
431	18 57 61	20.761	486	23 61 96	22.045
432	18 66 24	20.785	487	23 71 69	22.068
433	18 74 89	20.809	488	23 81 44	22.091
434	18 83 56	20.833	489	23 91 21	22.113
435	18 92 25	20.857	490	24 01 00	22.136
436	19 00 96	20.881	491	24 10 81	22.159
437	19 09 69	20.905	492	24 20 64	22.181
438	19 18 44	20.928	493	24 30 49	22.204
439	19 27 21	20.952	494	24 40 36	22.226
440	19 36 00	20.976	495	24 50 25	22.249
441	19 44 81	21.000	496	24 60 16	22.271
442	19 53 64	21.024	497	24 70 09	22.293
443	19 62 49	21.048	498	24 80 04	22.316
444	19 71 36	21.071	499	24 90 01	22.338
445	19 80 25	21.095	500	25 00 00	22.361
446	19 89 16	21.119	501	25 10 01	22.383
447	19 98 09	21.142	502	25 20 04	22.405
448	20 07 04	21.166	503	25 30 09	22.428
449	20 16 01	21.190	504	25 40 16	22.450
450	20 25 00	21.213	505	25 50 25	22.472
451	20 34 01	21.237	506	25 60 36	22.494
452	20 43 04	21.260	507	25 70 49	22.517
453	20 52 09	21.284	508	25 80 64	22.539
454	20 61 16	21.307	509	25 90 81	22.561
455	20 70 25	21.331	510	26 01 00	22.583
456	20 79 36	21.354	511	26 11 21	22.605
457	20 88 49	21.378	512	26 21 44	22.627
458	20 97 64	21.401	513	26 31 69	22.650
459	21 06 81	21.424	514	26 41 96	22.672
460	21 16 00	21.448	515	26 52 25	22.694
461	21 25 21	21.471	516	26 62 56	22.716
462	21 34 44	21.494	517	26 72 89	22.738
463	21 43 69	21.517	518	26 83 24	22.760
464	21 52 96	21.541	519	26 93 61	22.782
465	21 62 25	21.564	520	27 04 00	22.804

Number	Square	Square Root	Number	Square	Square Root
521	27 14 41	22.825	576	33 17 76	24.000
522	27 24 84	22.847	577	33 29 29	24.021
523	27 35 29	22.869	578	33 40 84	24.042
524	27 45 76	22.891	579	33 52 41	24.062
525	27 56 25	22.913	580	33 64 00	24.083
526	27 66 76	22.935	581	33 75 61	24.104
527	27 77 29	22.956	582	33 87 24	24.125
528	27 87 84	22.978	583	33 98 89	24.145
529	27 98 41	23.000	584	34 10 56	24.166
530	28 09 00	23.022	585	34 22 25	24.187
531	28 19 61	23.043	586	34 33 96	24.207
532	28 30 24	23.065	587	34 45 69	24.228
533	28 40 89	23.087	588	34 57 44	24.249
534	28 51 56	23.108	589	34 69 21	24.269
535	28 62 25	23.130	590	34 81 00	24.290
536	28 72 96	23.152	591	34 92 81	24.310
537	28 83 69	23.173	592	35 04 64	24.331
538	28 94 44	23.195	593	35 16 49	24.352
539	29 05 21	23.216	594	35 28 36	24.372
540	29 16 00	23.238	595	35 40 25	24.393
541	29 26 81	23.259	596	35 52 16	24.413
542	29 37 64	32.281	597	35 64 09	24.434
543	29 48 49	23.302	598	35 76 04	24.454
544	29 59 36	23.324	599	35 88 01	24.474
545	29 70 25	23.345	600	36 00 00	24.495
546	29 81 16	23.367	601	36 12 01	24.515
547	29 92 09	23.388	602	36 24 04	24.536
548	30 03 04	23.409	603	36 36 09	24.556
549	30 14 01	23.431	604	36 48 16	24.576
550	30 25 00	23.452	605	36 60 25	24.597
551	30 36 01	23.473	606	36 72 36	24.617
552	30 47 04	23.495	607	36 84 49	24.637
553	30 58 09	23.516	608	36 96 64	24.658
554	30 69 16	23.537	609	37 08 81	24.678
555	30 80 25	23.558	610	37 21 00	24.698
556	30 91 36	23.580	611	37 33 21	24.718
557	31 02 49	23.601	612	37 45 44	24.739
558	31 13 64	23.622	613	37 57 69	24.759
559	31 24 81	23.643	614	37 69 96	24.779
560	31 36 00	23.664	615	37 82 25	24.799
561	31 47 21	23.685	616	37 94 56	24.819
562	31 58 44	23.707	617	38 06 89	24.839
563	31 69 69	23.728	618	38 19 24	24.860
564	31 80 96	23.749	619	38 31 61	24.880
565	31 92 25	23.770	620	38 44 00	24.900
566	32 03 56	23.791	621	38 56 41	24.920
567	32 14 89	23.812	622	38 68 84	24.940
568	32 26 24	23.833	623	38 81 29	24.960
569	32 37 61	23.854	624	38 93 76	24.980
570	32 49 00	23.875	625	39 06 25	25.000
571	32 60 41	23.896	626	39 18 76	25.020
572	32 71 84	23.917	627	39 31 29	25.040
573	32 83 29	23.937	628	39 43 84	25.060
574	32 94 76	23.958	629	39 56 41	25.080
575	33 06 25	23.979	630	39 69 00	25.100

Number	Square	Square Root	Number	Square	Square Root
631	39 81 61	25.120	686	47 05 96	26.192
632	39 94 24	25.140	687	47 19 69	26.211
633	40 06 89	25.159	688	47 33 44	26.230
634	40 19 56	25.179	689	47 47 21	26.249
635	40 32 25	25.199	690	47 61 00	26.268
636	40 44 96	25.219	691	47 74 81	26.287
637	40 57 69	25.239	692	47 88 64	26.306
638	40 70 44	25.259	693	48 02 49	26.325
639	40 83 21	25.278	694	48 16 36	26.344
640	40 96 00	25.298	695	48 30 25	26.363
641	41 08 81	25.318	696	48 44 16	26.382
642	41 21 64	25.338	697	48 58 09	26.401
643	41 34 49	25.357	698	48 72 04	26.420
644	41 47 36	25.377	699	48 86 01	26.439
645	41 60 25	25.397	700	49 00 00	26.458
646	41 73 16	25.417	701	49 14 01	26.476
647	41 86 09	25.436	702	49 28 04	26.495
648	41 99 04	25.456	703	49 42 09	26.514
649	42 12 01	25.475	704	49 56 16	26.533
650	42 25 00	25.495	705	49 70 25	26.552
651	42 38 10	25.515	706	49 84 36	26.571
652	42 51 04	25.534	707	49 98 49	26.589
653	42 64 09	25.554	708	50 12 64	26.608
654	42 77 16	25.573	709	50 26 81	26.627
655	42 90 25	25.593	710	50 41 00	26.646
656	43 03 36	25.612	711	50 55 21	26.665
657	43 16 49	25.632	712	50 69 44	26.683
658	43 29 64	25.652	713	50 83 69	26.702
659	43 42 81	25.671	714	50 97 96	26.721
660	43 56 00	25.690	715	51 12 25	26.739
661	43 69 21	25.710	716	51 26 56	26.758
662	43 82 44	25.729	717	51 40 89	26.777
663	43 95 69	25.749	718	51 55 24	26.796
664	44 08 96	25.768	719	51 69 61	26.814
665	44 22 25	25.788	720	51 84 00	26.833
666	44 35 56	25.807	721	51 98 41	26.851
667	44 48 89	25.826	722	52 12 84	26.870
668	44 62 24	25.846	723	52 27 29	26.889
669	44 75 61	25.865	724	52 41 76	26.907
670	44 89 00	24.884	725	52 56 25	26.926
671	45 02 41	25.904	726	52 70 76	26.944
672	45 15 84	25.923	727	52 85 29	26.963
673	45 29 29	25.942	728	52 99 84	26.981
674	45 42 76	25.962	729	53 14 41	27.000
675	45 56 25	25.981	730	53 29 00	27.019
676	45 69 76	26.000	731	53 43 61	27.037
677	45 83 29	26.019	732	53 58 24	27.055
678	45 96 84	26.038	733	53 72 89	27.074
679	46 10 41	26.058	734	53 87 56	27.092
680	46 24 00	26.077	735	54 02 25	27.111
681	46 37 61	26.096	736	54 16 96	27.129
682	46 51 24	26.115	737	54 31 69	27.148
683	46 64 89	26.134	738	54 46 44	27.166
684	46 78 56	26.153	739	54 61 21	27.185
685	46 92 25	26.173	740	54 76 00	27.203

Number	Square	Square Root	Number	Square	Square Root
741	54 90 81	27.221	796	63 36 16	28.213
742	55 05 64	27.240	797	63 52 09	28.231
743	55 20 49	27.258	798	63 68 04	28.249
744	55 35 36	27.276	799	63 84 01	28.267
745	55 50 25	27.295	800	64 00 00	28.284
746	55 65 16	27.313	801	64 16 01	28.302
747	55 80 09	27.331	802	64 32 04	28.320
748	55 95 04	27.350	803	64 48 09	28.337
749	56 10 01	27.368	804	64 64 16	28.355
750	56 25 00	27.386	805	64 80 25	28.373
751	56 40 01	27.404	806	64 96 36	28.390
752	56 55 04	27.423	807	65 12 49	28.408
753	56 70 09	27.441	808	65 28 64	28.425
754	56 85 16	27.459	809	65 44 81	28.443
755	57 00 25	27.477	810	65 61 00	28.460
756	57 15 36	27.495	811	65 77 21	28.478
757	57 30 49	27.514	812	65 93 44	28.496
758	57 45 64	27.532	813	66 09 69	28.513
759	57 60 81	27.550	814	66 25 96	28.531
760	57 76 00	27.568	815	66 42 25	28.548
761	57 91 21	27.586	816	66 58 56	28.566
762	58 06 44	27.604	817	66 74 89	28.583
763	58 21 69	27.622	818	66 91 24	28.601
764	58 36 96	27.641	819	67 07 61	28.618
765	58 52 25	27.659	820	67 24 00	28.636
766	58 67 56	27.677	821	67 40 41	28.653
767	58 82 89	27.695	822	67 56 84	28.671
768	58 98 24	27.713	823	67 73 29	28.688
769	59 13 61	27.731	824	67 89 76	28.705
770	59 29 00	27.749	825	68 06 25	28.723
771	59 44 41	27.767	826	68 22 76	28.740
772	59 59 84	27.785	827	68 39 29	28.758
773	59 75 29	27.803	828	68 55 84	28.775
774	59 90 76	27.821	829	68 72 41	28.792
775	60 06 25	27.839	830	68 89 00	28.810
776	60 21 76	27.857	831	69 05 61	28.827
777	60 37 29	27.875	832	69 22 24	28.844
778	60 52 84	27.893	833	69 38 89	28.862
779	60 68 41	27.911	834	69 55 56	28.879
780	60 84 00	27.928	835	69 72 25	28.896
781	60 99 61	27.946	836	69 88 96	28.914
782	61 15 24	27.964	837	70 05 69	28.931
783	61 30 89	27.982	838	70 22 44	28.948
784	61 46 56	28.000	839	70 39 21	28.965
785	61 62 25	28.018	840	70 56 00	28.983
786	61 77 96	28.036	841	70 72 81	29.000
787	61 93 69	28.054	842	70 89 64	29.017
788	62 09 44	28.071	843	71 06 49	29.034
789	62 25 21	28.089	844	71 23 36	29.052
790	62 41 00	28.107	845	71 40 25	29.069
791	62 56 81	28.125	846	71 57 16	29.086
792	62 72 64	28.142	847	71 74 09	29.103
793	62 88 49	28.160	848	71 91 04	29.120
794	63 04 36	28.178	849	72 08 01	29.138
795	63 20 25	28.196	850	72 25 00	29.155

Number	Square	Square Root	Number	Square	Square Root
851	72 42 01	29.172	906	82 08 36	30.100
852	72 59 04	29.189	907	82 26 49	30.116
853	72 76 09	29.206	908	82 44 64	30.133
854	72 93 16	29.223	909	82 62 81	30.150
855	73 10 25	29.240	910	82 81 00	30.166
856	73 27 36	29.257	911	82 99 21	30.183
857	73 44 49	29.275	912	83 17 44	30.199
858	73 61 64	29.292	913	83 35 69	30.216
859	73 78 81	29.309	914	83 53 96	30.232
860	73 96 00	29.326	915	83 72 25	30.249
861	74 13 21	29.343	916	83 90 56	30.265
862	74 30 44	29.360	917	84 08 89	30.282
863	74 47 69	29.377	918	84 27 24	30.299
864	74 64 96	29.394	919	84 45 61	30.315
865	74 82 25	29.411	920	84 64 00	30.332
866	74 99 56	29.428	921	84 82 41	30.348
867	75 16 89	29.445	922	85 00 84	30.364
868	75 34 24	29.462	923	85 19 29	30.381
869	75 51 61	29.479	924	85 37 76	30.397
870	75 69 00	29.496	925	85 56 25	30.414
871	75 86 41	29.513	926	85 74 76	30.430
872	76 03 84	29.530	927	85 93 29	30.447
873	76 21 29	29.547	928	86 11 84	30.463
874	76 38 76	29.563	929	86 30 41	30.480
875	76 56 25	29.580	930	86 49 00	30.496
876	76 73 76	29.597	931	86 67 61	30.512
877	76 91 29	29.614	932	86 86 24	30.529
878	77 08 84	29.631	933	87 04 89	30.545
879	77 26 41	29.648	934	87 23 56	30.561
880	77 44 00	29.665	935	87 42 25	30.578
881	77 61 61	29.682	936	87 69 96	30.504
882	77 79 24	29.698	937	87 79 69	30.610
883	77 96 89	29.715	938	87 98 44	30.627
884	78 14 56	29.732	939	88 17 21	30.643
885	78 32 25	29.749	940	88 36 00	30.659
886	78 49 96	29.766	941	88 54 81	30.676
887	78 67 69	29.783	942	88 73 64	30.692
888	78 85 44	29.799	943	88 92 49	30.708
889	79 03 21	29.816	944	89 11 36	30.725
890	79 21 00	29.833	945	89 30 25	30.741
891	79 38 81	29.850	946	89 49 16	30.757
892	79 56 64	29.866	947	89 68 09	30.773
893	79 74 49	29.883	948	89 87 04	30.790
894	79 92 36	29.900	949	90 06 01	30.806
895	80 10 25	29.916	950	90 25 00	30.822
896	80 28 16	29.933	951	90 44 01	30.838
897	80 46 09	29.950	952	90 63 04	30.854
898	80 64 04	29.967	953	90 82 09	30.871
899	80 82 01	29.983	954	91 01 16	30.887
900	81 00 00	30.000	955	91 20 25	30.903
901	81 18 01	30.017	956	91 39 36	30.919
902	81 36 04	30.033	957	91 58 49	30.935
903	81 54 09	30.050	958	91 77 64	30.952
904	81 72 16	30.067	959	91 96 81	30.968
905	81 90 25	30.083	960	92 16 00	30.984

Number	Square	Square Root	Number	Square	Square Root
961	92 35 21	31.000	981	96 23 61	31.321
962	92 54 44	31.016	982	96 43 24	31.337
963	92 73 69	31.032	983	96 62 89	31.353
964	92 92 96	31.048	984	96 82 56	31.369
965	93 12 25	31.064	985	97 02 25	31.385
966	93 31 56	31.081	986	97 21 96	31.401
967	93 50 89	31.097	987	97 41 69	31.417
968	93 70 24	31.113	988	97 61 44	31.432
969	93 89 61	31.129	989	97 81 21	31.448
970	94 09 00	31.145	990	98 01 00	31.464
971	94 28 41	31.161	991	98 20 81	31.480
972	94 47 84	31.177	992	98 40 64	31.496
973	94 67 20	31.193	993	98 60 49	31.512
974	94 86 76	31.209	994	98 80 36	31.528
975	95 06 25	31.225	995	99 00 25	31.544
976	95 25 76	31.241	996	99 20 16	31.559
977	95 45 29	31.257	997	99 40 09	31.575
978	95 64 84	31.273	998	99 60 04	31.591
979	95 84 41	31.289	999	99 80 01	31.607
980	96 04 00	31.305	1000	100 00 00	31.623

Appendix F: Percentage of Cases within Standard Deviation Units of the Mean in a Normal Distribution Curve

σ	.00	.01	.02	.03	.04	.05	.06	.07	.08	.09
0.0	00.00	00.40	00.80	01.20	01.60	01.99	02.39	02.79	03.19	03.59
0.1	03.98	04.38	04.78	05.17	05.57	05.96	06.36	06.75	07.14	07.53
0.2	07.93	08.32	08.71	09.10	09.48	09.87	10.26	11.64	11.03	11.41
0.3	01.79	12.17	12.55	12.93	13.31	13.68	14.06	14.43	14.80	15.17
0.4	15.54	15.54	16.28	16.64	17.00	17.36	17.72	18.08	18.44	18.79
0.5	19.15	19.50	19.85	20.19	20.54	20.88	21.23	21.57	21.90	22.24
0.6	22.57	22.91	23.24	23.57	23.89	24.22	24.54	24.86	25.17	25.49
0.7	25.80	26.11	26.42	26.73	27.04	27.34	27.64	27.94	28.23	28.52
0.8	28.81	29.10	29.39	29.67	29.95	30.23	30.51	30.78	31.06	31.33
0.9	31.59	31.86	32.12	32.38	32.64	32.90	33.15	33.40	33.65	33.89
1.0	24.13	34.38	34.61	34.85	35.08	35.31	35.54	35.77	35.99	36.21
1.1	36.43	36.65	36.86	37.08	37.29	37.49	37.70	37.90	38.10	38.30
1.2	38.49	38.69	38.88	39.07	39.25	39.44	39.62	39.80	39.97	40.15
1.3	40.32	40.49	40.66	40.82	40.99	41.15	41.31	41.47	41.62	41.77
1.4	41.92	42.07	42.22	42.36	42.51	42.65	42.79	42.92	43.06	43.19
1.5	43.32	43.45	43.57	43.70	43.83	43.94	44.06	44.18	44.29	44.41
1.6	44.52	44.63	44.74	44.84	44.95	45.05	45.15	45.25	45.35	45.45
1.7	45.54	45.64	45.73	45.82	45.91	45.99	46.08	46.16	46.25	46.33
1.8	46.41	46.49	46.56	46.64	46.71	46.78	46.86	46.93	46.99	47.06
1.9	47.13	47.19	47.26	47.32	47.38	47.44	47.50	46.56	47.61	47.67
2.0	47.72	47.78	47.83	47.88	47.93	47.98	48.03	48.08	48.12	48.17
2.1	48.21	48.26	48.30	48.34	48.38	48.42	48.46	48.50	48.54	48.57
2.2	48.61	48.64	48.68	48.71	48.75	48.78	48.81	48.84	48.87	48.90
2.3	48.93	48.96	48.98	49.01	49.04	49.06	49.09	49.11	49.13	49.16
2.4	49.18	49.20	49.22	49.25	49.27	49.29	49.31	49.32	49.34	49.36
2.5	49.38	49.40	49.41	49.43	49.45	49.46	49.48	49.49	49.51	49.52
2.6	49.53	49.55	49.56	49.57	49.59	49.60	49.61	49.62	49.63	49.64
2.7	49.65	49.66	49.67	49.68	49.69	49.70	49.71	49.72	49.73	49.74
2.8	49.74	49.75	49.76	49.77	49.77	49.78	49.79	49.79	49.80	49.81
2.9	49.81	49.82	49.82	49.83	49.84	49.84	49.85	49.85	49.86	49.86
3.0	49.87									
3.5	49.98									
4.0	49.997									
5.0	49.99997									

* The data in this table were taken from *Tables for Statisticians and Biometricians*. Edited by Karl Pearson. Cambridge University Press.

Index